CERVICAL CANCER

Signaling Pathways, Molecular Mechanisms, Natural Products, and Therapeutic Approaches

Modern Trends in Molecular Biology

CERVICAL CANCER

Signaling Pathways, Molecular Mechanisms, Natural Products, and Therapeutic Approaches

by

Pratibha Pandey, PhD

Fahad Khan, PhD

Saher Islam, PhD

Devarajan Thangadurai, PhD

AAP | APPLE ACADEMIC PRESS

First edition published 2024

Apple Academic Press Inc.
1265 Goldenrod Circle, NE,
Palm Bay, FL 32905 USA

760 Laurentian Drive, Unit 19,
Burlington, ON L7N 0A4, CANADA

CRC Press
2385 NW Executive Center Drive,
Suite 320, Boca Raton FL 33431

4 Park Square, Milton Park,
Abingdon, Oxon, OX14 4RN UK

Library and Archives Canada Cataloguing in Publication

Title: Cervical cancer : signaling pathways, molecular mechanisms, natural products, and therapeutic approaches / by Pratibha Pandey, PhD, Fahad Khan, PhD, Saher Islam, PhD, Devarajan Thangadurai, PhD.
Names: Pandey, Pratibha, 1985- author | Khan, Fahad, 1987- author. | Islam, Saher, author. | Thangadurai, Devarajan, 1976- author.
Series: Modern trends in molecular biology.
Description: First edition. | Series statement: Modern trends in molecular biology | Includes bibliographical references and index.
Identifiers: Canadiana (print) 20230514081 | Canadiana (ebook) 20230514111 | ISBN 9781774915660 (hardcover) | ISBN 9781774915677 (softcover) | ISBN 9781032665832 (ebook)
Subjects: LCSH: Cervix uteri—Cancer. | LCSH: Cervix uteri—Cancer—Treatment.
Classification: LCC RC280.U8 P36 2024 | DDC 616.99/466—dc23

Library of Congress Cataloging-in-Publication Data

CIP data on file with US Library of Congress

ISBN: 978-1-77491-566-0 (hbk)
ISBN: 978-1-77491-567-7 (pbk)
ISBN: 978-1-03266-583-2 (ebk)

Modern Trends in Molecular Biology Book Series

ABOUT THE SERIES

Series Editor: Devarajan Thangadurai, PhD
Professor, Karnatak University, Dharwad, India
Email: drthangaduraid@gmail.com / drthanga.kud@gmail.com

Advancements in molecular biology have stimulated a great impact on all life sciences investigation to improve the trends in global biodiversity condition. This dynamic force involves the development of highly sophisticated experimental methods in molecular biology with broad interdisciplinary applications, the quickly expanding information flow of scientific discoveries and technical novelties across scientific community, and the development of precise computational tools with constantly updated biological databases for, respectively, analyzing gene expression level, cytogenetic profile, storing data for genotypes, and other molecular features. This has transformed the approach of scientific research allowing revolutionized discoveries in the area of molecular biology. Advances in high-throughput tools, recombinant technology, and NGS made it feasible to unveil genome complexity and to explain the detailed mechanisms for transmission of genetic information. Moreover disease analysis, treatment, and prevention; manipulation of animals and plants for improved phenotypic traits; and synthesis of new peptides and proteins are some of the applications of molecular biology that are frequently being adopted.

There are several approaches from which knowledge in the field of molecular biology is increasingly growing, and it could be challenging for researchers coming into life sciences field. Accordingly there is a need for a platform for preparing molecular biologists to keep themselves abreast of modern trends in molecular biology. Thus, this book series, Modern Trends in Molecular Biology includes the most of the dynamic pieces of research work being done across the globe on numerous themes associated with molecular biology. This book series attempts to enlighten readers regarding novel concepts and findings in the molecular biology field. The scope of this book series includes recent findings and advancements in the areas of transcriptomics, proteomics, genomics, micro RNA, molecular markers, DNA, RNA and protein isolation, CRISPR, gene editing molecular methods, gene cloning, construction of genome and cDNA library, DNA methylation role for gene expression analysis, AFLP, RAPD, RFLP, VNTRs, genome sequencing tools, phylogenetic analyses, protein modeling, restriction enzymes, metagenomics, metatranscriptomics, metaproteomics, DNA repair, replication and recombination, DNA forensics, pharmacogenomics, functional genomics, structural genomics, and computational analyses for proteins and genes.

This book series, Modern Trends in Molecular Biology, aims to relay state-of-the-art knowledge in field of molecular biology. This book series will provide important resources for college and university students, lecturers and professors, and researchers and scientists in almost all life sciences related disciplines. The book series will offer useful practical and theoretical basis with which to understand the knowledge gaps in relation to a wide range of scientific investigations exploiting molecular biology methods. Overall, presented in concise, organized, and simple format, this series allows smart access to highly considerate topics.

This book series will offer peer-reviewed resources on a variety of topics covering modern aspects of molecular biology, with the goal of helping to keep researchers, scientists, and students abreast of recent advances in the field. Topics will include:

- Molecular Biology: Fundamentals and Applications
- Molecular Parasitology
- Molecular Entomology
- Molecular Virology
- Molecular Phycology
- Molecular Ecology
- Molecular Nematology
- Molecular Physiology
- Molecular Epidemiology
- Molecular Breeding
- Molecular Agriculture
- Molecular Aquaculture
- Molecular Pathology
- Molecular Medicine
- Molecular Genetics
- Molecular Markers

- Molecular Diagnostics
- Molecular Evolution
- Molecular Immunology
- Molecular Microbiology
- Molecular Pharmacology
- Molecular Enzymology
- Molecular Phylogenetics

BOOKS IN THE SERIES

Hematopoiesis: Biochemical, Cellular, Molecular, and Genomic Perspectives
Editor: *Ravi Kumar Gutti, PhD*

Cervical Cancer: Signaling Pathways, Molecular Mechanisms, Natural Products, and Therapeutic Approaches
Authors: *Pratibha Pandey, PhD, Fahad Khan, PhD, Saher Islam, PhD, and Devarajan Thangadurai, PhD*

CRISPR-Based Gene Editing: A Solution for Global Food Security
Editors: *Shakeel Ahmad, PhD, Asif Ali Khan, PhD, and Muhammad Arshad Javed, PhD*

Other Books from AAP by Devarajan Thangadurai and Colleagues

Algal Farming Systems: From Production to Application for a Sustainable Future
Editors: *Jeyabalan Sangeetha, PhD, and Devarajan Thangadurai, PhD*

Algal Genetic Resources: Cosmeceuticals, Nutraceuticals, and Pharmaceuticals from Algae
Editors: *Jeyabalan Sangeetha, PhD, and Devarajan Thangadurai, PhD*

Algal Metabolites: Biotechnological, Commercial, and Industrial Applications
Editors: *Jeyabalan Sangeetha, PhD, Devarajan Thangadurai, PhD, Saher Islam, PhD, and Ravichandra Hospet, PhD*

Beneficial Microbes for Sustainable Agriculture and Environmental Management
Editors: *Jeyabalan Sangeetha, PhD, Devarajan Thangadurai, PhD, and Saher Islam, PhD*

Biodiversity and Conservation: Characterization and Utilization of Plants, Microbes, and Natural Resources for Sustainable Development and Ecosystem Management
Editors: *Jeyabalan Sangeetha, PhD, Devarajan Thangadurai, PhD, Hong Ching Goh, PhD, and Saher Islam, PhD*

Biogenic Nanomaterials: Structural Properties and Functional Applications
Editors: *Devarajan Thangadurai, PhD, Saher Islam, PhD, Jeyabalan Sangeetha, PhD, and Natália Cruz-Martins, PhD*

Biotechnology and Bioinformatics: Advances and Applications for Bioenergy, Bioremediation, and Biopharmaceutical Research
Editors: *Devarajan Thangadurai, PhD, and Jeyabalan Sangeetha, PhD*

Biotechnology of Microorganisms: Diversity, Improvement, and Application of Microbes for Food Processing, Healthcare, Environmental Safety, and Agriculture
Editors: *Jeyabalan Sangeetha, PhD, Devarajan Thangadurai, PhD, Somboon Tanasupawat, PhD, and Pradnya Pralhad Kanekar, PhD*

Cervical Cancer: Signaling Pathways, Molecular Mechanisms, Natural Products, and Therapeutic Approaches
Authors: *Pratibha Pandey, PhD, Fahad Khan, PhD, Saher Islam, PhD, and Devarajan Thangadurai, PhD*

Environmental Biotechnology: Biodegradation, Bioremediation, and Bioconversion of Xenobiotics for Sustainable Development
Editors: *Jeyabalan Sangeetha, PhD, Devarajan Thangadurai, PhD, Muniswamy David, PhD, and Mohd Azmuddin Abdullah, PhD*

Environmental Phycology: Climate Change Mitigation and Hazardous Pollutant Cleanup using Algal Resources
Editors: *Jeyabalan Sangeetha, PhD, and Devarajan Thangadurai, PhD*

Food Microbial and Molecular Biology: From Fundamentals to Applications
Editors: *Saher Islam, PhD, Devarajan Thangadurai, PhD, Jeyabalan Sangeetha, PhD, and Zaira Zaman Chowdhury, PhD*

Fundamentals of Molecular Mycology
Authors: *Devarajan Thangadurai, PhD, Jeyabalan Sangeetha, PhD, and Muniswamy David, PhD*

Genomics and Proteomics: Principles, Technologies, and Applications
Editors: *Devarajan Thangadurai, PhD, and Jeyabalan Sangeetha, PhD*

Global Food Safety: Microbial Interventions and Molecular Advancements
Editors: *Saher Islam, PhD, Devarajan Thangadurai, PhD, Jeyabalan Sangeetha, PhD, and Natália Cruz-Martins, PhD*

Industrial Biotechnology: Sustainable Production and Bioresource Utilization
Editors: *Devarajan Thangadurai, PhD, and Jeyabalan Sangeetha, PhD*

Microalgal Biotechnology: Bioprospecting Microalgae for Functional Metabolites towards Commercial and Sustainable Applications
Editors: *Jeyabalan Sangeetha, PhD, Svetlana Codreanu, PhD, and Devarajan Thangadurai, PhD*

Microbial Fertilizer Technology for Sustainable Crop Production
Editors: *Jeyabalan Sangeetha, PhD, Abdel Rahman Mohammad Al-Tawaha, PhD, and Devarajan Thangadurai, PhD*

Mycorrhizal Technology: Managing Plant Stress and Mitigating Climate Change using Mycorrhizae
Editors: *Jeyabalan Sangeetha, PhD, Abdel Rahman Mohammad Al-Tawaha, PhD, and Devarajan Thangadurai, PhD*

Organic Farming for Sustainable Development
Editors: *Jeyabalan Sangeetha, PhD, Kasem Soytong, PhD, Devarajan Thangadurai, PhD, and Abdel Rahman Mohammad Al-Tawaha, PhD*

Phycobiotechnology: Biodiversity and Biotechnology of Algae and Algal Products for Food, Feed, and Fuel
Editors: *Jeyabalan Sangeetha, PhD, Devarajan Thangadurai, PhD, Sanniyasi Elumalai, PhD, and Shivasharana Chandrabanda Thimmappa, PhD*

Seaweed Biotechnology: Biodiversity and Biotechnology of Seaweeds and Their Applications
Editors: *Jeyabalan Sangeetha, PhD, and Devarajan Thangadurai, PhD*

About the Authors

Pratibha Pandey, PhD

Assistant Professor, Department of Biotechnology, Noida Institute of Engineering and Technology, Greater Noida, India

Pratibha Pandey, PhD, is an Assistant Professor working in the Department of Biotechnology, Noida Institute of Engineering and Technology, Greater Noida, India. An ardent learner with a PhD in Bioengineering (Biotechnology), MTech (Silver Medalist, Biotechnology), MBA (HR), and BTech (Biotechnology), Dr. Pandey has been actively involved in research and development with seven years of teaching experience in the field of biotechnology and bioengineering. She has been awarded by various funding agencies like Young Women Scientist (WOS-A) from the Department of Science and Technology, Government of India, and CRIP Program of TEQIP III from Dr. A.P.J. Abdul Kalam Technical University, Lucknow. She is an editorial board member and reviewer for several journals, such as *Scientific Reports* (Springer Nature), *Cell Cycle* (Taylor and Francis), and *Frontiers in Pharmacology*. Her areas of research interest include cancer biology (biomarkers and signalosomes in gall bladder cancer, prostate cancer, lung cancer, and cervical cancer) and chemoprevention using natural products via in silico and in vitro techniques.

Fahad Khan, PhD

Assistant Professor, Department of Biotechnology, Noida Institute of Engineering and Technology, Greater Noida, India

Fahad Khan, PhD, is an Assistant Professor in the Department of Biotechnology at Noida Institute of Engineering and Technology, Greater Noida, India. He has more than four years of experience as an academic in the areas of bioengineering and biotechnology. He is an editorial board member and reviewer for several journals, such as *Molecules, Healthcare, Computers in Biology and Medicine*, and *Gene Reports*. Dr. Khan's research investigates the effects of natural compounds against different types of cancers. His main focus is the cell signaling pathways by which the natural compounds could induce apoptosis in cancer cells and thus inhibits cancer metastasis and angiogenesis in in-vitro models. He also has a keen interest in computational biology-based therapeutic approaches for disease prevention and exploration of the underlying mechanism. His research findings have received extensive coverage in national and international journals. His work has also been funded by Dr. APJ Abdul Kalam Technical University, Lucknow, India.

Saher Islam, PhD

Postdoctoral Researcher, University of Texas Southwestern Medical Center, Dallas, Texas, USA

Saher Islam, PhD, is a Postdoctoral Researcher at the University of Texas Southwestern Medical Center, Dallas, USA. She has worked at Cornell University and West Virginia State University in the USA for her doctoral research. She has keen research interests in genetics, oncology, molecular biology, biotechnology, and bioinformatics, and has ample hands-on experience in molecular marker analysis, whole genome sequencing, and RNA sequencing. She has visited the USA, UK, Singapore, Germany, Italy, and Russia for academic and scientific training, courses, and meetings. She is the recipient of the 2016 Boehringer Ingelheim Fonds Travel Grant from the European Molecular Biology Laboratory, Germany. She is an author/coauthor of 70 publications, including journal articles, book chapters, books, and conference presentations.

Devarajan Thangadurai, PhD

Professor, Karnatak University, Dharwad, India

Devarajan Thangadurai, PhD, is a Professor at Karnatak University, Dharwad in India, and did his postdoctoral research at the University of Madeira, Portugal, University of Delhi, India, and ICAR National Research Centre for Banana, India. He is the recipient of the Best Young Scientist Award with Gold Medal from Acharya Nagarjuna University, India, and the VGST-SMYSR Young Scientist Award of the Government of Karnataka, India. He has authored/edited more than 30 books with international publishers in USA, Canada, Switzerland, India and the Netherlands. He has authored/coauthored 250 publications, inclusive of journal articles, book chapters, books, and invited presentations. He has extensively traveled to many universities and institutes in Africa, Asia, Europe, and the Middle East for academic works, scientific meetings, and international collaborations. He is also a peer reviewer for several reputed journals, including *Comprehensive Reviews in Food Science and Food Safety, Food Science and Technology International, Journal of Agricultural and Food Chemistry, Journal of Food Science,* and *Journal of the Science of Food and Agriculture.*

Contents

Abbreviations .... *xix*

Foreword .... *xxvii*

Preface .... *xxix*

1. Cervical Cancer: Global Incidences and Progression 1

2. Wnt Signaling Pathway in Cervical Cancer 33

3. TLR Signaling Pathway in Cervical Cancer 49

4. PI3K-Akt-mTOR Signaling Pathways 71

5. Notch Signaling Pathway 91

6. Apoptotic Pathways in Cervical Cancer Management 117

7. NF-kB in Cervical Cancer Management 135

8. JAK-STAT Pathway in Cervical Cancer Management 153

9. Role of Micro-RNA in Cervical Cancer Progression and Its Therapeutic Implications 175

10. Cervical Cancer and Natural Products: Anticancerous Efficacy and Mechanism 215

11. Therapeutic Approaches for Cervical Cancer Management 257

Index* *279

Abbreviations

4E-BP1	4E binding protein 1
ACA	1'S-1'-acetoxychavicol
ACCS	1-aminocyclopropane-1-carboxylate synthase
ADAM	a disintegrin and metalloprotease
AID	activation-induced cytodine deaminase
AIDS	acquired immunodeficiency syndrome
AIF	apoptosis-inducing factor
ALL	acute lymphoblastic leukemia
AMKL	acute megakaryoblastic leukemia
AML	acute myeloid leukemia
AP-1	activator protein-1
APOBEC	apolipoprotein B mRNA editing catalytic polypeptide-like
ARID3B	AT-rich interaction domain 3B
BAFF	B cell activating factor
BAK	BCL2 antagonist/killer
BAX	Bcl-2-associated X-protein
BBC3	BCL2 binding component 3
BCG	Bacillus Calmette-Guérin
BCLL	B-cell chronic lymphoid leukemia
Bcl-xL	B-cell lymphoma-extra large
BDLNR	baicalein suppressed long non-coding RNA
CAR T	chimeric antigen receptor T-cell
CAR	chimeric antigen receptor
CAT	catalase
Cav-1	caveolin-1
CBFB	core-binding factor beta
CC	cervical cancer
CCND1	cyclin D1
CCSCC	cervical cancer squamous cell carcinomas
CDK	cyclin-dependent kinase
CDKN2A	cyclin-dependent kinase inhibitor 2A
CEM	2-cyanoethoxymethyl
CFTR	cystic fibrosis transmembrane conductance regulator

cIAP	cellular inhibitor of apoptosis protein
CIN	cervical intraepithelial neoplasia
CKIs	cyclin-dependent protein kinase inhibitors
CLDN1	claudin 1
CLL	chronic lymphocytic leukemia
CML	chronic myelogenous leukemia
c-MYC	master regulator of cell cycle entry and proliferative metabolism
COX-2	cyclooxygenase-2
CRE	cyclic adenosine monophosphate-responsive element
CSCC	cervical squamous cervical carcinoma
CSCs	cancer stem cells
CTLA-4	cytotoxic T lymphocyte-associated antigen
CTLs	cytotoxic T lymphocytes
CTNNB1	catenin beta 1
CUL5	Cullin 5
CXCR4	C-X-C motif chemokine receptor 4
CYR61	cysteine-rich angiogenic inducer 61
DC	dendritic cell
DIM	3,3-diindolylmethane
DISC	death-inducing signaling complex
DKK	Dickkopf
Dll	delta-like
DNA	deoxyribonucleic acid
DNMT1	DNA methyltransferase 1
DR5	death receptor 5
DSH	disheveled
EDA	extra domain A
EGCG	epigallocatechin gallate
EGF	epidermal growth factor
EGFR	epidermal growth factor receptor
EMT	epithelial-mesenchymal transition
ER	endoplasmic reticulum
ERK	extracellular-signal-regulated kinase
ET-1	endothelin-1
ETC	electron transport chain
FADD	Fas-associated death domain
FasL	Fas ligand

FDA	US Food and Drug Administration
FGF9	fibroblast growth factor 9
FLICE	FADD-like ICE
FLIPs	FADD-like interleukin-1β converting enzyme-like protease
FLT3	Fms-like tyrosine kinase 3
FOXM1	forkhead box protein M1
FOXO	forkhead box O protein
FZD7	frizzled class receptor 7
GHET1	gastric carcinoma proliferation enhancing transcript 1
GLUT1	glucose transporter protein type 1
GOG	gynecologic oncology group
GOLM1	Golgi membrane protein 1
GRP78	glucose-regulated protein of 78
GSH	glutathione
GSH-PX	glutathione peroxidase
GSK3	glycogen synthase kinase-3
HAS2	hyaluronan synthase 2
HCCR1	human cervical cancer oncogene 1
HDAC	histone deacetylase
HDGF	heparin-binding growth factor
HDI	human development index
HECW2	HECT domain ligase W2
HER2	human epidermal growth factor receptor 2
HES	hairy enhancer of split
HFKs	human foreskin keratinocytes
HIF-1	hypoxia-inducible factor-1
HIF-1α	hypoxia-inducible factor 1 alpha
HLTF	helicase like transcription factor
HMGB1	high mobility group box 1
HPV	human papillomavirus
HR-HPV	high risk HPV
HSP70	heat shock protein 70
hTERT	human telomerase reverse transcriptase
ICI	immune checkpoint inhibitor
IFNs	interferons
IFN-γ	interferon γ
IGFBP7	insulin-like growth factor-binding protein 7

IkB	inhibitor of kB
IKK	IkappaB kinase
IKZF4	IKAROS family zinc finger 4
ILs	interleukins
iNOS	inducible nitric oxide synthase
IR	immune response
IRF3	interferon regulatory factor 3
ISREs	IFN-stimulated response elements
JAK2	janus kinase 2
JAK-STAT	janus kinases-signal transducer and activated transcription proteins
JNK	c-Jun N-terminal kinase
KIR	kinase inhibitory region
KLK10	kallikrein related peptidase 10
LCR	long control region
LDH	lactate dehydrogenase
LEF	lymphoid enhancer factor
LIN28B	lin-28 homolog B
LIPA	lipase A, lysosomal acid type
LKB1	liver kinase B1
lncRNA	long non-coding RNA
LPS	lipopolysaccharides
LRP	low density lipoprotein receptor-related proteins
MACC1	metastasis-associated colon cancer 1
MAPK	mitogen activated protein kinase
MCM2	minichromosome maintenance complex II
MCP1	monocyte chemoattractant protein 1
MDR	multidrug resistance
METTL3	methyltransferase-like 3
MHC	major histocompatibility complex
miRNA	microRNA
MKI67	marker of proliferation Ki-67
MM	multiple myeloma
MMC	mitomycin C
MMP	mitochondrial membrane potential
MMP2	matrix metalloproteinase 2
MMPs	metalloproteinases
MPL	monophosphoryl lipid A

MRE	magnetic resonance elastography
MRI	magnetic resonance imaging
mRNA	messenger RNA
MRP	multidrug resistance-associated protein
MST2	mammalian sterile 20-like kinase
MTDH	metadherin
mTOR	mammalian target of rapamycin
MyD88	myeloid differentiation factor 88
MZF1	myeloid zinc finger 1
NCDB	National Cancer Database
NCI	National Cancer Institute
NCR	non-coding region
NFkB	nuclear factor kappa B
NICD	notch intracellular domain
NKX2–1	NK2 homeobox 1
NO	nitric oxide
NSCLC	non-small cell lung cancer
oncomiRs	oncogenic mRNAs
ORF	open reading frames
OS	overall survival
PARP	poly(ADP-ribose) polymerase
PCP	planar cell polarity
PCTP	phosphatidylcholine transfer protein
PD-1	programmed cell death protein 1
PDCD4	programmed cell death 4
PDGF	platelet-derived growth factor
PDGFR	platelet-derived growth factor receptors
PD-L1	programmed death-ligand 1
PDX	patient-derived xenograft
PET	positron emission tomography
PFS	progression-free survival
PGE2	prostaglandin E2
PI3K	phosphatidylinositol-3 kinase
PI3K/Akt	phosphatidylinositol-3 kinase/Akt
PIAS	protein inhibitor of activated STAT
PIK3CD	phosphoinositide-3-kinase catalytic subunit delta
PIP2	phosphatidylinositol-4,5-bisphosphate
PIP3	phosphatidylinositol-3,4,5-triphosphate

PKA	protein kinase A
PLSCR1	phospholipid scramblase 1
PP2A	phosphoprotein phosphatase 2A
pRB	retinoblastoma protein
PRDM1	PR/SET domain 1
PTEN	phosphatase and tensin homolog
PTK	protein tyrosine kinase
PTPN9	protein tyrosine phosphatase non-receptor type 9
PTPs	protein tyrosine phosphatases
PUMA	p53-upregulated modulator of apoptosis
RANKL	receptor activator of NF-kB ligand
RCTs	randomized controlled trials
RHD	Rel homology domain
RHOA	Ras homolog gene family member A
RISC	RNA-induced silencing complex
RNA	ribose nucleic acid
RUNX3	runt-related transcription factor 3
S6k-1	ribosomal protein S6 kinase-1
SCC	squamous cell carcinoma
SCD1	stearoyl-CoA desaturase 1
SCJ	squamous columnar junction
siRNA	small interfering RNA
SOCS	suppressor of cytokine signaling
STARD13	StAR related lipid transfer domain containing 13
STAT	signal transducer and activator of transcription
TACE	TNF-alpha converting enzyme
TCF	T-cell factor
TCGA	the cancer genome atlas
TFCP2	transcription factor CP2
TILs	tumor-infiltrating lymphocytes
TIMP1	tissue inhibitor of metalloproteinase-1
TIRAP	TIR-containing adaptor protein
TLRs	toll-like receptors
TME	tumor microenvironment
TNF	tumor necrosis factor
TNF-α	tumor necrosis factor-alpha
TNKS2	tyrosine kinase nonreceptor-2
TOP2	topoisomerase II protein

TP53INP1	tumor protein P53 inducible nuclear protein 1
TRADD	TNF receptor-associated death domain
TRAF1	tumor expression necrosis factor-associated receptor factor 1
TRAIL	TNF-related apoptosis-inducing ligand
tsmiRs	tumor suppressor miRNAs
UHFR1	ubiquitin-like with PHD and ring finger domains 1
UPR	unfolded protein response
URR	upstream regulatory region
UTR	untranslated region
UV	ultraviolet
VASP	vasodilator-stimulated phosphoprotein
VDAC1	voltage-dependent anion channel 1
VEGF	vascular endothelial growth factor
VLPs	virus-like particles
WHO	World Health Organization
WIF1	Wnt inhibitory factor 1
Wnt	wingless-type
XIAP	X-linked inhibitor of apoptosis protein
YAP1	yes-associated protein 1
YBX1	Y-box binding protein 1
ZEB1	zinc finger E-box binding homeobox 1

Foreword

Driven by the intense research in the field of oncology, and by the increasing incidence and high mortality rates associated with cancer, this book aims to provide an up-to-date view of the epidemiology related to cervical cancer. Indeed, and alarmingly, current estimates point to 6,04,000 new cases and 3,42,000 deaths in 2020, with an age-standardized death rate among women of 13.3/1,00,000. Recent data also underlined that the adoption of effective therapeutic interventions suited to the woman's life cycle would promote a marked reduction in mortality rates, particularly in low- and middle-income countries, where the incidence is more notorious.

The intense research in the area has boosted marked advances in the understanding of cervical cancer pathogenesis, suggesting, as a result of several researches, that the modulation of several signaling pathways constitutes a promising therapeutic approach in its control, monitoring, and even treatment, and more importantly in preventing the disease's onset.

Thus, this book is an asset for students, researchers in the area, and even oncologists who are dedicated to research, but also to clinicians that are directly in contact with patients to deepen knowledge on the signaling pathways directly related to the onset of cervical cancer, the molecular biology techniques used for its identification (such as DNA replication and transcription, as well as protein activity), the pharmacological approaches that have been developed to date to prevent the outcomes related to the alterations in signaling pathways, culminating in a brushstroke on the anticancer potential of natural products and their mode of action, while highly promising matrices and a source of outstanding molecules with therapeutic properties.

Taken together, all aspects highlighted above and addressed throughout this book make it of greatest interest and importance, being, therefore, an extremely valuable tool for students, researchers, and even health professionals who wish to design their future research studies, promote the continuous development of the area and even contribute to a marked progress in the area of oncology, insofar as some signaling pathways identified here may contribute to a deepening of knowledge and innovation in other sub-areas of oncology.

—Prof. Dr. Natália Cruz-Martins, PhD
Cooperativa de Ensino Superior Politécnico e Universitário (CESPU)
Faculdade de Medicina, Universidade do Porto (FMUP)
Porto, Portugal

Preface

The prime aim of this book is to connect exigent medical issues, including cancer, with different plausible solutions via a description of an array of research possibilities in this field. This book provides a concise yet thorough outline of the signaling cascade operating between cellular machinery, which will definitely help and motivate future and emerging researchers. The scientists and researchers will also be inspired by this book to navigate the maze of signaling pathways and the plethora of signals, receptors, effectors, and transducers that promote carcinogenesis.

Presentation of every signaling pathway would be accompanied by a brief summary of the modifications reported in malignancies and the targeted pharmaceutical strategies that can be employed to prevent the outcomes associated with these oncogenic alterations. Mechanisms of molecular biology at different cellular levels (DNA replication, transcription, and translation phases) are displayed in a sequence of pedagogic annexes, aiding readers to better recognize the aberrations in signaling pathways. Hence, this book will undoubtedly provide a thorough introduction to cell signaling, the transformations it encounters in cancer, and the compounds that are emerging as potential targets for drug development in cervical cancer. In addition, it would present various therapies that are being utilized for the efficient treatment and management of cervical cancer.

The book comprises of 11 chapters. Chapter 1 discusses the global incidences and progression of cervical cancer. Chapter 2 utilizes the association of Wnt signaling pathway in cervical cancer progression. Chapter 3 provides detailed insights about the involvement of the aberrated TLR signaling pathway in cervical cancer development. Chapter 4 unravels the role of P13K-Akt-mTOR signaling pathways in cervical cancer development and progression. Chapter 5 focuses on the role of a Notch signaling pathway in the development and progression of cervical cancer. Chapter 6 represents apoptotic pathways implicated in cervical cancer progression. Chapter 7 targets the NF-kB signaling pathway and its aberrant elements associated with cervical cancer. Chapter 8 describes the crucial targets of JAK-STAT signaling pathway responsible for cervical cancer development. Chapter 9 explains the emerging role of natural bioactive compounds from plants against cervical cancer. Chapter 10 focuses on the role of micro-RNA in cervical cancer development and progression. Finally, Chapter 11 explains several therapeutic approaches utilized for elucidating better therapeutic approaches for cervical cancer management.

Our main focus was to present a comprehensive introduction to cell signaling, its alterations in cancer, and molecules that have been emerging as potential targets for drug development in cervical cancer. This book would definitely help students and researchers understand the crucial involvement of these aberrated signaling pathways in the progression of cervical cancer. This would help researchers in elucidating novel approaches for the better management of cervical cancer. Additionally, this book would help researchers explore these pathways, thereby adding to the existing implications of these pathways in cancer.

First and foremost, we would like to thank Ashish Kumar and Sandra Sickels at Apple Academic Press for their invaluable advice and guidance throughout the preparation of this book. We thank our family and friends for their motivation, help, and continuous support. Without that, we could not have succeeded in completing this book. Last but not least, we would like to express our gratitude to everyone who inspired us to work on this most influential and necessary publication and assisted us along the way.

—Authors

CHAPTER 1

Cervical Cancer: Global Incidences and Progression

1.1 INTRODUCTION

Cervical cancer has been one of the fourth most deadly malignancies amongst women globally. The discovery that chronic infection with oncogenic *human papillomavirus* (HPV) forms is the principal cause of cervical cancer paved the way for innovative primary and secondary preventive strategies (Petry, 2014). Cervical cancer occurrence and death can be greatly reduced if both strategies of prevention are used. In the United States, its mortality and incidence rates have been reducing due to the wider implementation of cytological screening programs (Hogarth et al., 2012). However, there have been geographical disparities in cervical carcinoma patients, predominantly in the US. This chapter outlines the global prevalence of cancer of cervix and reported the factors associated with disparities in the mortality and incidence rates of cervical cancer. We have conducted a literature search between the years 1999 and 2020 regarding the disparities associated with incidence and mortality rates of cervical cancer. Ethnic and racial minorities, socio-economically disenfranchised, and populations residing in rural regions have dissimilar vaccination rates, treatment, and screening for cervical cancer, thereby leading to worst outcomes (Musselwhite et al., 2016). Thus, it can be determined that incidences and mortality rates of cervical cancer can be achieved by addressing these discrepancies by providing education, easy access to health care and wider implementation of vaccination and screening programs.

Cervical Cancer: Signaling Pathways, Molecular Mechanisms, Natural Products, and Therapeutic Approaches. Pratibha Pandey, Fahad Khan, Saher Islam, and Devarajan Thangadurai, (Eds.)

Cervical cancer is the fourth most common malignancy in women globally, behind breast cancer, colorectal cancer, and lung cancer (Small et al., 2017). In the year 2018, there were almost 5,70,000 instances of cervical carcinoma in the United States, as per the National Cancer Institute, and a total of 3,11,000 people were killed. Cervical cancer affected 13.1 out of every 1,00,000 women worldwide (Alter et al., 2018). Together, China and India made an impact. More than a third of all cervical cancer cases occur in developing countries. In China, there were 1,06,000 instances and 48,000 fatalities, and in the United States, there were 1,06,000 instances and 48,000 fatalities. In India, 97,000 people have been diagnosed with the disease, with 60,000 people dying as a result (Arbyn et al., 2020). Across the board, cervical cancer was diagnosed on average at 53 years old and the average age of death in the world was 59 years. While cancer incidence and death have decreased in Western, affluent countries as a result of lifestyle changes such as smoking cessation and advances in screening and treatment techniques, cancer incidence and death have increased in low-income and developing countries. Infectious agents, including *Human papillomavirus* (HPV), hepatitis B/C viruses, and *Helicobacter pylori*, inexplicably distress underdeveloped countries and they recurrently lack the financial and institutional ways to implement widespread screening programs.

Since the 1970s, the incidence and death of cervical cancer in the United States have gradually decreased, owing largely to the widespread implementation of cytological screening programs based on the Papanicolaou test (Koss et al., 1989). Despite these gains, it is anticipated that 13,800 women in the United States would be freshly reported with cervical malignancy in 2020, with 4,290 women dying as a result of their illness. The most preventable types of cancer, such as cervical cancer, show the greatest geographic disparities in cancer rates in the US. This gap was documented between 2012 and 2016, when the total incidence rate for cervical cancer in the United States was 7.6 instances per 1,00,000 people, with the highest rate of 9.8 instances per 1,00,000 people in Arkansas and the lowest rate of 4.1 per 1,00,000 people in Vermont. These regional variations are expected to persist, with new cervical cancer cases in California (1630), Texas (1410), Florida (1130), and New York (930) expected to be among the highest in 2020. The process of carcinogenesis of HPV has been studied for more than 30 years, with several low and high-risk strains being identified and associated with the most common kinds of cervical cancer. HPV-16 and -18 are the most high-risk HPV types, contributing to greater than 70% of cervical malignancies. There are 15 high-risk HPV strains identified so far, with seven of them (HPV 16/18/31/33/45/52/58) protected by the commercial HPV vaccine Gardasil-9 (Kirby et al., 2015). The vaccination was found to be 97% effective only against these high-risk variants in the randomized experiment that led to FDA clearance (Silver et al., 2020). Prior to its approval, various safety investigations were completed, and continuous safety monitoring systems continue to show that the product is safe.

1.2 VACCINATION AND WHO STRATEGY

The HPV vaccine is prescribed for regular immunization of teenage children aged 11 or 12, with catch-up vaccines available until age 26 for individuals who have not been immunized, and shared decision-making for those aged 27 to 45 (Mix et al., 2021). Despite these advancements in cervical cancer screening and inhibition, the US susceptible population continues to trail behind other developed nations, with only about half of adolescent girls receiving full vaccination and only 43% of women at the age of 30 encounter recent HPV DNA screening tests in 2015 (Beavis et al., 2016). Although overall cervical cancer incidence and mortality have reduced, there may be disparities in screening, immunization, treatment, and overall mortality among the most vulnerable populations, such as racial and ethnic minorities, the poor, and women living in rural and isolated locations.

The global strategy of the WHO (World Health Organization) for the eradication of cervical cancer by 2030 mainly comprises three primary pillars: screening, prevention, and treatment. According to the WHO, in order to meet global elimination targets by this date, every country must achieve 90% HPV vaccination coverage among girls (at the age of 15), 70% screening, 90% precancerous lesions therapy, and 90% management of invasive cancer cases (Sriplung et al., 2014; Canfell et al., 2020). There are several differences in each of these areas that have the potential to jeopardize the fulfillment of these objectives and must be highlighted. Screening and immunization are the first steps toward preventing and/or intervening in cervical cancer before it develops. Although the vaccination to prevent oncogenic variants of HPV has been widely accessible since

2006, vaccine uptake has been modest in the United States and varies greatly within various geographical, racial, and ethnic groups (Trottier et al., 2006). Overall, 48.6% of adolescents aged 13 to 17 were up to date on their HPV vaccine series in 2017. Initially, it was stated that blacks, Asians, and Latinas in the United States had lower vaccination rates than whites. Recent research, on the other hand, has revealed a sharper increase in vaccination uptake among racial and ethnic adolescents, emerging in greater coverage compared to their white counterparts. In 2017, whites had a vaccination rate of 44.7%, blacks had a rate of 50.2%, Hispanics had a rate of 56.4%, and Asians had a rate of 52.5%.

Vaccination coverage varies greatly by region, with non-metropolitan areas and women without health insurance having the lowest rates. In 2018, HPV vaccination rates among adolescents aged 13 to 17 years girls ranged between 38% in Kansas and Mississippi area to about 70% in Washington DC, and Rhode Island, while for boys, it was between 27% in Mississippi to about 70% in Massachusetts and Rhode Island (Chen et al., 2020). Strong physician recommendations and better patient knowledge and comprehension of HPV are likely to have contributed to augmented vaccination among minorities over time. Knowledge of the virus and strong clinicians' endorsements have had a significant impact on HPV vaccination initiation and could be crucial in raising uptake and reducing geographic disparities. The disparity in cervical malignancy screening frequencies is a contributing element, as well as a potential exacerbating factor, in the differences in cervical cancer incidence and mortality (Bao et al., 2018). There was a significant drop in pap smear test diagnoses amongst women aged 21–65 years between 2000 and 2015. The link between insufficient screening and an increased risk of cervical cancer is well supported by this research. Women with low educational attainment or who are uninsured, as well as immigrants, have the lowest rates of cervical cancer screening. Asian and Hispanic women had lower screening rates than white and black non-Hispanic women (Jørgensen et al., 2022).

1.3 EPIDEMIOLOGY OF CERVICAL CANCER

Furthermore, geographic location has been linked to differences in cervical cancer screening, with women in rural locations being less prone to have their cervical cancer checked than those in urban or suburban areas. In addition, southern states in the United States have reported a much greater percentage of women who had not had a cervical cancer screening in the previous five years. This was sadly connected with the fact that the South had the greatest incidence rate of recently detected cervical carcinoma (8.5 per 1,00,000) and the maximum mortality (relative to other census regions) (2.7 per 1,00,000). These geographical inequalities in screening are assumed to be linked to a scarcity of clinicians in rural locations and an increase in the uninsured population (Figure 1.1). Cervical cancer screening challenges can be individual and, secondary to structural barriers to care. Personal barriers to screening have been identified, including ignorance of screening and risk factors, anxiety about cancer detection, shame, and mistrust of the healthcare system. Furthermore, transportation, expense, time away from work, language hurdles and a lack of physician availability or advice have all been linked to insufficient screening among our most vulnerable populations. The development of cervical cancer is directly linked to limited possibilities for inhibition through immunization and screening. However, not only disparities in cervical cancer prevention options, but there are also disparities in cervical cancer treatment and mortality rates for the most susceptible communities once the disease has been diagnosed.

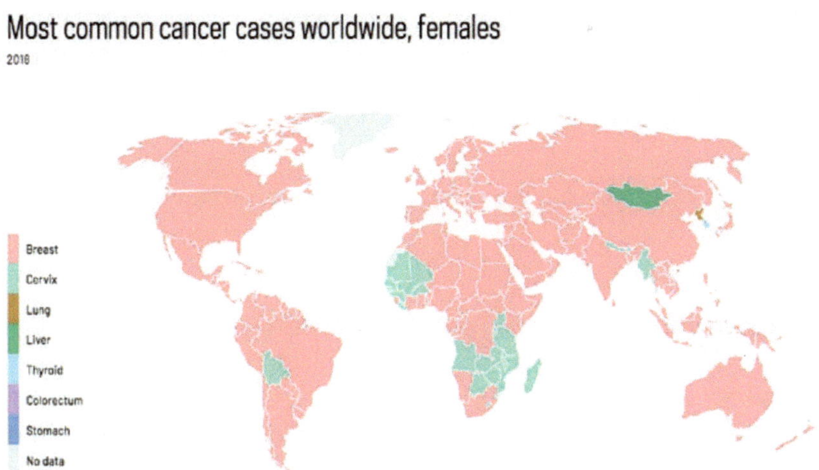

FIGURE 1.1 Worldwide representation of cervical cancer cases in comparison to other cancer in females.

Source: Extracted from The Cancer Genome Atlas.

Black women still had a 19% higher probability of dying from their disease than white women, even after adjusting for age, phase, histology, and the type of first therapy (Table 1.1). However, more current data showing mortality rates adjusted for hysterectomy rates has revealed that the apparent mortality discrepancy among black and white females may have been understated by 44%. The corrected death rate for black women was 10.1 cases per 1,00,000 (uncorrected 5.7 instances per 1,00,000) vs. 4.7 per 1,00,000 for white women (uncorrected 3.2 instances per 1,00,000). Furthermore, the adjusted death rates among black women climbed dramatically with age, reaching 29.7 per 1,00,000 for those 75–79 years old, 33.4 for those 80–84 years old, and 37.2 for those 85 years old (Figure 1.2). Differences in adherence to treatment and accessibility to healthcare have been linked to racial and ethnic variations in morbidity. Recent studies have found that discrepancies in the treatment standard for females with primary disease stage (IA1-IIA) have decreased in recent years as more black women have undergone the necessary surgery or chemo-radiotherapy. However, black women were less likely than other women to receive chemo-radiotherapy for later-stage illness (stage IIB-IVA) (75.6% versus 80.4%) (Beavis et al., 2017). Despite the fact that the extent of the discrepancy has diminished over time, black women had a 35% lower chance of obtaining chemo-radiotherapy after accounting for known confounders. There has been a mixed bag of research on how access to care contributes to disparities in results. According to recent NCDB research on later-stage IB2-IVA illness, differences in guideline-based care were greatest at high-volume hospitals, indicating that access was not the primary issue (Gill et al., 2014). Other studies, on the other hand, have found that having equal access to care results in equivalent survival rates.

1.4 CERVICAL CANCER AND ITS DEVELOPMENT

Cervical cancer emerged second over breast cancer in women globally. There is a constant increase in cervical cancer incidences, although this malignancy has been reported to be one of the best preventable human carcinomas (Waggoner et al., 2003). Cervical cancer genesis has been mainly associated with uterine cervix infection with HPV (*Human papillomavirus*) that persists for several decades (Cohen et al., 2019). Numerous

TABLE 1.1 International Federation of Gynecology and Obstetrics (FIGO) Staging

FIGO Stages	Definition
IA	Invasive carcinoma is diagnosed only by microscopy, with a maximum depth of invasion <5 mm.
IA1	Measured stromal invasion <3 mm in depth.
IA2	Measured stromal invasion ≥3 mm and <5 mm in depth.
IB	Clinically visible lesion confined to the cervix or microscopic lesion greater than IA2.
IB1	Invasive carcinoma ≥5 mm depth of stromal invasion, and <2 cm in greatest dimension.
IB2	Invasive carcinoma ≥2 cm and <4 cm in greatest dimension.
IB3	Invasive carcinoma ≥4 cm in greatest dimension.
II	Cervical carcinoma invades beyond the uterus but not to the pelvic wall or to lower third of vagina.
IIA	Tumor without parametrial invasion or involvement of the lower one-third of the vagina.
IIA1	Clinically visible lesion <4 cm in greatest dimension with involvement of less than the upper two-thirds of the vagina.
IIA2	Clinically visible lesion >4 cm in greatest dimension with involvement of less than the upper two-thirds of the vagina.
IIB	Tumor with parametrial invasion but not up to the pelvic wall.
III	Tumor extends to pelvic wall and/or involves lower third of vagina, and/or causes hydronephrosis or nonfunctioning kidney, and/or involves pelvic and/or para-aortic lymph nodes.
IIIA	Tumor involves lower third of vagina, no extension to the pelvic wall.
IIIB	Tumor extends to pelvic wall and/or causes hydronephrosis or nonfunctioning kidney.
IIIC	Tumor involves pelvic and/or para-aortic lymph nodes, irrespective of tumor size and extent.
IV	Tumor invades mucosa of bladder or rectum (biopsy proven), and/or extends beyond true pelvis.
IVA	Tumor has spread to adjacent pelvic organs.
IVB	Tumor has spread to distant organs.

Source: Reproduced with permission from Burmeister et al. (2022); Copyright © Elsevier (2022).

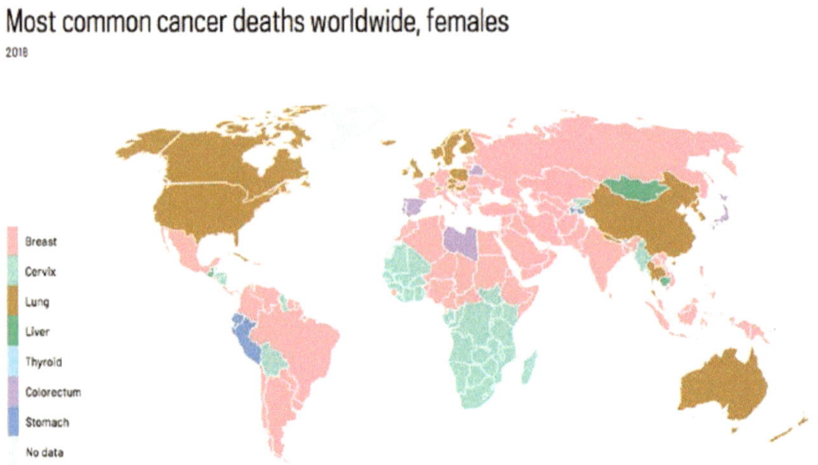

FIGURE 1.2 Worldwide representation of cervical cancer death rate in comparison to other cancer in females.

Source: Extracted from The Cancer Genome Atlas.

investigations have found significant oncogenic cell transformation in the SCJ (squamous columnar junction) cell population. These specifications facilitate primary prevention with HPV vaccination along with the detection and treatment of precursor lesions. Apart from some unusual exceptions, cervical carcinoma is the accidental endpoint of persisting HPV infections (Sankaranarayanan et al., 2016). The complete cancer genesis from persistent HPV infection to invasive cancer seems to need several years and, in most cases, approximately seven years. The elucidation of better precursors and cervical cancer seems to be dependent on infection of cells located at SCJ (border between endo and ecto cervix) (Figure 1.3).

1.4.1 CERVICAL CANCER AND HPV

Uterine cancer of the cervix is the second foremost basis of cancer fatalities in women, and it kills the most people in areas where there are no screening programs to detect precursor lesions. Persistent infection with 'high risk' *Human papillomavirus* (HPV) genotypes is essential, but not adequate for cervical cancer to develop. There are more than 120 different types of HPV that infect human mucosa and skin (Neels et al., 2013).

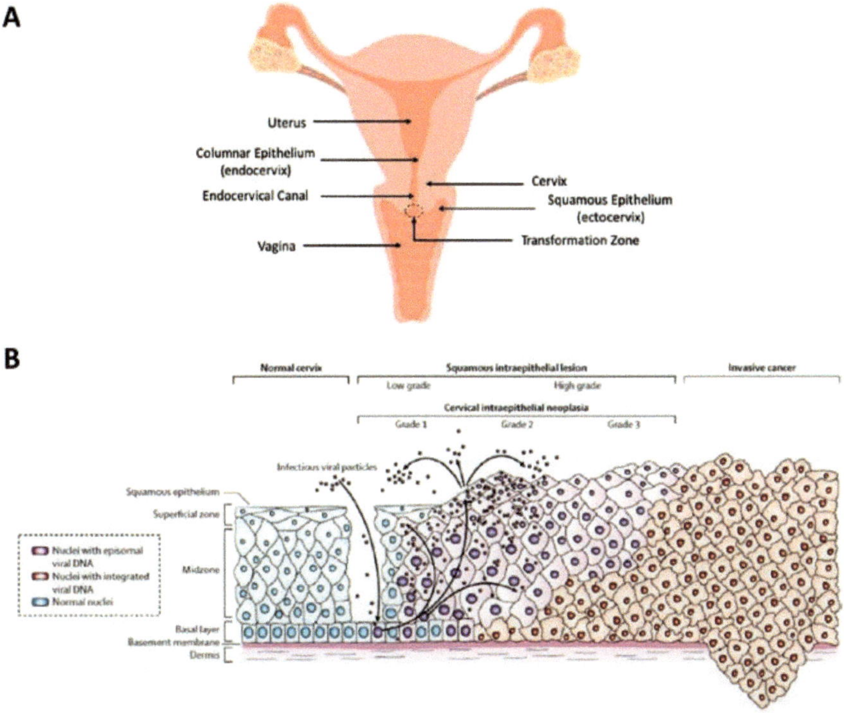

FIGURE 1.3 Anatomical location of cervical cancer origin and progression from a normal cervix to invasive squamous cell carcinoma mediated by HPV. (A) Anatomical diagram representing the female reproductive organs; **(B)** Schematic representation of HPV infection and cervical cancer development. Post-infection, HPV oncoproteins are overexpressed and play key roles in altering host cellular function. This results in precursor lesions, and cervical intraepithelial neoplasia, which progresses over time to invasive cancer.

Source: Reproduced with permission from Burmeister et al. (2022); Copyright © Elsevier (2022).

Human mucosa and skin can become infected by more than 120 different strains of HPV (Neels et al., 2013). HPV16 is one of the most crucial high risks HPV that has been linked to about 50% of cervical cancers globally. HPV18 and HPV16 have been associated with 2/3rd of all cervical cancer (Maheshwari et al., 2020).

Papillomavirus particles have a double-stranded DNA genome of about 7,000–8,000 base pairs and have a tiny diameter of 55 nm (McCarthy et al., 1998). The viral capsid is made up of 72 capsomeres, each of which contains two capsid proteins: L1 (major) and L2 (minor) (Pereira et al., 2009). The regulative mechanism of viral gene expression is complicated, and it is influenced by a number of cellular and viral transcription factors. High-risk HPV is distinguished from other forms of HPV by the carcinogenic potential of two key proteins, E7 and E6, which may disrupt cell development and control (Sen et al., 2018). Uterine cervix with HPV infection is very common, specifically in women of early 20s. Almost HPV infections would get clear rapidly with only a very few persisting for decades or several years (Senapati et al., 2016). Thus, high-risk HPV prevalence rates decline with increasing age. According to the findings, there are four crucial phases and cofactors involved in the genesis of cancer, commencing with the initial infection and continuing through persistent infection with CIN3 precursor development, which leads to cancer progression in more than 30% of cancer cases (Wentzensen et al., 2012) (Figure 1.4).

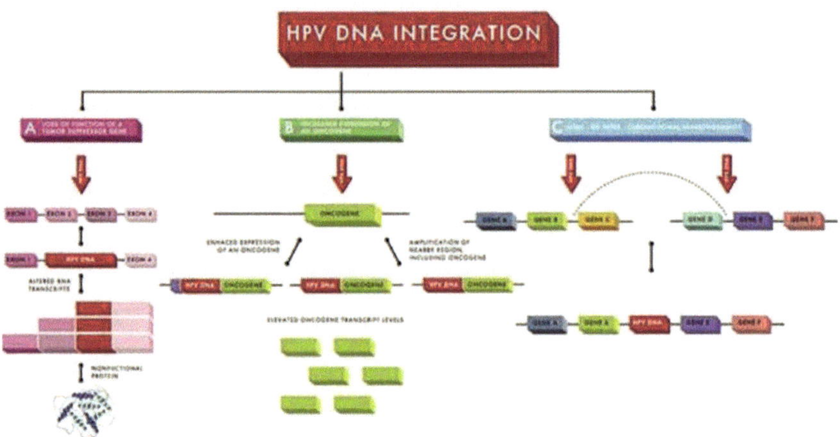

FIGURE 1.4 Alterations produced by viral integration in the host genome. These integration mechanisms can lead to alterations in key genes. (A) Loss of function of a tumor suppressor gene, with transcripts producing truncated or non-functional proteins. (B) Increased expression of an oncogene can occur when the virus integrates upstream of an oncogene in the host cell or when the site of integration stimulates the promoters of viral oncogenes. And (C) intra- or inter-chromosomal rearrangements can result in altered expression of multiple genes in the regions affected by the viral integration site.

Source: Reproduced with permission from: Oyervides-Muñoz et al. (2018); Copyright © Elsevier (2018).

HPV causes basal and Para basal cell proliferation, which leads to epithelial hyperplasia or papillomatosis with various extensions. The activity of E5, E6, and E7 viral proteins is responsible for this oncogenicity (Haller et al., 1995; McLaughlin-Drubin & Münger, 2009). These oncoproteins cause continuous cell growth and an inability to repair possible genetic damage, resulting in the accumulation of rearrangements, aneuploidies, and mutations that can lead to cancer (Vousden, 1993). A number of typical cell pathways and proteins are disrupted, including those involved in cell division and apoptosis (Sandal, 2002; Jayshree et al., 2009).

The E7 protein, for example, binds to pRB family tumor suppressor proteins and degrades them to allow uncontrolled expression of the E2F transcription factor, which increases the expression of genes involved in the synthesis stage (S) of the cell cycle. E7 also interacts with p21 and p27, which are key cyclin-dependent kinase inhibitors (CDK). In human keratinocytes, CDK proteins primarily target cyclin-CDK2, which governs the transition from G1 to S phase (Eichten et al., 2004). The E6 protein also inhibits the pro-apoptotic actions of proteins like Bak, Bax, c-myc, and p53, which are required for the neoplastic phenotype to be maintained. The incorporation of HPV genome into the host genetic material is thought to be a critical step in the progression of cervical cancer. This stage occurs when the viral DNA is cleaved at the E1/E2 gene cleavage site (Finzer et al., 2002), resulting in the loss of the E2 gene, and neighboring sections of the E4, E5, and L2 genes (Motoyama et al., 2004). As a result, E2's transcriptional regulation is disrupted, leading to E6 and E7 overexpression and severe malignancy (Park et al., 1997). Telomerase, centrosome duplication factors and signaling proteins have all been identified as targets for the E6 and E7 oncoproteins in other research (Cai et al., 2013; Scarth et al., 2021). Despite the fact that the HPV E6 and E7 proteins are critical for HPV transforming properties, the significance of the E5 protein in the development of cervical cancer is increasingly being investigated (Malla & Kamal, 2021). Because the E5 gene is deleted after the viral DNA has been integrated into the host genome, the activities of this oncoprotein promote tumor formation, especially in the early stages of the disease. E5 is involved in a variety of mechanisms involving multiple signaling pathways for cell proliferation, angiogenesis, and death (Liao et al., 2013; Ren et al., 2020). The association of E5 with the epidermal growth factor receptor (EGFR), which leads to cell proliferation, is one of the most well-known E5-mediated tumorigenic actions. Modulation of host miRNAs is another recently found mechanism linked to HPV oncogenesis (Liu et al., 2015). More than half of miRNA genes are found in the fragile regions or integration sites of hrHPVs, causing HPV interference in miRNA production (Calin et al., 2004). Integration can change miRNA expression by deleting, amplification, or rearranging the genome. However, certain functional investigations have demonstrated that the functions of E5, E6, and E7 oncoproteins cause abnormal profiles of specific miRNAs (Greco et al., 2011). A more detailed description of miRNA role in cervical cancer progression and therapeutics is provided in a subsequent chapter.

1.4.2 HPV STRUCTURE AND GENOME

HPV belongs to the small and non-enveloped, dsDNA virus family *Papillomaviridae* family having the capability to target epithelial cells of anogenital, oral, and skin mucosa. HPV group of viruses can spread via numerous routes such as anal, vaginal, or oral sex and may cause numerous carcinomas, including vulvar, cervical, oral, anal, penile, and vaginal cancer in the human body (Furomoto et al., 2002) (Figure 1.5).

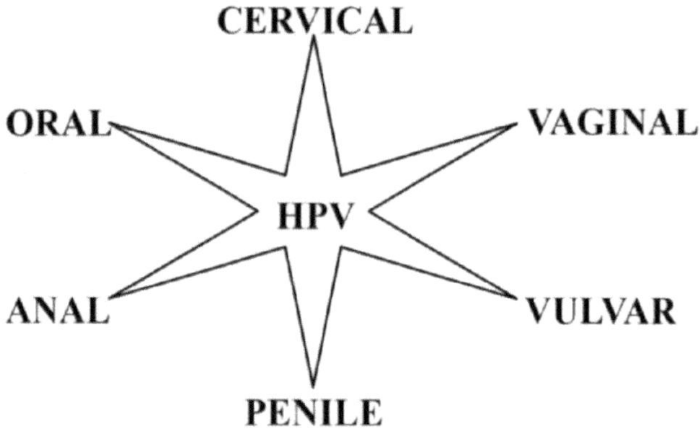

FIGURE 1.5 HPV-induced carcinomas in the human body.

HPV (sexually transmitted) may be categorized as a high-risk or low-risk cancer type. Low-risk HPV may lead to warts either on or around the anus, genitals, throat, and mouth. High-risk HPV, including HPV18 and HPV 16 may lead to numerous carcinomas (Stanley et al., 2007). Viral genome constitutes three regions, namely E (early) region having numerous ORF (open reading frames) that encode E1, E2, and E4 (replication proteins) and E5, E6, and E7 (oncoproteins); L (late) region with L1 and L2 late genes encoding L1 (major) and L2 (minor) capsid proteins of virus. HPV capsid has 50–60 nm diameter and icosahedral formation (72 L1 protein pentamers). Major L2 protein is found in the center region of pentamers (L2:L1 ratio of 1:5–1:10); and URR (upstream regulatory region)/NCR (non-coding region)/LCR (long control region), located between E6 and L1 open reading frames containing regulatory elements responsible for DNA replication and transcription in virus (Scudellari, 2013) (Table 1.2 and Figure 1.6).

Several studies have described various approaches for developing HPV vaccines, with a focus on the L1 (or major) capsid protein, which self-assembles to empty VLPs (virus-like particles) that are extremely immunogenic when administered intramuscularly, and which have been accepted and licensed in several countries since 2006. These vaccines have shown significant efficacy against HPV-16 or 18-related cervical intraepithelial neoplasia, with acceptable safety and tolerability, long protective duration, and high immunogenicity (Wang et al., 2006). Other preventive approach includes prevention mechanism based upon the detection of surgically excised precursor lesions. Therefore, natural carcinogenesis is interrupted, and cervical cancer development is actively prevented. There is a low risk of invasive cervical cancer in case of complete excision of pre-cancer cells. Since the 1990s, HPV testing has emerged as a possible screening test due to HPV's essential involvement in cervical cancer genesis (Franco et al., 2003). For numerous years, a negative HPV test ruled out any chance of cervical cancer. In comparison to Pap smear-based screening, HPV screening resulted in a higher detection rate of high-grade precursors, according to six RCTs (randomized controlled trials) and numerous high-quality cohort studies (Petry, 2014).

1.5 MOLECULAR TARGETS OF HPV ONCOPROTEINS

Presently, there has been an upsurge in the studies looking into the genes or proteins, that are linked to cervical tumorigenesis, with the goal of finding a biomarker that can substitute or enhance cytohistological assays

TABLE 1.2 Synopsis of the Role of HPV Early Proteins in CC and Their Therapeutic Targets

Early Protein	*Preclinical*	Pathways	Cancer Hallmark	Mechanisms	Therapeutic Potential	References
E1	*In vitro* and *in vivo*	NF-κB	NA	Helps in initiation and regulation of HPV replication. Acts as a helicase and recruits replication factors.	ATP acts as an allosteric modulator of E1-E2 interactions. Indandione is a small class of molecules that act as a potential inhibitor of the E1-E2 interaction.	Berg & Stenlund (1997); Goodwin & DiMaio (2000); White et al. (2001, 2003); Moody & Laimins (2010); D'Abramo & Archambault (2011); Bergvall et al. (2013); Chojnacki & Melendy (2018); Castro-Muñoz et al. (2019)
E2	*In vitro* and *in vivo*	NA	NA	Aids in initiation and regulation of HPV replication. Enable the binding of E1 protein. Disruption of E2 leads to CC progression. Negative transcription regulator of E6.	ATP acts as an allosteric modulator of E1-E2 interactions. Indandione is a small class of molecules that act as a potential inhibitor of the E1-E2 interaction.	Berg & Stenlund (1997); Goodwin & DiMaio (2000); White et al. (2001, 2003); Moody & Laimins (2010); D'Abramo & Archambault (2011); Chojnacki & Melendy (2018); Cruz-Gregorio et al. (2018); Zahra et al. (2021)
E4	*In vitro* and *in vivo*	NA	NA	Involved in viral release, transmission, and PTM. Associates with keratin and could manipulate cytokeratin network, essential in the release of the virus.	Controlling the phosphorylation of E4 modulates its activity and is unable to affect the host.	Rogel-Gaillard et al. (1993); Doorbar et al. (1996); Roberts et al. (2003); Kim et al. (2009); Wang et al. (2009); McIntosh et al. (2010); Khan et al. (2011); Doorbar (2013)

TABLE 1.2 *(Continued)*

Early Protein	*Preclinical*	Pathways	Cancer Hallmark	Mechanisms	Therapeutic Potential	References
E5	*In vitro*	MAPK-ERK pathways	Angiogenesis, evading cell death, cellular proliferation	Major oncoprotein in HPV mediated carcinogenesis. Supportive role in E6 and E7 modulation. Suppresses p21 expression and initiates CC progression.	E5 inhibition by inhibiting the NF-kB pathway with inhibitors like narasin or flurosalan or celecoxib. Specific cytotoxic T cells are designed specifically for HPV E5 proteins with CpG-oligodeoxynucleotide and targets and degrade them so that their function is lost permanently.	Crook et al. (1991); Jones and Münger (1996); Stöppler et al. (1996); Kabsch & Alonso (2002); Dinneen & Ceresa (2004); DeMasi et al. (2005); Farley et al. (2006); Kim et al. (2006); Regan & Laimins (2008); Sima et al. (2008); Wang et al. (2010); Ganguly (2012)
E6	*In vitro* and *in vivo*	PI3K, AKT, Wnt, Notch pathways, and EMT	Cellular proliferation, invasion metastasis, genomic instability, cellular immortality, cell cycle arrest, tumor-promoting inflammation, resisting cell death	Neoplastic effect on HPV-infected cells by promoting ubiquitin-dependent proteasome degradation of p53 and evades cell death. Targets degradation of apoptotic signaling cascade molecules through the ubiquitin-proteasome pathway leading to tumor development by inhibiting apoptosis. Causes dysregulated cell proliferation by downregulating transcriptional co-activator p300/CBP, essential for cell cycle. E6 is associated with the production of ROS that induces DNA breakdown and downregulates tumor suppressor genes. Downregulates IRF-3 of IFN-β and makes the immune response vulnerable against antigens of HPV. E6 inhibits the X-ray repair cross-complementing 1 is a scaffold DNA repair protein leading to increased mutation.	PDZ domains proteins including HDL protein, MUPP1, MAGI-1,2,3 are useful as therapeutic targets. Replacement of Lxx Φ Lsh leucine motifs with alanine results in E6 binding being terminated. RNA interference (RNAi) technology simultaneously knockdown both E6 and E7 expression.	Lee et al. (1997); Sanchez-Perez et al. (1997); Brehm et al. (1999); Li et al. (1999); Patel et al. (1999); Nakagawa & Huibregtse (2000); Be et al. (2001); Filippova et al. (2002); Nguyen et al. (2002); Thomas et al. (2002); Al Moustafa et al. (2004); Kelley et al. (2005); Baleja et al. (2006); Brennan et al. (2009); Jung et al. (2013); Henderson et al. (2014); Manzo-Merino et al. (2014); Vieira et al. (2014); Shah et al. (2015); Warren et al. (2017)

TABLE 1.2 *(Continued)*

Early Protein	*Preclinical*	Pathways	Cancer Hallmark	Mechanisms	Therapeutic Potential	References
E7	*In vitro*	PI3K/AKT, EMT	Replicative immortality, activating invasion and metastasis, evading growth suppressors, cell invasion, genomic instability, chronic inflammation	Promotes cervical dysplasia causing dysregulated cell cycle. Inactivates pRb and downregulates E2F for CC progression through conserved LXCXE motif of amino terminus 9. Causes deregulation of cyclin A/CDK2 and cyclin E/CDK2 by inactivation of p21 and p27 leading to increases in the spindle formation rate, which brings uncontrollable cell cycle formation. Facilitates cell invasion by overexpression of MMP-9 leading to degradation of ECM. Binds to TLR9 leading to disrupted IFN-γ signaling and inhibiting the cyclic GMP-AMP-synthase, causing inflammation.	Various HDAC inhibitors inactivate E7. p600 induces anchorage-dependent integrin-modulated cellular interaction and is an important target for targeted therapy. RNAi technology simultaneously knockdowns both E6 and E7 expression.	Hinds et al. (1992); Brehm et al. (1999); Duensing et al. (2001); Kabsch & Alonso (2002); Nguyen et al. (2002); Dinneen & Ceresa (2004); DeMasi et al. (2005); Huh et al. (2005); Brennan et al. (2009); Cardeal et al. (2012); Hasan et al. (2013); Akagi et al. (2014); Ivashkiv & Donlin (2014); Songock et al. (2017)

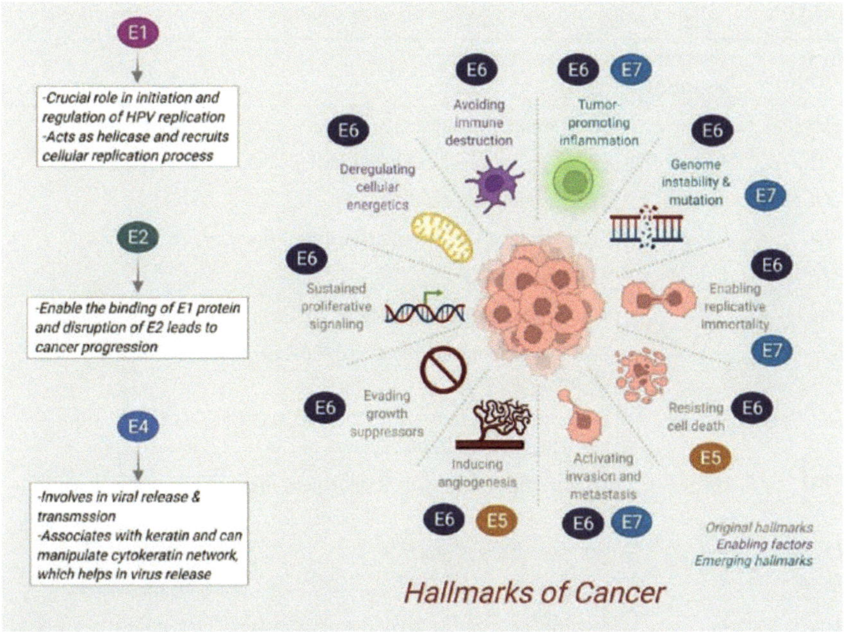

FIGURE 1.6 Role of early proteins and its characteristics as cancer hallmarks.

Source: Adapted from Bhattacharjee et al. (2022); https://creativecommons.org/licenses/by/4.0/

and HPV diagnosis (Laengsri et al., 2018). The majority of putative biomarkers are associated with cell cycle regulation, which is disturbed by hrHPV E5, E6, and E7 oncoprotein production. Some of these potent biomarkers have been shown to be critical for genital keratinocyte immortalization and are engaged in the p53 and pRb cascades, which are often damaged by E6 and E7 HPV oncoprotein (Sano et al., 1998) (Table 1.3). The molecular targets of HPV E5 and their potential utility as biomarkers are still in the early stages of development and warranted to be further explored. In transgenic mice models of cervical carcinogenesis, studies have shown that the E5 oncoprotein can produce tumors, particularly in the early phases of cervical carcinogenesis (Basukala & Banks, 2021). E5 appears to play a role in cervical carcinogenesis later on, since it has been discovered to be expressed by episomal viral genomes that coexist with integrated viral genomes in 26% to 76% of cervical cancer patients (Chang et al., 2001; Hafner et al., 2008).

TABLE 1.3 Major Genes Affected by Viral Integration and Their Cellular Functions

Gene	Integrations Reported	Cellular Function
C9orf156	15	Nucleosomes assembly.
MYC	13	Cell cycle, apoptosis, cellular transformation.
POU5F1B	10	Transcription factor.
FHIT	9	Purine metabolism; associated with translocations in cancer.
KLF12	8	Transcription factor.
HMGA2	8	Transcriptional regulation factor.
KLF5	7	Post-translational modifications; suppressor/promoter of cell proliferation.
DIAPH2	7	Development and normal function of the ovaries; associated with premature ovarian insufficiency.
TP63	6	Transcription factor, skin development, maintenance, and premature aging.
LRP1B	6	Normal cell development.
NFIB	6	Transcription factor, regulates cellular and viral gene transcription.
MACROD2	6	Modifies proteins involved with gene transcription and regulates cell signaling.
PVT1	5	c-Myc activator, binding site of many transcription factors.
LEPREL1	5	Assembly, stability, and chain crosslinking; decreased in breast cancer.
DLG2	5	Cellular signaling.
SEMAD	5	Receptor activity.
TMEM49	5	Cellular adhesion, cell death.
FANCC	4	DNA repair.
MSX2	4	Transcriptional receptor; balance between survival and apoptosis.
CPNE8	4	Regulator of molecular events in the interphase of the cell membrane and cytoplasm.
HS3ST4	4	Enzyme expressed during HPV-1 pathogenesis.
DCC	4	Tumor suppressor.
CDH7	4	Cadherin; ERK pathway.
AGTR2	4	Angiotensin receptor; mediator of cell death.
RAD51B	3	DNA repair by homologous recombination; associated with other types of cancer, such as breast, ovary, prostate, and colorectal.

Source: Reproduced with permission from Oyervides-Muñoz et al. (2018); Copyright © Elsevier (2018).

1.5.1 p16 INK4a

The tumor suppressor protein p16INK4a is encoded by the CDKN2A gene and delays cell cycle progression by inactivating the cyclin D-CDK4/6 complex, which promotes pRb phosphorylation for cell cycle progression. HPV E7 oncoprotein drives cell cycle progression to S phase in carcinogenic HPV-infected cells by inactivating pRb and releasing E2F transcription factor, resulting in p16INK4a overexpression. HPV E7-induced up-regulation of p16INK4a makes this protein a viable biomarker for cervical cancer (Klaes et al., 2001; Murphy et al., 2003).

1.5.2 Ki-67

The MKI67 gene encodes the Ki-67 antigen, a nuclear protein associated with cell proliferation that is produced in all the phases of the cell cycle. The release of E2F transcription factor (HPV E7-mediated) has been shown to increase Ki-67 expression in the cervical epithelium by several authors. Overexpression of Ki-67 was linked to increased expression of cyclins D and E and decreased expression of the tumor suppressor's p21 and p27 in one study. Because of its relationship with different CIN degrees and HPV infection, Ki-67 is regarded as a proliferation marker in basal cells, as well as intermediate and superficial squamous cells (Kruse et al., 2001; Zhang & Shen, 2018).

1.5.3 ProEx C

Topoisomerase II protein (TOP2) and the minichromosome maintenance complex II (MCM2) proteins are found in ProEx C. TOP2 is an enzyme that is involved in DNA replication as well as packaging. MCM2 is a protein that is implicated in the creation of replication forks as well as the recruitment of other DNA replication proteins. Both proteins are important throughout the S phase of the cell cycle and are overexpressed in HPV-infected cells due to aberrant gene transcription and abnormal stimulation of the S phase in these cells (Malinowski, 2005; Santin et al., 2005).

1.5.4 p21 AND p27

p21 and p27 are tumor suppressor proteins that inhibit cyclin-dependent kinase (cyclin-dependent protein kinase inhibitors: CKIs) and cause cell cycle arrest. When these proteins are blocked by HPV E5, cell cycle progression is stimulated indefinitely. The transcriptional inhibition of p21 by E5 has been discovered in immortalized human keratinocytes. HPV E5, on the other hand, decreased the half-life of the p27 protein. Activation of EGRF enhances the action of E5 on p27 KIP1 (Tsao et al., 1996; Van de Putte et al., 2003).

1.5.5 CELL SURFACE RECEPTORS

One of the most well-known pathways involving HPV E5 protein is its engagement with the epidermal growth factor receptor (EGFR). EGFR is a tyrosine kinase cell surface receptor for epidermal growth factor (EGF) that can be present in the epithelial cells of the cervix, including mucosal cells. The E5 protein binds to the endosome's vacuolar ATPase, which is involved in receptor degradation, and suppresses its activity. As a result, EGFR recycling to the cell surface is boosted, and receptor signaling is improved. E5 also increases EGF phosphorylation, which intensifies EGRF activity (Gutiérrez-Hoya et al., 2019). These E5-mediated processes stimulate signaling pathways implicated in cell proliferation, angiogenesis, and apoptosis, such as Ras-Raf-MAP kinase and PI3K-Akt. HPV16 E5 protein promotes mitogenesis, angiogenesis, and cell invasion by activating G-protein-coupled receptors such as ETAR. When E5 is present in growth factor-depleted keratinocytes, it boosts the mitogenic activity of the ETAR ligand, endothelin-1 (ET-1), and causes E5-transfected cells to proliferate more than untransfected cells (Soonthornthum et al., 2001).

1.5.6 COX-2, VEGF, AND Cav-1

HPV E5 upregulates cellular proteins such as cyclooxygenase-2 (COX-2), vascular endothelial growth factor (VEGF), and caveolin-1 (Cav-1). COX-2 is an enzyme that catalyzes the conversion of arachidonic acid to prostaglandins and other eicosanoids, resulting in cell cycle regulation, apoptosis suppression, extracellular matrix formation, and angiogenesis. As a result, COX-2 plays a function in a variety of cancers at diverse stages of carcinogenesis. VEGF is a cytokine that is involved in both healthy and pathological angiogenesis, as well as lymph angiogenesis (Myong, 2012). COX-2 and VEGF are both induced by the E5 oncoprotein, which triggers the EGFR signaling cascade. As a result, the E5 oncoprotein promotes angiogenesis in cervical carcinogenesis, which is an important stage in tumor invasion and metastasis. Caveolin-1 (Cav-1) is a membrane protein that has a role in cell proliferation and differentiation. Cav-1 overexpression by E5 is poorly understood; nevertheless, this host protein may play a role in cell transformation by changing EGFR signaling (Suprynowicz et al., 2008; Fukazawa et al., 2014).

1.6 CONCLUSION

Cervical cancer is the fourth most frequent malignancy among women globally, and it remains a root cause of mortality and morbidity in the USA. The most susceptible populations, including ethnic and racial minorities, and living in isolated or rural areas, have uneven screening, vaccination, and treatment rates (Tabibi et al., 2022). WHO has projected to eliminate cervical cancer by 2030 by taking these issues as a serious concern. Because the average age at diagnosis of this malignancy is much lower in comparison to other types, it causes slightly larger life loss years. Age-specific analyses made it abundantly evident that cervical cancer might be found in adult women of all ages, including those who are heavily burdened with domestic and financial duties. The lack of a further escalation in instances after the age of 40 in high-resource nations could be due to malignancies averted by screening, while hysterectomy may have also contributed to the decreased incidence of cervical cancer. There were significant rate fluctuations, with frequencies ranging from lesser than 3 per 1,00,000 women to more than 70 per 1,00,000 women. Cervical cancer mortality has the most range of variation among all malignancies in terms of inter-country variation (Vu et al., 2018; Arbyn et al., 2020). In 42 low-resource nations, cervical cancer is still the biggest cause of cancer death in women, despite being the 19th most prevalent reason in Finland (a high resource nation). Such striking geographic disparities reflect variances in risk factor exposure as well as significant disparities in access to adequate cancer screening and treatment facilities. The key etiological cause for cervical cancer is sexually transmitted infection with high-risk HPV strains. Other cofactors, such as sexually transmitted illnesses (HIV and *Chlamydia trachomatis*), conventional contraceptives, and smoking, may potentially play a role in worldwide cervical cancer burden changes and differences. The observation of an upswing in cervical cancer instances in various countries with established preventative programs, which could be explained by increased HPV exposure not adequately balanced by cytological screening, is a major and novel public health problem (Simms et al., 2019; Buskwofie et al., 2020). HPV prevalence is low in regions of western Asia and northern Africa where cervical cancer is common, which is most likely explained by social variables connected to sexual behavior. Other sexually transmitted illnesses, such as HIV, are similarly uncommon in these nations. The high cervical cancer rates in Latin America, Sub-Saharan Africa, and South Asia, on the other hand, are most likely due to an elevated background risk, which can be explained by greater instances of HPV and HIV infection. The lower prevalence of cervical carcinoma in North America, some regions of Europe, as well as Australia and New Zealand, are most likely due to effective cytological screening (Mahantshetty et al., 2021; Zhang et al., 2021). This can be eradicated via educational reforms, access to better care and screening facilities, and, lastly, by the expansion of both vaccination and screening programs at both local as well as global levels.

KEYWORDS

- **cervical cancer**
- ***Chlamydia trachomatis***
- **cytological screening**
- **HIV infection**
- ***Human papillomavirus***
- **mortality**

REFERENCES

Akagi, K., Li, J., & Broutian, T. R., (2014). Genome-wide analysis of HPV integration in human cancers reveals recurrent, focal genomic instability. *Genome Research, 24*(2), 185–199.

Al Moustafa, A. E., Foulkes, W. D., Benlimame, N., et al., (2004). E6/E7 proteins of HPV type 16 and ErbB-2 cooperate to induce neoplastic transformation of primary normal oral epithelial cells. *Oncogene, 23*(2), 350–358.

Alter, B. P., Giri, N., Savage, S. A., & Rosenberg, P. S., (2018). Cancer in the National Cancer Institute inherited bone marrow failure syndrome cohort after fifteen years of follow-up. *Haematologica, 103*(1), 30.

Arbyn, M., Weiderpass, E., Bruni, L., De Sanjosé, S., Saraiya, M., Ferlay, J., & Bray, F., (2020). Estimates of incidence and mortality of cervical cancer in 2018: A worldwide analysis. *The Lancet Global Health, 8*(2), e191–e203.

Baleja, J. D., Cherry, J. J., & Liu, Z., (2006). Identification of inhibitors to papillomavirus type 16 E6 protein based on three-dimensional structures of interacting proteins. *Antiviral Research, 72*(1), 49–59.

Bao, H., Zhang, L., Wang, L., et al., (2018). Significant variations in the cervical cancer screening rate in China by individual-level and geographical measures of socioeconomic status: A multilevel model analysis of a nationally representative survey dataset. *Cancer Medicine, 7*(5), 2089–2100.

Basukala, O., & Banks, L., (2021). The not-so-good, the bad and the ugly: HPV E5, E6 and E7 oncoproteins in the orchestration of carcinogenesis. *Viruses, 13*(10), 1892.

Be, X., Hong, Y., Wei, J., Androphy, E. J., Chen, J. J., & Baleja, J. D., (2001). Solution structure determination and mutational analysis of the papillomavirus E6 interacting peptide of E6AP. *Biochemistry, 40*(5), 1293–1299.

Beavis, A. L., & Levinson, K. L., (2016). Preventing cervical cancer in the United States: Barriers and resolutions for HPV vaccination. *Frontiers in Oncology, 6*, 19.

Beavis, A. L., Gravitt, P. E., & Rositch, A. F., (2017). Hysterectomy-corrected cervical cancer mortality rates reveal a larger racial disparity in the United States. *Cancer, 123*(6), 1044–1050.

Berg, M., & Stenlund, A., (1997). Functional interaction between papillomavirus E1 and E2 protein. *Journal of Virology, 71*, 3853–3863.

Bhattacharjee, R., Smruti, S. S., Biswal, S., et al., (2022). Mechanistic role of HPV-associated early proteins in cervical cancer: Molecular pathways and targeted therapeutic strategies. *Critical Reviews in Oncology/Hematology, 174*, 103675.

Brehm, A., Nielsen, S. J., Miska, E. A., McCance, D. J., Reid, J. L., Bannister, A. J., & Kouzarides, T., (1999). The E7 oncoprotein associates with Mi2 and histone deacetylase activity to promote cell growth. *EMBO J., 18*(9), 2449–2458.

Brennan, K., Offiah, G., McSherry, E. A., & Hopkins, A. M., (2009). Tight junctions: A barrier to the initiation and progression of breast cancer? *J. Biomed. Biotechnol., 2010*, 16.

Burmeister, C. A., Khan, S. F., Schäfer, G., Mbatani, N., Adams, T., Moodley, J., & Prince, S., (2022). Cervical cancer therapies: Current challenges and future perspectives. *Tumour Virus Research, 13*, 200238. https://doi.org/10.1016/j.tvr.2022.200238.

Buskwofie, A., David-West, G., & Clare, C. A., (2020). A review of cervical cancer: Incidence and disparities. *Journal of the National Medical Association, 112*(2), 229–232.

Cai, Q., Lv, L., Shao, Q., Li, X., & Dian, A., (2013). Human papillomavirus early proteins and apoptosis. *Archives of Gynecology and Obstetrics, 287*(3), 541–548.

Calin, G. A., Sevignani, C., Dumitru, C. D., et al., (2004). Human microRNA genes are frequently located at fragile sites and genomic regions involved in cancers. *Proceedings of the National Academy of Sciences of the United States of America, 101*(9), 2999–3004.

Canfell, K., Kim, J. J., Brisson, M., et al., (2020). Mortality impact of achieving WHO cervical cancer elimination targets: A comparative modeling analysis in 78 low-income and lower-middle-income countries. *The Lancet, 395*(10224), 591–603.

Cardeal, L. Bd. S., Boccardo, E., & Termini, L., (2012). HPV16 oncoproteins induce MMPs/RECK-TIMP-2 imbalance in primary keratinocytes: Possible implications in cervical carcinogenesis. *PLoS One, 7*(3), e33585.

Carlos De, F. A., Da Conceicao, G. L., M., & Campos, C. E., (2015). Prospects of molecularly-targeted therapies for cervical cancer treatment. *Current Drug Targets, 16*(1), 77–91.

Castro-Muñoz, L. J., Manzo-Merino, J., Muñoz-Bello, J. O., et al., (2019). The human papillomavirus (HPV) E1 protein regulates the expression of cellular genes involved in immune response. *Scientific Reports, 9*, 13620. https://doi.org/10.1038/s41598-019-49886-4.

Chang, J. L., Tsao, Y. P., Liu, D. W., Huang, S. J., Lee, W. H., & Chen, S. L., (2001). The expression of HPV-16 E5 protein in squamous neoplastic changes in the uterine cervix. *Journal of Biomedical Science, 8*(2), 206–213.

Chen, S. T., Huybrechts, K. F., Bateman, B. T., & Hernández-Díaz, S., (2020). Trends in human papillomavirus vaccination in commercially insured children in the United States. *Pediatrics, 146*(4).

Chojnacki, M., & Melendy, T., (2018). The human papillomavirus DNA helicase E1 binds, stimulates, and confers processivity to cellular DNA polymerase epsilon. *Nucleic Acids Research, 46*(1), 229–241. doi: 10.1093/nar/gkx1103.

Cohen, P. A., Jhingran, A., Oaknin, A., & Denny, L., (2019). Cervical cancer. *Lancet, 393*(10167), 169–182.

Crook, T., Vousden, K. H., & Tidy, J. A., (1991). Degradation of p53 can be targeted by HPV E6 sequences distinct from those required for p53 binding and trans-activation. *Cell, 67*(3), 547–556.

Cruz-Gregorio, A., Manzo-Merino, J., Gonzaléz-García, et al., (2018). Human papillomavirus types 16 and 18 early-expressed proteins differentially modulate the cellular redox state and DNA damage. *International Journal of Biological Science, 14*(1), 21.

D'Abramo, C., & Archambault, J., (2011). Small molecule inhibitors of human papillomavirus protein-protein interactions. *The Open Virology Journal, 5*, 80–95.

DeMasi, J., Huh, K. W., Nakatani, Y., Münger, K., & Howley, P. M., (2005). Bovine papillomavirus E7 transformation function correlates with cellular p600 protein binding. *Proceedings of the National Academy of Sciences of the United States of America, 102*(32), 11486–11491.

Dinneen, J. L., & Ceresa, B. P., (2004). Continual expression of rab5 (Q79L) causes a ligand-independent EGFR internalization and diminishes EGFR activity. *Traffic, 5*(8), 606–615.

Doorbar, J., (2013). The E4 protein; structure, function and patterns of expression. *Virology, 445*(1, 2), 80–98.

Doorbar, J., Medcalf, E., & Napthine, S., (1996). Analysis of HPV1 E4 complexes and their association with keratins *in vivo*. *Virology, 218*(1), 114–126.

Duensing, S., Duensing, A., Crum, C. P., & Münger, K., (2001). Human papillomavirus type 16 E7 oncoprotein-induced abnormal centrosome synthesis is an early event in the evolving malignant phenotype. *Cancer Research, 61*(6), 2356–2360.

Eichten, A., Rud, D. S., Grace, M., Piboonniyom, S. O., Zacny, V., & Münger, K., (2004). Molecular pathways executing the "trophic sentinel" response in HPV-16 E7-expressing normal human diploid fibroblasts upon growth factor deprivation. *Virology, 319*(1), 81–93.

Farley, J. H., Truong, V., Goo, E., Uyehara, C., Belnap, C., & Larsen, W. I., (2006). A randomized double-blind placebo-controlled phase II trial of the cyclooxygenase-2 inhibitor celecoxib in the treatment of cervical dysplasia. *Gynecologic Oncology, 103*(2), 425–430.

Ferlay, J., Ervik, M., Lam, F., et al., (2018). *Global Cancer Observatory: Cancer Today* (pp. 1–6). Lyon, France: International Agency for Research on Cancer.

Filippova, M., Song, H., Connolly, J. L., Dermody, T. S., & Duerksen-Hughes, P. J., (2002). The human papillomavirus 16 E6 protein binds to tumor necrosis factor (TNF) R1 and protects cells from TNF-induced apoptosis. *Journal of Biological Chemistry, 277*(24), 21730–21739.

Finzer, P., Aguilar-Lemarroy, A., & Rösl, F., (2002). The role of human papillomavirus oncoproteins E6 and E7 in apoptosis. *Cancer Letters, 188*(1, 2), 15–24.

Franco, E. L., Schlecht, N. F., & Saslow, D., (2003). The epidemiology of cervical cancer. *The Cancer Journal, 9*(5), 348–359.

Fukazawa, E. M., Baiocchi, G., Soares, F. A., et al., (2014). Cox-2, EGFR, and ERBB-2 expression in cervical intraepithelial neoplasia and cervical cancer using an automated imaging system. *International Journal of Gynecological Pathology, 33*(3), 225–234.

Furumoto, H., & Irahara, M., (2002). Human papilloma virus (HPV) and cervical cancer. *Journal of Medical Investigation, 49*(3/4), 124–133.

Ganguly, N., (2012). Human papillomavirus-16 E5 protein: Oncogenic role and therapeutic value. *Cell Oncology, 35*(2), 67–76.

Gill, B. S., Lin, J. F., Krivak, T. C., et al., (2014). National cancer data base analysis of radiation therapy consolidation modality for cervical cancer: The impact of new technological advancements. *International Journal of Radiation Oncology, Biology, Physics, 90*(5), 1083–1090.

Goodwin, E. C., & DiMaio, D., (2000). Repression of human papillomavirus oncogenes in HeLa cervical carcinoma cells causes the orderly reactivation of dormant tumor suppressor pathways. *Proceedings of the National Academy of Sciences of the United States of America, 97*(23), 12513–12518.

Greco, D., Kivi, N., Qian, K., Leivonen, S. K., Auvinen, P., & Auvinen, E., (2011). Human papillomavirus 16 E5 modulates the expression of host microRNAs. *PLoS One, 6*(7), e21646.

Gutiérrez-Hoya, A., Zerecero-Carreón, O., Valle-Mendiola, A., Moreno-Lafont, M., López-Santiago, R., Weiss-Steider, B., & Soto-Cruz, I., (2019). Cervical cancer cells express markers associated with immunesurveillance. *Journal of Immunology Research, 2019*, 1242979.

Häfner, N., Driesch, C., Gajda, M., Jansen, L., Kirchmayr, R., Runnebaum, I. B., & Dürst, M., (2008). Integration of the HPV16 genome does not invariably result in high levels of viral oncogene transcripts. *Oncogene, 27*(11), 1610–1617.

Haller, K., Stubenrauch, F., & Pfister, H., (1995). Differentiation-dependent transcription of the epidermodysplasia verruciformis-associated human papillomavirus type 5 in benign lesions. *Virology, 214*(1), 245–255.

Hasan, U. A., Zannetti, C., & Parroche, P., (2013). The human papillomavirus type 16 E7 oncoprotein induces a transcriptional repressor complex on the toll-like receptor 9 promoter. *J. Exp. Med., 210*(7), 1369–1387.

Henderson, S., Chakravarthy, A., Su, X., Boshoff, C., & Fenton, T. R., (2014). APOBEC-mediated cytosine deamination links PIK3CA helical domain mutations to human papillomavirus-driven tumor development. *Cell Reports, 7*(6), 1833–1840.

Hinds, P. W., Mittnacht, S., Dulic, V., Arnold, A., Reed, S. I., & Weinberg, R. A., (1992). Regulation of retinoblastoma protein functions by ectopic expression of human cyclins. *Cell, 70*(6), 993–1006.

Hogarth, S., Hopkins, M. M., & Rodriguez, V., (2012). A molecular monopoly? HPV testing, the Pap smear and the molecularization of cervical cancer screening in the USA. *Sociology of Health and Illness, 34*(2), 234–250.

Huh, K. W., DeMasi, J., Ogawa, H., Nakatani, Y., Howley, P. M., & Münger, K., (2005). Association of the human papillomavirus type 16 E7 oncoprotein with the 600-kDa retinoblastoma protein-associated factor, p600. *Proceedings of the National Academy of Sciences of the United States of America, 102*(32), 11492–11497.

Ivashkiv, L. B., & Donlin, L. T., (2014). Regulation of type I interferon responses. *Nat. Rev. Immunol., 14*(1), 36–49.

Jayshree, R. S., Sreenivas, A., Tessy, M., & Krishna, S., (2009). Cell intrinsic and extrinsic factors in cervical carcinogenesis. *The Indian Journal of Medical Research, 130*(3), 286–295.

Jones, D. L., & Münger, K., (1996). Interactions of the human papillomavirus E7 protein with cell cycle regulators. *Seminars in Cancer Biology*, 327–337.

Jørgensen, S. F., Andersen, B., Petersen, L. K., Rebolj, M., & Njor, S. H., (2022). Adherence to follow-up after the exit cervical cancer screening test at age 60–64: A nationwide register-based study. *Cancer Medicine, 11*(1), 224–237.

Jung, Y. S., Kato, I., & Kim, H. R. C., (2013). A novel function of HPV16-E6/E7 in epithelial–mesenchymal transition. *Biochemical and Biophysics Research Communication, 435*(3), 339–344.

Kabsch, K., & Alonso, A., (2002). The human papillomavirus type 16 E5 protein impairs TRAIL– and FasL-mediated apoptosis in HaCaT cells by different mechanisms. *Journal of Virology, 76* (23), 12162–12172.

Kelley, M. L., Keiger, K. E., Lee, C. J., & Huibregtse, J. M., (2005). The global transcriptional effects of the human papillomavirus E6 protein in cervical carcinoma cell lines are mediated by the E6AP ubiquitin ligase. *Journal of Virology, 79*(6), 3737–3747.

Khan, J., Davy, C. J., McIntosh, P. .B, Jackson, D. J., Hinz, S., Wang, Q., & Doorbar, J. (2011). Role of calpain in the formation of human papillomavirus type 16 E1^ E4 amyloid fibers and reorganization of the keratin network. *Journal of Virology, 85*(19), 9984–9997.

Kim, S. H., Juhnn, Y. S., Kang, S., Park, S. W., Sung, M. W., Bang, Y. J., & Song, Y. S., (2006). Human papillomavirus 16 E5 up-regulates the expression of vascular endothelial growth factor through the activation of epidermal growth factor receptor, MEK/ERK1, 2 and PI3K/Akt. *Cell. Mol. Life Sci., 63*(7), 930–938.

Kim, S. H., Oh, J. M., No, J. H., Bang, Y. J., Juhnn, Y. S., & Song, Y. S., (2009). Involvement of NF-κB and AP-1 in COX-2 upregulation by human papillomavirus 16 E5 oncoprotein. *Carcinogenesis, 30*(5), 753–757.

Kirby, T., (2015). FDA approves new upgraded Gardasil 9. *The Lancet Oncology, 16*(2), e56.

Klaes, R., Friedrich, T., Spitkovsky, D., et al., (2001). Overexpression of p16(INK4A) as a specific marker for dysplastic and neoplastic epithelial cells of the cervix uteri. *International Journal of Cancer, 92*(2), 276–284.

Koss, L. G., (1989). The Papanicolaou test for cervical cancer detection: A triumph and a tragedy. *JAMA, 261*(5), 737–743.

Kruse, A. J., Baak, J. P., De Bruin, P. C., et al., (2001). Ki-67 immunoquantitation in cervical intraepithelial neoplasia (CIN): A sensitive marker for grading. *The Journal of Pathology, 193*(1), 48–54.

Laengsri, V., Kerdpin, U., Plabplueng, C., Treeratanapiboon, L., & Nuchnoi, P., (2018). Cervical cancer markers: Epigenetics and microRNAs. *Laboratory Medicine, 49*(2), 97–111.

Lee, S. S., Weiss, R. S., & Javier, R. T., (1997). Binding of human virus oncoproteins to hDlg/SAP97, a mammalian homolog of the Drosophila discs large tumor suppressor protein. *Proceedings of the National Academy of Sciences of the United States of America, 94*(13), 6670–6675.

Li, S., Labrecque, S., Gauzzi, M. C., et al., (1999). The human papilloma virus (HPV)-18 E6 oncoprotein physically associates with Tyk2 and impairs Jak-STAT activation by interferon-α. *Oncogene, 18*(42), 5727–5737.

Liao, S., Deng, D., Zhang, W., et al., (2013). Human papillomavirus 16/18 E5 promotes cervical cancer cell proliferation, migration and invasion *in vitro* and accelerates tumor growth *in vivo*. *Oncology Reports, 29*(1), 95–102.

Liu, C., Lin, J., Li, L., et al., (2015). HPV16 early gene E5 specifically reduces miRNA-196a in cervical cancer cells. *Scientific Reports, 5*, 7653.

Mahantshetty, U., Lavanya, G., Grover, S., Akinfenwa, C. A., Carvalho, H., & Amornwichet, N., (2021). Incidence, treatment and outcomes of cervical cancer in low– and middle-income countries. *Clinical Oncology, 33*(9), e363–e371.

Maheshwari, S., Nautiyal, R., Kotwal, A., & Chandra, S., (2020). Prevalence and distribution of various human papillomavirus genotypes in women with high risk for cervical carcinoma. *International Journal of Reproduction, Contraception, Obstetrics and Gynecology, 9*(6), 2498–2504.

Malinowski, D. P., (2005). Molecular diagnostic assays for cervical neoplasia: Emerging markers for the detection of high-grade cervical disease. *Biotechniques, 38*(S4), S17–S23.

Malla, R., & Kamal, M. A., (2021). E6 and E7 oncoproteins: Potential targets of cervical cancer. *Current Medicinal Chemistry, 28*(39), 8163–8181.

Manzo-Merino, J., Contreras-Paredes, A., Vázquez-Ulloa, E., Rocha-Zavaleta, L., Fuentes-Gonzalez, A. M., & Lizano, M., (2014). The role of signaling pathways in cervical cancer and molecular therapeutic targets. *Arch. Med. Res., 45*(7), 525–539.

McCarthy, M. P., White, W. I., Palmer-Hill, F., Koenig, S., & Suzich, J. A., (1998). Quantitative disassembly and reassembly of human papillomavirus type 11 virus like particles *in vitro*. *Journal of Virology, 72*(1), 32–41.

McIntosh, P. B., Laskey, P., Sullivan, K., Davy, C., Wang, Q., Jackson, D. J., Griffin, H. .M., & Doorbar, J. (2010). E1-E4-mediated keratin phosphorylation and ubiquitylation: A mechanism for keratin depletion in HPV16-infected epithelium. *Journal of Cell Science, 123*(16), 2810–2822.

McLaughlin-Drubin, M. E., & Münger, K., (2009). Oncogenic activities of human papillomaviruses. *Virus Research, 143*(2), 195–208.

Mix, J. M., Van, D. E. A., Saraiya, M., Hallowell, B. D., & Thomas, C. C., (2021). Assessing impact of HPV vaccination on cervical cancer incidence among women aged 15–29 years in the United States, 1999–2017: An ecologic study. *Cancer Epidemiology and Prevention Biomarkers, 30*(1), 30–37.

Monika, B., Thomas, M., & Jacques, A., (2013). The E1 protein. *Virology, 445*, 35–56.

Moody, C. A., & Laimins, L. A., (2010). Human papillomavirus oncoproteins: Pathways to transformation. *Nat. Rev. Cancer, 10*(8), 550–560.

Motoyama, S., Ladines-Llave, C. A., Luis, V. S., & Maruo, T., (2004). The role of human papilloma virus in the molecular biology of cervical carcinogenesis. *The Kobe Journal of Medical Sciences, 50*(1, 2), 9–19.

Murphy, N., Ring, M., Killalea, A. G., et al., (2003). p16INK4A as a marker for cervical dyskaryosis: CIN and cGIN in cervical biopsies and ThinPrep smears. *Journal of Clinical Pathology, 56*(1), 56–63.

Musselwhite, L. W., Oliveira, C. M., Kwaramba, T., et al., (2016). Racial/ethnic disparities in cervical cancer screening and outcomes. *Acta Cytologica, 60*(6), 518–526.

Myong, N. H., (2012). Loss of E-cadherin and acquisition of vimentin in epithelial-mesenchymal transition are noble indicators of uterine cervix cancer progression. *Korean Journal of Pathology, 46*(4), 341.

Nakagawa, S., & Huibregtse, J. M., (2000). Human scribble (vartul) is targeted for ubiquitin-mediated degradation by the high-risk papillomavirus E6 proteins and the E6AP ubiquitin-protein ligase. *Molecular and Cell Biology, 20*(21), 8244–8253.

Neels, P., Van, D. P., Van, R. M., & Dogné, J. M., (2013). Human papillomavirus vaccines: Understanding the benefit-risk. *Annals of Medicine, 45*(3), 203–205.

Nguyen, M., Song, S., Liem, A., Androphy, E., Liu, Y., & Lambert, P. F., (2002). A mutant of human papillomavirus type 16 E6 deficient in binding α-helix partners displays reduced oncogenic potential *in vivo*. *Journal of Virology, 76*(24), 13039–13048.

Oyervides-Muñoz, M. A., Pérez-Maya, A., Rodríguez-Gutiérrez, H. F., et al., (2018). Understanding the HPV integration and its progression to cervical cancer. *Infection Genetics and Evolution, 61*, 134–140.

Park, J. S., Hwang, E. S., Park, S. N., et al., (1997). Physical status and expression of HPV genes in cervical cancers. *Gynecologic Oncology, 65*(1), 121–129.

Patel, D., Huang, S. M., Baglia, L. A., & McCance, D. J., (1999). The E6 protein of human papillomavirus type 16 binds to and inhibits co-activation by CBP and p300. *EMBO J., 18*(18), 5061–5072.

Pereira, R., Hitzeroth, I. I., & Rybicki, E. P., (2009). Insights into the role and function of L2, the minor capsid protein of papillomaviruses. *Archives of Virology, 154*(2), 187–197.

Petry, K. U., (2014). HPV and cervical cancer. *Scandinavian Journal of Clinical and Laboratory Investigation, 74*(S244), 59–62.

Rahul, B., Sabya, S. D., Smuruti, S. D., et al., (2022). Mechanistic role of HPV-associated early proteins in cervical cancer: Molecular pathways and targeted therapeutic strategies. *Critical Reviews in Oncology/Hematology, 174*, 103675.

Regan, J. A., & Laimins, L. A., (2008). Bap31 is a novel target of the human papillomavirus E5 protein. *Journal of Virology, 82*(20), 10042–10051.

Ren, S., Gaykalova, D. A., Guo, T., et al., (2020). HPV E2, E4, E5 drive alternative carcinogenic pathways in HPV positive cancers. *Oncogene, 39*(40), 6327–6339.

Roberts, S., Hillman, M. L., Knight, G. L., & Gallimore, P. H., (2013). The ND10 component promyelocytic leukemia protein relocates to human papillomavirus type 1 E4 intranuclear inclusion bodies in cultured keratinocytes and in warts. *Journal of Virology, 77*(1), 673–684.

Rogel-Gaillard, C., Pehau-Arnaudet, G., Breitburd, F., & Orth, G., (1993). Cytopathic effect in human papillomavirus type 1–induced inclusion warts: *In vitro* analysis of the contribution of two forms of the viral E4 protein. *Journal of Investigative Dermatology, 101*(6), 843–851.

Sanchez-Perez, A. M., Soriano, S., Clarke, A. R., & Gaston, K., (1997). Disruption of the human papillomavirus type 16 E2 gene protects cervical carcinoma cells from E2F-induced apoptosis. *J. Gen. Virol., 78*(Pt 11), 3009–3018.

Sandal, T., (2002). Molecular aspects of the mammalian cell cycle and cancer. *The Oncologist, 7*(1), 73–81.

Sankaranarayanan, R., Bhatla, N., & Basu, P., (2016). Current global status and impact of human papillomavirus vaccination: Implications for India. *The Indian Journal of Medical Research, 144*(2), 169–180.

Sano, T., Oyama, T., Kashiwabara, K., Fukuda, T., & Nakajima, T., (1998). Expression status of p16 protein is associated with human papillomavirus oncogenic potential in cervical and genital lesions. *The American Journal of Pathology, 153*(6), 1741–1748.

Santin, A. D., Zhan, F., Bignotti, E., et al., (2005). Gene expression profiles of primary HPV16- and HPV18-infected early stage cervical cancers and normal cervical epithelium: Identification of novel candidate molecular markers for cervical cancer diagnosis and therapy. *Virology, 331*(2), 269–291.

Scarth, J. A., Patterson, M. R., Morgan, E. L., & Macdonald, A., (2021). The human papillomavirus oncoproteins: A review of the host pathways targeted on the road to transformation. *The Journal of General Virology, 102*(3), 001540.

Scudellari, M., (2013). Sex, cancer and a virus: Human papillomavirus is causing a new form of head and neck cancer – leaving researchers scrambling to understand risk factors, tests and treatments. *Nature, 503*(7476), 330–333.

Sen, P., Ganguly, P., & Ganguly, N., (2018). Modulation of DNA methylation by human papillomavirus E6 and E7 oncoproteins in cervical cancer. *Oncology Letters, 15*(1), 11–22.

Senapati, R., Senapati, N. N., & Dwibedi, B., (2016). Molecular mechanisms of HPV mediated neoplastic progression. *Infectious Agents and Cancer, 11*(1), 1–11.

Shah, M., Anwar, M. A., Park, S., Jafri, S. S., & Choi, S., (2015). In silico mechanistic analysis of IRF3 inactivation and high-risk HPV E6 species-dependent drug response. *Scientific Reports, 5*(1), 1–14.

Silver, M. I., & Kobrin, S., (2020). Exacerbating disparities?: Cervical cancer screening and HPV vaccination. *Preventive Medicine, 130*, 105902.

Sima, N., Wang, W., Kong, D., et al., (2008). RNA interference against HPV16 E7 oncogene leads to viral E6 and E7 suppression in cervical cancer cells and apoptosis via upregulation of Rb and p53. *Apoptosis, 13*(2), 273–281.

Simms, K. T., Steinberg, J., Caruana, M., et al., (2019). Impact of scaled up human papillomavirus vaccination and cervical screening and the potential for global elimination of cervical cancer in 181 countries, 2020–99: A modeling study. *The Lancet Oncology, 20*(3), 394–407.

Small, Jr. W., Bacon, M. A., Bajaj, A., et al., (2017). Cervical cancer: A global health crisis. *Cancer, 123*(13), 2404–2412.

Songock, W. K., Kim, S. M., & Bodily, J. M., (2017). The human papillomavirus E7 oncoprotein as a regulator of transcription. *Virus Res., 231*, 56–75.

Soonthornthum, T., Arias-Pulido, H., Joste, N., Lomo, L., Muller, C., Rutledge, T., & Verschraegen, C., (2011). Epidermal growth factor receptor as a biomarker for cervical cancer. *Annals of Oncology, 22*(10), 2166–2178.

Sriplung, H., Singkham, P., Iamsirithaworn, S., Jiraphongsa, C., & Bilheem, S., (2014). Success of a cervical cancer screening program: Trends in incidence in Songkhla, Southern Thailand, 1989–2010, and prediction of future incidences to 2030. *Asian Pacific Journal of Cancer Prevention, 15*(22), 10003–10008.

Stanley, M. A., Pett, M. R., & Coleman, N., (2007). HPV: From infection to cancer. *Biochemical Society Transactions, 35*(6), 1456–1460.

Stöppler, M. C., Straight, S. W., Tsao, G., Schlegel, R., & Mccance, D. J., (1996). The E5 gene of HPV-16 enhances keratinocyte immortalization by full-length DNA. *Virology, 223*(1), 251–254.

Suprynowicz, F. A., Disbrow, G. L., Krawczyk, E., Simic, V., Lantzky, K., & Schlegel, R., (2008). HPV-16 E5 oncoprotein upregulates lipid raft components caveolin-1 and ganglioside GM1 at the plasma membrane of cervical cells. *Oncogene, 27*(8), 1071–1078.

Tabibi, T., Barnes, J. M., Shah, A., Osazuwa-Peters, N., Johnson, K. J., & Brown, D. S., (2022). Human papillomavirus vaccination and trends in cervical cancer incidence and mortality in the US. *JAMA Pediatrics, 176*(3), 313–316.

Thomas, M., Laura, R., Hepner, K., Guccione, E., Sawyers, C., Lasky, L., & Banks, L., (2002). Oncogenic human papillomavirus E6 proteins target the MAGI-2 and MAGI-3 proteins for degradation. *Oncogene, 21*(33), 5088–5096.

Trottier, H., & Franco, E. L., (2006). The epidemiology of genital human papillomavirus infection. *Vaccine, 24*, S4–S15.

Tsao, Y. P., Li, L. Y., Tsai, T. C., & Chen, S. L., (1996). Human papillomavirus type 11 and 16 E5 represses p21(WafI/SdiI/CipI) gene expression in fibroblasts and keratinocytes. *Journal of Virology, 70*(11), 7535–7539.

Van De, P. G., Holm, R., Lie, A. K., Tropé, C. G., & Kristensen, G. B., (2003). Expression of p27, p21, and p16 protein in early squamous cervical cancer and its relation to prognosis. *Gynecologic Oncology, 89*(1), 140–147.

Vieira, V. C., Leonard, B., White, E. A., et al., (2014). Human papillomavirus E6 triggers upregulation of the antiviral and cancer genomic DNA deaminase APOBEC3B. *MBio, 5*(6), e02234.

Vousden, K., (1993). Interactions of human papillomavirus transforming proteins with the products of tumor suppressor genes. *FASEB Journal, 7*(10), 872–879.

Vu, M., Yu, J., Awolude, O. A., & Chuang, L., (2018). Cervical cancer worldwide. *Current Problems in Cancer, 42*(5), 457–465.

Waggoner, S. E., (2003). Cervical cancer. *Lancet, 361*(9376), 2217–2225.

Wang, J., Zhao, C. A., Wang, K., Zheng, J., Wang, Y. L., & Si, L. S., (2006). Enhanced immunization after intranasal coadministration of *Escherichia coli* heat-labile enterotoxin B subunit and human papillomavirus 16-L1 DNA vaccine. *Chinese Medical Journal, 119*(05), 408–411.

Wang, Q., Kennedy, A., Das, P., et al., (2009). Phosphorylation of the human papillomavirus type 16 E1^ E4 protein at T57 by ERK triggers a structural change that enhances keratin binding and protein stability. *Journal of Virology, 83*(8), 3668–3683.

Wang, W., Sima, N., Kong, D., et al., (2010). Selective targeting of HPV-16 E6/E7 in cervical cancer cells with a potent oncolytic adenovirus and its enhanced effect with radiotherapy *in vitro* and vivo. *Cancer Letters, 291*(1), 67–75.

Warren, C. J., Westrich, J. A., Doorslaer, K. V., & Pyeon, D., (2017). Roles of APOBEC3A and APOBEC3B in human papillomavirus infection and disease progression. *Viruses, 9*(8), 233.

Wentzensen, N., Schwartz, L., Zuna, R. E., et al., (2012). Performance of p16/Ki-67 Immunostaining to detect cervical cancer precursors in a colposcopy referral population p16/Ki-67 for cervical cancer screening. *Clinical Cancer Research, 18*(15), 4154–4162.

Werness, B. A., Levine, A. J., & Howley, P. M., (1990). Association of human papillomavirus types 16 and 18 E6 proteins with p53. *Science, 248*(4951), 76–79.

White, P. W., Faucher, A. M., Massariol, M. J., et al., (2005). Biphenylsulfonacetic acid inhibitors of the human papillomavirus type 6 E1 helicase inhibit ATP hydrolysis by an allosteric mechanism involving tyrosine 486. *Antimicrobial Agents and Chemotherapy, 49*(12), 4834–4842.

White, P. W., Pelletier, A., Brault, K., et al., (2001). Characterization of recombinant HPV6 and 11 E1 helicases: Effect of ATP on the interaction of E1 with E2 and mapping of a minimal helicase domain. *Journal of Biological Chemistry, 276*(25), 22426–22438.

Zahra, K., Patel, S., Dey, T., Pandey, U., & Mishra, S. P., (2021). A study of oxidative stress in cervical cancer – an institutional study. *Biochemical Biophysics Reports, 25*, 100881.

Zhang, X., & Shen, D., (2018). p16INK4a and Ki-67 measurement predict progression of cervical low-grade squamous intraepithelial lesion. *International Journal of Clinical and Experimental Pathology, 11*(8), 4109–4116.

Zhang, X., Zeng, Q., Cai, W., & Ruan, W., (2021). Trends of cervical cancer at global, regional, and national level: Data from the global burden of disease study 2019. *BMC Public Health, 21*(1), 1–10.

CHAPTER 2

Wnt Signaling Pathway in Cervical Cancer

2.1 ABERRANT SIGNALING PATHWAYS AS EMERGING TARGETS IN CERVICAL CANCER

Conventional treatment methods used for cervical cancer management include radiation, surgery, and chemotherapy (either in combination or alone). However, these treatment approaches remain suboptimal, with residual tumors observed in approximately 50% of advanced cancer patients (Kuo et al., 2003; Liang et al., 2021). Cancer cells have the inherent ability to grow and divide uncontrollably, generally via genetic alterations in specific genes (Hanahan & Weinberg, 2011). Recent advances in DNA sequencing over the past several years have made it approachable to systematically identify and study these genetic alterations and present a better and more detailed understanding of involved signaling pathways and their processes. There are several variations reported in these signaling pathways in numerous tumor types. Hence a complete and detailed understanding of these genetic alterations in signaling pathways in all cancer types is crucial to elucidate potent therapeutic vulnerabilities and options (Figure 2.1). The dependence of transformed cells on the activation of survival signaling pathways has gained wider recognition in the management of numerous malignancies. Elucidation of various mutant oncoproteins such as STAT5, AKT, and NF-kB ignited the discovery of kinase inhibitors, including nilotinib and imatinib, for the treatment of chronic leukemia (Grant, 2008).

Cervical Cancer: Signaling Pathways, Molecular Mechanisms, Natural Products, and Therapeutic Approaches. Pratibha Pandey, Fahad Khan, Saher Islam, and Devarajan Thangadurai, (Eds.)

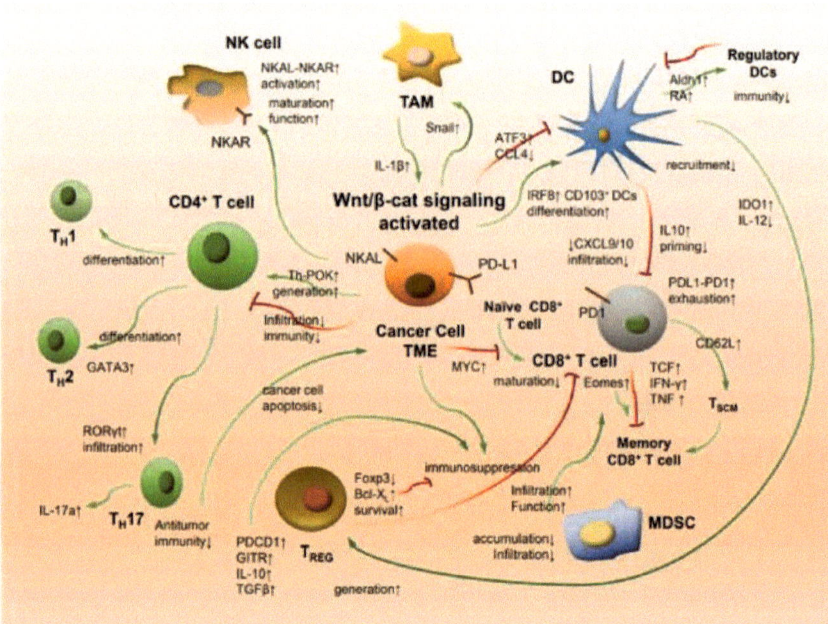

FIGURE 2.1. Wnt/β-cat signaling in vital immunooncological components. Activated Wnt/β-cat signaling in cancer cells can deplete DC recruitment by downregulating CCL4 expression, thereby decreasing CXCL9/10 and IL-10 secretion to limit CD8+ T-cell infiltration and priming. Wnt-active DCs can also restrain CD8+ T cells, thus benefiting Treg function and enhancing immunosuppression. The differentiation of CD4+ T cells into TH1 and TH2 can be enforced by β-cat activity. TAMs can interact with Wnt-active cancer cells through IL-1β and Snail, while MDSCs regulate CD8+ T-cell infiltration and function. PD-L1 and NKAL on cancer cells are upregulated, ligand-receptor interactions are enhanced, and PDL1-PD1-induced CD8+ T-cell exhaustion is triggered to form a non-T-cell-inflamed TME.

Source: Reproduced with permission from Zhou et al. (2022); Copyright © Elsevier (2022).

The apoptosis and proliferation of cervical cancer cells need the cooperation and positive involvement of various signaling molecules. Genetic alterations in these crucial signaling pathways that control apoptosis, cell-cycle progression, and growth are major hallmarks of cancer, but the mechanisms and extent of these alterations differ from individual tumor types (Sanchez-Vega et al., 2018). Thus, there is a strong need for elucidating more potent and novel therapeutic approaches which could increase the overall survival rate and life quality of cervical cancer patients. Numerous altered signaling pathways have been positively correlated with cervical cancer progression (Pandita et al., 2017). Hence, understanding of the associated mechanism behind cervical cancer progression would be highly beneficial in elucidating and developing better therapeutic approaches for cervical cancer management.

One of the most promising treatment targets has been identified as the molecular signaling pathways involved in cervical malignant transformation (Gupta et al., 2018; Sanchez-Vega et al., 2018) such as PI3K/AKT (phosphatidylinositol-3 kinase/AKT), RAF/MEK/ERK, apoptosis, Wnt/β-catenin, Notch, JAK/STAT, NF Kappa B, EGFR, and Toll-like receptor signaling. Overexpression of several components of these pathways, in particular, is thought to have a role in carcinogenesis, progression, and metastasis in a variety of solid tumors.

2.2 Wnt SIGNALING PATHWAY

The wingless form of the Wnt signaling pathway has been implicated in a variety of regulatory activities, including cell differentiation, migration, proliferation, and polarity. Embryonic development, stem cell maintenance, tissue regeneration, and homeostasis all require these regulatory systems (Anstas & Moon, 2013). Few studies have shown that ectopic DNA methylation and mutations in the Wnt signaling pathway might cause molecular alterations in the signaling system. Deregulated Wnt pathway has been reported in numerous carcinomas, including cervical cancer, breast cancer, osteosarcoma, colorectal cancer, bone cancer, nasopharyngeal cancer, and oral cavity cancer (Zhan et al., 2017). Wnt signaling is important for proper keratinocyte growth, and inhibiting the Wnt pathway appears to be a vital stage in cervical carcinogenesis. Numerous studies have suggested that, in cervical cancer, the aberrated Wnt pathway stimulates cancer cell differentiation, proliferation, and invasion (Chatterjee et al., 2022). This chapter has been mainly focused towards projecting the association of deregulated Wnt signaling pathway and cervical cancer progression.

2.3 Wnt (WINGLESS TYPE) SIGNALING PATHWAY TYPES

The Wnt signaling pathway, also known as the Wingless signaling system, is made up of a number of proteins that are essential for cell development and differentiation in a variety of tissues (Bahrami et al., 2017). Protein binding to the Fz (Frizzled) family receptor controls the activation of the Wnt pathway. When the Fz receptor is activated, it sends a signal to the phosphoprotein disheveled.

Wnt signaling is divided into two types: canonical and non-canonical pathways (Ackers & Malgor, 2018). Canonical Wnt signaling pathway gets activated when seven pass transmembrane receptors and LRP5/6 coreceptors obtain secreted Wnts and recruit Disheveled (Dsh/Dvl) cytoplasmic phosphoprotein. Phosphorylated Disheveled leads to β-catenin translocation into the nucleus, causing biological response via gene transduction via TCF/LEF transcription factors in the canonical Wnt signaling pathway (Moradi et al., 2017). GSK3β is a significant negative regulator of signaling pathways, forming a multiprotein complex with Axin and APC in the absence of Wnts (adenomatous polyposis coli). This is referred to as the 'destruction complex,' and it phosphorylates β-catenin while keeping cytoplasmic catenin expression low. The phosphorylated β-catenin is then targeted by proteasomes for destruction (Metcalfe & Bienz, 2011). Despite this, in the absence of Wnt ligands, β-catenin is typically found at cellular junctions. The destruction complex is broken during Wnt signaling start, and GSK3β is phosphorylated to its inactive state, preventing β-catenin phosphorylation. The non-canonical Wnt signaling (or catenin-independent pathway) is divided into two categories: Wnt/PCP (planar cell polarity) and Wnt/Ca^{2+}. Convergent extension movements, planar cell polarity, and cell migration were all influenced by both pathways (Lehoczky & Tabin, 2018). Wnt ligands (WNT4, WNT5A, and WNT11) must bind to the Fzd receptor before Dsh/Dvl protein may be activated in these pathways. Both polarized cell migration and asymmetric cytoskeletal assembly need the Wnt/PCP pathway (or Wnt/JNK pathway). The JNK (c-Jun N-terminal kinase) cascade is stimulated by Wnt-mediated activation of RhoA (GTPase Ras homolog gene family member A) and Rac (Ciani & Salinas, 2007). Various endogenously produced Wnt antagonists have been found to control the Wnt signaling pathway. DKK (Dickkopf) family members also interact with LRP 5/6 coreceptors to inhibit canonical Wnt signaling. Finally, by generating a TCF/β-catenin complex, RUNX3 (Runt-related transcription factor 3) blocked the Wnt signaling pathway (Li et al., 2018).

Wnt signaling is also thought to play a role in tumor proliferation and tumorigenesis, according to several studies (Brookes et al., 2008). Wnt signaling that is activated promotes cell proliferation and metastasis, whereas Wnt signaling that is inhibited stops tumor propagation and cancer stemness (Maftouh et al., 2014). The Wnt signaling pathway has also been linked to chemosensitivity and radioresistance (Dandekar et al., 2014). Several studies have shown that the Wnt signaling pathway has a role in the progression and invasion of cervical cancer. Pérez-Plasencia et al. (2012) proposed that cervical carcinogenesis is a multi-step process that begins with the activation of the Wnt/β-catenin pathway. Activation of the β-catenin pathway is also essential for the maintenance of EMT-associated cervical cancer cells, according to Li & Zhou (2011). WIF1 (Wnt inhibitory factor 1) was proposed by Ramachandran et al. (2012) as an upstream secreted Wnt antagonist that triggered apoptosis and reduced tumor growth, development, and angiogenesis in cervical cancer. In SiHa cells, Chang et al. (2012) found that Klotho (Wnt antagonist) expression reduced cancer cell motility and invasiveness by downregulating EMT and increasing E-cadherin levels. Variations in β-catenin-associated cell adherence have been found to be contributing to cervical carcinogenesis (Fadare et al., 2005).

2.4 DYSREGULATED Wnt SIGNALING COMPONENTS IN CERVICAL CANCER

Aberrantly activated Wnt signaling pathway is reported in numerous carcinomas such as breast cancer, lung cancer, cervical cancer, and so on (Li et al., 2015). Epigenetic or genetic alterations can lead to mutations in several Wnt signaling components, including Wnt inhibitors, Wnt ligands, intracellular mediators, and membrane receptors, that can result in abnormal activation of the Wnt pathway. Some Wnt signaling genes have been linked to cervical carcinogenesis in numerous studies (Figure 2.2). In cervical cancer, mutated Wnt ligands have been extensively characterized among all Wnt signaling components (Coopes et al., 2018).

Wnt ligands and their associated pathway have been involved in regulating cellular differentiation and proliferation processes, tissue homeostasis, and cancer progression. Wnt pathway activation resulted in β-catenin accumulation which in turn resulted in increased transcription of several genes for cell proliferation (Ayala Calvillo et al., 2018). Inactivated Wnt pathway (β-catenin) forms degradation complex with several other proteins such as GSK3β (glycogen synthase kinase-3β), polyposis coli, casein kinases, and Axin2 and gets phosphorylated at threonine and

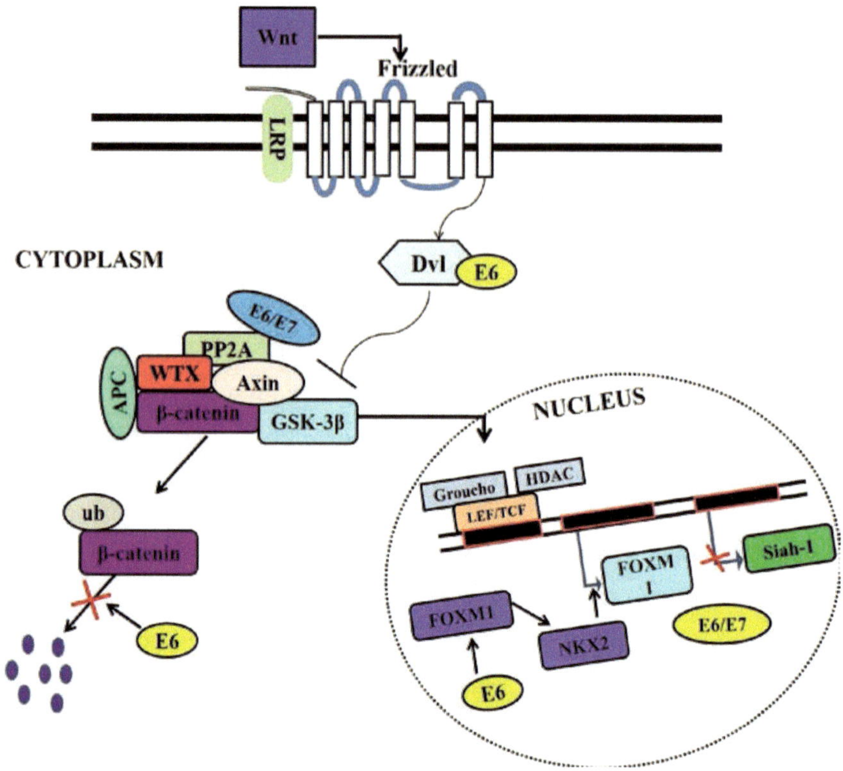

FIGURE 2.2 Wnt signaling pathway in cervical cancer progression.

serine and residues. β-catenin phosphorylation induces ubiquitination via β-TcRP (ubiquitin ligase) which further leads to degradation (Dao et al., 2007). During the activated state of the Wnt signaling pathway, disheveled protein (intracellular) gets phosphorylated and then interacts with Axin2 leading to deregulation of degradation complex and β-catenin accumulation. Thereafter accumulated β-catenin gets translocated into nucleus and binds with T-cell or lymphoid enhancer family of transcription factors for regulating target genes such as c-jun, cyclin D1, c-myc, multidrug resistance, VEGF (vascular endothelial growth factor), Axin2, matrilysine, survivin, matrix metalloproteinases, and COX-2 (Cheng et al., 2017; Liu et al., 2018; Zheng et al., 2019). Accumulated β-catenin (nuclear) has not only been reported in invasive HPV16 +ve human cancer samples but has also been reported in early dysplastic lesions, validating Wnt pathway activation by HPV oncogenes. β-catenin accumulation correlates with cervical cancer progression and HPV infection in several cell lines such as HPV16 +ve 147T and 090 (oropharyngeal) cancer cell lines, HPV –ve cell line 040T and SiHa cancer cell lines (Wang et al., 2020). In HPV +ve cancer cells, silencing the E6 gene resulted in a significant reduction of nuclear β-catenin, implying that E6 is important for Wnt pathway activation (Bello et al., 2015).

Downregulated Wnt7A expression was significantly reported in biopsies and cell lines derived from cervical cancer (Barreto-Vargas et al., 2020). In Hela S3 cancer cells, Wnt10B mRNA was shown to be significantly expressed. In comparison to nearby normal cervical tissues, Lin et al. found overexpressed Wnt5A in cervical cancer tissue (Lin et al., 2014). Wnt8A and Wnt4 levels were also higher in HPV16 cervical cancer cells compared to normal cervical epithelia cells, according to Yang et al. (2018). They also discovered that cervical cancer patients had changed the expression of many receptors, including increased Fzd10 and Fzd2 expression and decreased Fzd7 expression (Terasaki et al., 2002). One of the recurrent events in several human carcinomas is dysregulation of the Wnt signaling pathway via beta-catenin. In HPV-positive cells, beta-catenin expression is mostly found in the nucleus and cytoplasm, whereas in HPV-negative cells, beta-catenin expression is primarily found in the cell membrane (Hu et al., 2015). Rath et al. reported reduced expression of active GSK3β in precancerous and cancerous lesions in different stages of cervical cancer (Prasad et al., 2009; Rath et al., 2015). Furthermore, malignant and precancerous tissues had significant nuclear and cytoplasmic inactive GSK3 immunoreactivity, whereas normal cervical lesions did not. Dvl-1 overexpression has also been detected in cervical cancer cell lines (Kwan et al., 2013). Furthermore, against cervical cancer tissues, PP2A (phosphoprotein phosphatase 2A) is actively expressed in normal cervical epithelia (Elgenaidi & Spiers, 2019). In cervical cancer, Wnt signaling components are increased while Wnt pathway inhibitors are decreased. As a result of this event, it's possible that Wnt signaling is stimulated in cervical cancer (Ford et al., 2016). Several studies have found decreased levels of a few Wnt signaling components, such as Fzd7 and Wnt7A, in malignant and precancerous tumors (Sompel et al., 2021). Depending on the binding receptor, the Wnt7A component can activate both non-canonical and canonical pathways. Wnt7A also reduces tumors in CCRCC patients (clear cell renal cell carcinomas) (Kruck et al., 2013).

The activation of the canonical Wnt pathway is enough to convert HPV immortalized cells. Furthermore, only a few studies have found that the viral oncogenes E6 and E7 are actively overexpressed in cervical cancer tissues (Nishida et al., 2016). Activation of the canonical Wnt pathway has been indicated as a secondary need for the onset of malignant transformation in a number of studies (Wei et al., 2016).

The viral oncogenes E6 and E7 both increased beta-catenin expression and TCF-mediated transcription. This causes a reduction in the protein ubiquitin ligase type 3 Siah-1, which causes beta-catenin degradation (Matsuzawa et al., 2001). Another possibility is that E6 promotes NKX2-1 (NK2 homeobox 1) transcription by inducing MZF1 (Myeloid zinc finger 1) expression (Wang et al., 2020). E6 indirectly activated the Wnt signaling pathway since the FOXM1 (Forkhead box protein M1) promoter has three potential sites for NK2 homeobox 1, and FOXM1 could stimulate translocation of beta-catenin into nucleus through beta-catenin binding (Scarth et al., 2021). Dvl2 and E6 interaction also boosts TCF transcriptional activity, according to *in vivo* research (Bonilla-Delgado et al., 2012). E7 binds to the PP2A subunit and inhibits its enzymatic activity, resulting in the cytoplasmic stability of β-catenin. As previously stated, the Wnt signaling pathway aids cell proliferation, differentiation, migration, and polarity, and so plays an important role in embryonic development, tissue regeneration, homeostasis, and stem cell maintenance. Overall, these studies have confirmed the important role of inhibitors, ligands, receptors, and other Wnt signaling pathway components in cervical cancer. In addition, three CpG islands within the Wnt7A promoter were found to be methylated in SiHa and Hela cancer cells. WIF1 also inhibited tumor progression by causing G2/M growth arrest, which was aided by the suppression of the Wnt/-β-catenin pathway and concomitant downregulation of cyclin D1, c-Myc, and CD44. WIF1 also limits invasion by upregulating E-cadherin expression, decreasing angiogenesis by downregulating Wnt1 and VEGF, and inducing apoptosis by downregulating Wnt1 and VEGF.

Later, a non-canonical kind of Wnt pathway was discovered to be linked to a number of malignancies. Other studies have found a relationship between the Wnt/Ca^{2+} pathway and cancer stem cells and progression. Similarly, in cervical cancer, the non-canonical Wnt pathway plays an important carcinogenic function (Krishnamurthy et al., 2018). Wei et al. found a link between Wnt11 and P-JNK1 levels and discovered that Wnt11 is involved in tumor cell proliferation and invasion in cervical cancer patients via the Wnt/JNK pathway. Overall, activation of the Wnt pathway is required for HPV-mediated carcinogenesis in humans. Furthermore, tumor cell growth, proliferation, metastasis, and death can be induced by activated canonical and non-canonical Wnt signaling alone or in combination with a variety of other mechanisms (Wei et al., 2016).

A recent study has also identified a promising biological target that could help in improving the prognosis of cervical cancer. GHET1 (Gastric carcinoma proliferation enhancing transcript 1) has been recently explored in cervical cancer and reported to be positively associated with the progression of cervical cancer. It has also been found that GHET1 downregulation resulted in the suppression of cervical cancer via regulating Wnt/β-catenin and AKT/mTOR signaling pathways. Modern tests (HPV and Papanikolaou tests) employed for cervical cancer screening are credited with reduced death incidences associated with invasive cervical cancer (Zhang et al., 2019). Papanikolaou test helps in the early detection of cancerous and precancerous cellular lesions, while HPV test helps in the detection of HPV infection type. PET-CTs and pelvic MRIs have been widely used for the diagnosis of localized and advanced cervical cancer cases.

In contrast, GSK3β and Wnt11 expression has not only been reported in normal cervical tissues but also found to be enhanced in cancerous and precancerous lesions, which clearly indicates the correlation between expression patterns and cervical cancer progression. Biomarkers in combination with biopsies might lead to an increase in diagnosis efficacy and further facilitate division of cervical cancer stages. Unfortunately, these conventional (surgery, radiation, and chemotherapy) treatments have been failed in several advanced-stage cervical cancer patients.

Usage of chemotherapeutic agents results in drug resistance through activating these cells signaling pathway. Therefore, a combination of target therapy and chemotherapy could be more effective in cancer management. Medicinal drugs targeting Wnt signaling have displayed significant therapeutic efficiency in numerous carcinomas (Blagodatski et al., 2014). Few drugs have shifted to phase II oncology trials. Furthermore, increased Wnt signaling activity may make malignant cells more susceptible to certain chemotherapeutic drugs (Table 2.1). Therefore, different components of the Wnt signaling pathway can be utilized as prognostic and diagnostic biomarkers of cervical cancer.

TABLE 2.1 Current Wnt Inhibitors under Development

Agent	Target	Stage/ Phase	Illustration
		Upstream	
LGK974	PORCN	I/II	–
ETC1922159	PORCN	I	–
C59	PORCN	Pre	Synergizes with $CTLA_4$
IWP-2	PORCN/DVL_2	Pre	CD8+T/CD4+T cells infiltration ↑; TREGs infiltration ↓
NSC669036	DVL	Pre	–
Jo1-017a	DVL	Pre	–
Niclosamide	DVL2	App	–
Sulindac	DVL	App	–
CGX1321	DVL	I	–
OTSA101	Fzd10	I	–
OMP-18R5 (Vantictumab)	Fzd	I/Ib	–
OMP-54F28 (Ipafricept)	Wnt/Fzd8	I/Ib	–
Foxy-5	Fzd5/Wnt5a	I/Ib	–
Wnt5a trap	Wnt5a	Pre	Doxorubicin-induced cell death ↑
DKN-01	DKK	I/II	TME MDSCs ↓; CD8+T/CD4+T infiltration ↑
CGX1321	GSK3	Pre	NK maturation ↑
SB415286	GSK3	Pre	PD-1 ↓; NK maturation in leukemia ↑
TWS119	GSK3	Pre	CD8+memory cells ↑
IWR1	Axin/Tankyrase	Pre	–
XAV939	Axin1	Pre	CD8+T infiltration ↑; TREGs infiltration ↓
JW74	Axin/Tankyrase	Pre	–
NVP-TNKS656	Axin/Tankyrase	Pre	–
Pyrivinium	CK1α	App	–
Lenalidomide	CK1α	App	CD8+T/CD4+T cells infiltration ↑; TREGs infiltration ↓
		Downstream	
CWP232291	β-catenin	I	–
PKF118-310	β-catenin/TCF	Pre	–
PKF115-584	β-catenin/LEF-1	Pre	CTLs activation ↑
iCRT3/5/14	β-catenin-TCF	Pre	–

TABLE 2.1 *(Continued)*

Agent	Target	Stage/ Phase	Illustration
PNU-74654	β-catenin/TCF	Pre	–
NCB-0846	TCF/ LEF(TNIK)	Pre	–
PRI-724	CBP/β-catenin	Ia/Ib/II	–
ICG-001	CBP	Pre	–
SAH-BCL9B	BCL9	Pre	–
		Crosstalk	
		Notch	
MK0752 (+docetaxel/+ Gemcitabine)	γ-sectetase	I/II	–
RO4929097	γ-sectetase	II	–
PF-03084014	γ-sectetase	I	–
MEDI0639	DLL4	I	–
Shh			
Vismodogib	SMO	App	–
Erismodegib	SMO	App	–
IPI-926	SMO	App	–
		Others	
CWP232291	SAM68	I	TCF alternative splicing, NF-KB ↑
Celecoxib	COX2	App	IDO1 ↓, TREG ↓; DCs vaccine ↑

Source: Reproduced with permission from Zhou et al. (2022); Copyright © Elsevier (2022).

KEYWORDS

- **cervical cancer**
- **chemotherapeutic drugs**
- **chemotherapy**
- **conventional treatment methods**
- **diagnostic biomarkers**
- **therapeutic efficiency**

REFERENCES

Ackers, I., & Malgor, R., (2018). Interrelationship of canonical and non-canonical Wnt signaling pathways in chronic metabolic diseases. *Diabetes and Vascular Disease Research, 15*(1), 3–13.

Anastas, J. N., & Moon, R. T., (2013). WNT signaling pathways as therapeutic targets in cancer. *Nature Reviews Cancer, 13*(1), 11–26.

Ayala, C. E., Mojica, V. L. H., García, C. A., & González, M. L., (2018). Wnt/β catenin pathway activation and silencing of the APC gene in HPV positive human cervical cancer derived cells. *Molecular Medicine Reports, 17*(1), 200–208.

Bahrami, A., Amerizadeh, F., ShahidSales, S., et al., (2017a). Therapeutic potential of targeting Wnt/β-catenin pathway in treatment of colorectal cancer: Rational and progress. *Journal of Cellular Biochemistry, 118*(8), 1979–1983.

Bahrami, A., Hasanzadeh, M., ShahidSales, S., et al., (2017b). Clinical significance and prognosis value of Wnt signaling pathway in cervical cancer. *Journal of Cellular Biochemistry, 118*(10), 3028–3033.

Barreto-Vargas, C., Alvarez-Zavala, M., Garcia-Chagollan, M., Hernandez-Flores, G., Aguilar-Lemarroy, A., & Jave-Suarez, L. F., (2020). WNT7A expression is downregulated in T lymphocytes after T-cell receptor activation due to histone modifications and in T-ALL by DNA methylation. *Archivum Immunologiae et Therapiae Experimentalis, 68*, 1–14.

Bello, J. O. M., Nieva, L. O., Paredes, A. C., Gonzalez, A. M. F., Zavaleta, L. R., & Lizano, M., (2015). Regulation of the Wnt/β-catenin signaling pathway by human papillomavirus E6 and E7 oncoproteins. *Viruses, 7*(8), 4734–4755.

Blagodatski, A., Klimenko, A., Jia, L., & Katanaev, V. L., (2020). Small molecule Wnt pathway modulators from natural sources: History, state of the art and perspectives. *Cells, 9*(3), 589.

Bonilla-Delgado, J., Bulut, G., Liu, X., et al., (2012). The E6 oncoprotein from HPV16 enhances the canonical Wnt/β-catenin pathway in skin epidermis *in vivo*. *Molecular Cancer Research, 10*(2), 250–258.

Bosch, F. X., & De Sanjosé, S., (2007). The epidemiology of human papillomavirus infection and cervical cancer. *Disease Markers, 23*(4), 213–227.

Bosch, X., & Harper, D., (2006). Prevention strategies of cervical cancer in the HPV vaccine era. *Gynecologic Oncology, 103*(1), 21–24.

Brookes, M. J., Boult, J., Roberts, K., et al., (2008). A role for iron in Wnt signaling. *Oncogene, 27*(7), 966–975.

Chang, B., Kim, J., Jeong, D., et al., (2012). Klotho inhibits the capacity of cell migration and invasion in cervical cancer. *Oncology Reports, 28*(3), 1022–1028.

Chatterjee, A., Paul, S., Bisht, B., Bhattacharya, S., Sivasubramaniam, S., & Paul, M. K., (2022). Advances in targeting the WNT/β-catenin signaling pathway in cancer. *Drug Discovery Today, 27*(1), 82–101.

Chatzistamatiou, K., Moysiadis, T., Moschaki, V., Panteleris, N., & Agorastos, T., (2016). Comparison of cytology, HPV DNA testing and HPV 16/18 genotyping alone or combined targeting to the more balanced methodology for cervical cancer screening. *Gynecologic Oncology, 142*(1), 120–127.

Cheng, Y., Geng, L., Zhao, L., Zuo, P., & Wang, J., (2017). Human papillomavirus E6-regulated microRNA-20b promotes invasion in cervical cancer by targeting tissue inhibitor of metalloproteinase 2. *Molecular Medicine Reports, 16*(4), 5464–5470.

Ciani, L., & Salinas, P. C., (2007). c-Jun N-terminal kinase (JNK) cooperates with Gsk3β to regulate dishevelled-mediated microtubule stability. *BMC Cell Biology, 8*(1), 1–14.

Cohen, P. A., Jhingran, A., Oaknin, A., & Denny, L., (2019). Cervical cancer. *The Lancet, 393*(10167), 169–182.

Coopes, A., Henry, C. E., Llamosas, E., & Ford, C. E., (2018). An update of Wnt signaling in endometrial cancer and its potential as a therapeutic target. *Endocrine-Related Cancer, 25*(12), R647–R662.

Dandekar, S., Romanos-Sirakis, E., Pais, F., et al., (2014). Wnt inhibition leads to improved chemosensitivity in paediatric acute lymphoblastic leukaemia. *British Journal of Haematology, 167*(1), 87–99.

Dao, D. Y., Yang, X. U. E., Di, C., Zuscik, M., & O'Keefe, R. J., (2007). Axin1 and Axin2 are regulated by TGF-β and mediate crosstalk between TGF-β and Wnt signaling pathways. *Annals of the New York Academy of Sciences, 1116*, 82.

Elgenaidi, I. S., & Spiers, J. P., (2019). Regulation of the phosphoprotein phosphatase 2A system and its modulation during oxidative stress: A potential therapeutic target? *Pharmacology and Therapeutics, 198*, 68–89.

Evans, M. F., & Cooper, K., (2004). Human papillomavirus integration: Detection by in situ hybridization and potential clinical application. *The Journal of Pathology, 202*(1), 1–4.

Fadare, O., Reddy, H., Wang, J., Hileeto, D., Schwartz, P. E., & Zheng, W., (2005). E-cadherin and β-catenin expression in early stage cervical carcinoma: A tissue microarray study of 147 cases. *World Journal of Surgical Oncology, 3*(1), 1–11.

Ford, C. E., Henry, C., Llamosas, E., Djordjevic, A., & Hacker, N., (2016). Wnt signaling in gynaecological cancers: A future target for personalized medicine? *Gynecologic Oncology, 140*(2), 345–351.

Franco, E. L., (2003). Primary screening of cervical cancer with human papillomavirus tests. *JNCI Monographs, 2003*(31), 89–96.

Furumoto, H., & Irahara, M., (2002). Human papilloma virus (HPV) and cervical cancer. *Journal of Medical Investigation, 49*(3, 4), 124–133.

Grant, S., (2008). Cotargeting survival signaling pathways in cancer. *The Journal of Clinical Investigation, 118*(9), 3003–3006.

Gupta, S., Kumar, P., & Das, B. C., (2018). HPV: Molecular pathways and targets. *Current Problems in Cancer, 42*(2), 161–174.

Hanahan, D., & Weinberg, R. A., (2011). Hallmarks of cancer: The next generation. *Cell, 144*(5), 646–674.

Hu, Z., Müller, S., Qian, G., et al., (2015). Human papillomavirus 16 oncoprotein regulates the translocation of β-catenin via the activation of epidermal growth factor receptor. *Cancer, 121*(2), 214–225.

Ishii, Y., Ozaki, S., Tanaka, K., & Kanda, T., (2005). Human papillomavirus 16 minor capsid protein L2 helps capsomeres assemble independently of intercapsomeric disulfide bonding. *Virus Genes, 31*(3), 321–328.

Krishnamurthy, N., & Kurzrock, R., (2018). Targeting the Wnt/beta-catenin pathway in cancer: Update on effectors and inhibitors. *Cancer Treatment Reviews, 62*, 50–60.

Kruck, S., Eyrich, C., Scharpf, M., Sievert, K. D., Fend, F., Stenzl, A., & Bedke, J., (2013). Impact of an altered Wnt1/β-catenin expression on clinicopathology and prognosis in clear cell renal cell carcinoma. *International Journal of Molecular Sciences, 14*(6), 10944–10957.

Kuo, D. Y. S., & Goldberg, G. L., (2003). Screening of cervical cancer: Where do we go from here? *Cancer Investigation, 21*(1), 157–161.

Kwan, H. T., Chan, D. W., Cai, P. C., et al., (2013). AMPK activators suppress cervical cancer cell growth through inhibition of DVL3 mediated Wnt/β-catenin signaling activity. *PLoS One, 8*(1), e53597.

Lehoczky, J. A., & Tabin, C. J., (2018). Rethinking WNT signaling. *Nature, 557*(7706), 495–496.

Li, C., Zheng, Z., Jiang, J., et al., (2018). Neural EGFL-like 1 regulates cartilage maturation through Runt-related transcription factor 3–mediated Indian hedgehog signaling. *The American Journal of Pathology, 188*(2), 392–403.

Li, H., Jiao, S., Li, X., Banu, H., Hamal, S., & Wang, X., (2015). Therapeutic effects of antibiotic drug tigecycline against cervical squamous cell carcinoma by inhibiting Wnt/β-catenin signaling. *Biochemical and Biophysical Research Communications, 467*(1), 14–20.

Li, J., & Zhou, B. P., (2011). Activation of β-catenin and Akt pathways by Twist are critical for the maintenance of EMT associated cancer stem cell-like characters. *BMC Cancer, 11*(1), 1–11.

Liang, L. A., Einzmann, T., Franzen, A., et al., (2021). Cervical cancer screening: Comparison of conventional pap smear test, liquid-based cytology, and human papillomavirus testing as stand-alone or cotesting strategies. *Cancer Epidemiology and Prevention Biomarkers, 30*(3), 474–484.

Lin, L., Liu, Y., Zhao, W., Sun, B., & Chen, Q., (2014). Wnt5A expression is associated with tumor metastasis and clinical survival in cervical cancer. *International Journal of Clinical and Experimental Pathology, 7*(9), 6072–6078.

Liu, X. F., Li, X. Y., Zheng, P. S., & Yang, W. T., (2018). DAX1 promotes cervical cancer cell growth and tumorigenicity through activation of Wnt/β-catenin pathway via GSK3β. *Cell Death and Disease, 9*(3), 1–13.

Maftouh, M., Belo, A. I., Avan, A., Funel, N., Peters, G. J., Giovannetti, E., & Van, D. I., (2014). Galectin-4 expression is associated with reduced lymph node metastasis and modulation of Wnt/β-catenin signaling in pancreatic adenocarcinoma. *Oncotarget, 5*(14), 5335.

Maheshwari, S., Nautiyal, R., Kotwal, A., & Chandra, S., (2020). Prevalence and distribution of various human papillomavirus genotypes in women with high risk for cervical carcinoma. *International Journal of Reproduction, Contraception, Obstetrics and Gynecology, 9*(6), 2498–2504.

Matsuzawa, S. I., & Reed, J. C., (2001). Siah-1, SIP, and Ebi collaborate in a novel pathway for β-catenin degradation linked to p53 responses. *Molecular Cell, 7*(5), 915–926.

McCarthy, M. P., White, W. I., Palmer-Hill, F., Koenig, S., & Suzich, J. A., (1998). Quantitative disassembly and reassembly of human papillomavirus type 11 virus like particles *in vitro*. *Journal of Virology, 72*(1), 32–41.

Metcalfe, C., & Bienz, M., (2011). Inhibition of GSK3 by Wnt signaling–two contrasting models. *Journal of Cell Science, 124*(21), 3537–3544.

Moradi, A., Ghasemi, F., Anvari, K., et al., (2017). The cross-regulation between SOX15 and Wnt signaling pathway. *Journal of Cellular Physiology, 232*(12), 3221–3225.

Narisawa-Saito, M., & Kiyono, T., (2007). Basic mechanisms of high-risk human papillomavirus-induced carcinogenesis: Roles of E6 and E7 proteins. *Cancer Science, 98*(10), 1505–1511.

Neels, P., Van, D. P., Van, R. M., & Dogne, J. M., (2013). Human papillomavirus vaccines: Understanding the benefit–risk. *Annals of Medicine, 45*(3), 203–205.

Nishida, H., Matsumoto, Y., Kawana, K., et al., (2016). Systemic delivery of siRNA by actively targeted polyion complex micelles for silencing the E6 and E7 human papillomavirus oncogenes. *Journal of Controlled Release, 231*, 29–37.

Pandita, S., Deshpande, R., Aphale, S., & Kaul-Ghanekar, R., (2017). Role of medicinal plants in targeting important signaling pathways in cervical cancer. In: George, A., Oluwafemi, O. S., Joseph, B., Thomas, S., Mathew, S., & Raji, V., (eds.), *Holistic Healthcare: Possibilities and Challenges*. Apple Academic Press, Florida, USA.

Pedroza-Torres, A., López-Urrutia, E., García-Castillo, V., et al., (2014). MicroRNAs in cervical cancer: Evidences for a miRNA profile deregulated by HPV and its impact on radio-resistance. *Molecules, 19*(5), 6263–6281.

Pereira, R., Hitzeroth, I. I., & Rybicki, E. P., (2009). Insights into the role and function of L2, the minor capsid protein of papillomaviruses. *Archives of Virology, 154*(2), 187–197.

Pérez-Plasencia, C., Piña-Sánchez, P., Vaca-Paniagua, F., Fragoso-Ontiveros, V., Jacobo-Herrera, N., López-Camarillo, C., & Vargas-Hernández, O., (2012). Molecular events towards Wnt pathway activation in cervical cancer: Changing the balance on NKD/DVL signals. In: Broeck, D. V., (ed.), *Human Papillomavirus and Related Diseases – From Bench to Bedside – Research Aspects* (pp. 325–346). IntechOpen, London.

Petry, K. U., (2014). HPV and cervical cancer. *Scandinavian Journal of Clinical and Laboratory Investigation, 74*(S244), 59–62.

Prasad, C. P., Rath, G., Mathur, S., Bhatnagar, D., Parshad, R., & Ralhan, R., (2009). Expression analysis of E-cadherin, Slug and GSK3β in invasive ductal carcinoma of breast. *BMC Cancer, 9*(1), 1–10.

Ramachandran, I., Thavathiru, E., Ramalingam, S., et al., (2012). Wnt inhibitory factor 1 induces apoptosis and inhibits cervical cancer growth, invasion and angiogenesis *in vivo*. *Oncogene, 31*(22), 2725–2737.

Rath, G., Jawanjal, P., Salhan, S., Nalliah, M., & Dhawan, I., (2015). Clinical significance of inactivated glycogen synthase kinase 3β in HPV-associated cervical cancer: Relationship with W nt/β-C atenin pathway activation. American *Journal of Reproductive Immunology, 73*(5), 460–478.

Sanchez-Vega, F., Mina, M., Armenia, J., et al., (2018). Oncogenic signaling pathways in the cancer genome atlas. *Cell, 173*(2), 321–337.

Sankaranarayanan, R., Bhatla, N., & Basu, P., (2016). Current global status and impact of human papillomavirus vaccination: Implications for India. *The Indian Journal of Medical Research, 144*(2), 169.

Scarth, J. A., Patterson, M. R., Morgan, E. L., & Macdonald, A., (2021). The human papillomavirus oncoproteins: A review of the host pathways targeted on the road to transformation. *The Journal of General Virology, 102*(3).

Scudellari, M., (2013). HPV: Sex, cancer and a virus. *Nature News, 503*(7476), 330.

Sen, P., Ganguly, P., & Ganguly, N., (2018). Modulation of DNA methylation by human papillomavirus E6 and E7 oncoproteins in cervical cancer. *Oncology Letters, 15*(1), 11–22.

Senapati, R., Senapati, N. N., & Dwibedi, B., (2016). Molecular mechanisms of HPV mediated neoplastic progression. *Infectious Agents and Cancer, 11*(1), 1–11.

Sompel, K., Elango, A., Smith, A. J., & Tennis, M. A., (2021). Cancer chemoprevention through frizzled receptors and EMT. *Discover Oncology, 12*(1), 1–15.

Stanley, M. A., Pett, M. R., & Coleman, N., (2007). HPV: From infection to cancer. *Biochemical Society Transactions, 35*(6), 1456–1460.

Terasaki, H., Saitoh, T., Shiokawa, K., & Katoh, M., (2002). Frizzled-10, up-regulated in primary colorectal cancer, is a positive regulator of the WNT-β-catenin-TCF signaling pathway. *International Journal of Molecular Medicine, 9*(2), 107–112.

Üren, A., Fallen, S., Yuan, H., Usubütün, A., Küçükali, T., Schlegel, R., & Toretsky, J. A., (2005). Activation of the canonical Wnt pathway during genital keratinocyte transformation: A model for cervical cancer progression. *Cancer Research, 65*(14), 6199–6206.

Waggoner, S. E., (2003). Cervical cancer. *The Lancet, 361*(9376), 2217–2225.

Wang, B., Li, X., Liu, L., & Wang, M., (2020). β-catenin: Oncogenic role and therapeutic target in cervical cancer. *Biological Research, 53*(1), 1–11.

Wang, R., Pan, W., Jin, L., et al., (2020). Human papillomavirus vaccine against cervical cancer: Opportunity and challenge. *Cancer Letters, 471*, 88–102.

Wei, H., Wang, N., Zhang, Y., Wang, S., Pang, X., & Zhang, S., (2016). Wnt-11 overexpression promotes the invasion of cervical cancer cells. *Tumor Biology, 37*(9), 11789–11798.

Wentzensen, N., Schwartz, L., Zuna, R. E., et al., (2012). Performance of p16/Ki-67 immunostaining to detect cervical cancer precursors in a colposcopy referral population. *Clinical Cancer Research, 18*(15), 4154–4162.

Yang, M., Wang, M., Li, X., et al., (2018). Wnt signaling in cervical cancer? *Journal of Cancer, 9*(7), 1277.

Zhan, T., Rindtorff, N., & Boutros, M., (2017). Wnt signaling in cancer. *Oncogene, 36*(11), 1461–1473.

Zheng, M., Zhou, Q., Liu, X., Wang, C., & Liu, G., (2019). CTHRC1 overexpression promotes cervical carcinoma progression by activating the Wnt/PCP signaling pathway. *Oncology Reports, 41*(3), 1531–1538.

CHAPTER 3

TLR Signaling Pathway in Cervical Cancer

3.1 WHAT ARE TLRs?

Toll-like receptors (TLRs), also recognized as Pattern Recognition Receptors, are considered the first line of defense against innate immunity, leading to the activation of cellular signaling pathways. These cellular pathways control the expression of genes associated with inflammation and immunity, including the tumor microenvironment (Kawai & Akira, 2007). Activation of TLR signaling in tumor cells by their specific ligands promotes the synthesis of various soluble factors and proteins together with proinflammatory cytokines (TNF-α, interleukins, chemokines, and type 1 IFNs), inducible nitric oxides synthase, B7-H1, and B7-H2, and activating apoptotic cascade (caspases, Bax, Bcl-2 and p53), which results in resistance of tumor cells to immunological attack. TLRs stand as an advance guard of immunological defense, serving as the instant components of a multitier signaling cascade that plays a major role in cellular immune regulation, cell proliferation and survival, apoptosis, cell migration, metastasis, angiogenesis, inflammation, and finally, cancer (Takeda & Akira, 2005; Vijay, 2018). The TLR family is the best-characterized group of innate immune receptors in terms of identified ligands, downstream signaling pathways, and functional significance. It consists of 10 members (TLR1–TLR10). The mammalian immune system detects invasion by pathogens by the identification of their microbial components through TLRs (Mukherjee et al., 2019). Each TLR has been known to recognize specific components of pathogens, as shown in Table 3.1.

Cervical Cancer: Signaling Pathways, Molecular Mechanisms, Natural Products, and Therapeutic Approaches. Pratibha Pandey, Fahad Khan, Saher Islam, and Devarajan Thangadurai, (Eds.)

TABLE 3.1 Human TLRs and Their Related Ligands and Their Function in Immunity

TLRs	Ligand	Function
TLR1	Triacyl lipopeptides, Modulin, Pam3Cys-Ser-(Lys)4 (synthetic lipoprotein).	Stimulate production of IL-6 in human tonsillar B-cells.
TLR2	Peptidoglycan, lipoprotein, lipopeptides, atypical LPS, lipoteichoic acid, phenol-soluble modulin (bacteria) zymozan, lipoarabinomannan (fungi) GPI anchors, glycolipids (protozoa) envelope protein (virus) Pam3Cys-Ser-(Lys)4 (synthetic lipoprotein).	Activation of NF-κB and apoptosis induction in THP-1 monocytice cells; induction of proinflammatory cytokine IL-6 in monocytic cells and surface expression of CD150.
TLR3	dsRNA (virus) mRNA (host) poly(I:C) (synthetic dsRNA).	Activates type I interferon, NK cells, CTLs, inflammatory cytokine production and dendritic cell (DC) maturation.
TLR4	Lipopolysachcharide, flavolipin, mannuronic acid mannan, glucoronoxylomannan (fungi) heat-shock protein 60, glycoinositolphospholipids (protozoa) envelope F protein (virus) HSP60, HSP70, polysaccharide fragments of heparin sulfate, hyaluronic acid, fibrinogen, fibronectin DA domain (host), taxol.	Induction of TNF-α, NF-κB, and up-regulate the expression of proinflammatory cytokines in human monocytes.
TLR5	Flagellin	Stimulate production of chemokines, cytokines, and co-stimulatory molecules from T cells.
TLR6	Lipoproteins	Induce NF-κB and apoptosis.
TLR7	ssRNA, imidazoquinolines (synthetic antiviral compound), bropirimine, guanosine analog isatoribine.	Stimulate secretion of inflammatory cytokines (IFNα), decreases plasma virus concentration in chronic hepatitis C infection.
TLR8	ssRNA	Stimulate secretion of inflammatory cytokines.
TLR9	Unmethylated CpG DNA, chromatin-IgG complex	Stimulate secretion of inflammatory cytokines.
TLR10	Unknown	–

3.2 TLR SIGNALING PATHWAYS

TLRs signaling pathways are grouped into the MyD88 (human myeloid differentiation factor 88)-dependent and MyD88-independent pathways.

The signaling pathways associated with TLR1, TLR2, TLR5, TLR6, TLR7, TLR8, and TLR9 are moderated by MyD88-dependent pathway, while TLR3 signaling pathway is activated by the MyD88-independent pathway (Calich et al., 2008; Lim & Staudt, 2013). The TLR4 signaling cascade, on the other hand, can be mediated by both pathways at the same time (O'Neill et al., 2003; O'Neill & Bowie, 2007). In case of MyD88 independent pathway, TLR3 and TLR4 can induce activation of NF-κB, IRF-3 and stimulate IFN-stimulated regulatory elements. After binding to its ligands, TLRs gets activated that resulted in the recruitment of a variety of adaptor molecules and induction of signaling cascades causing the stimulation of various transcriptional factors, such as the nuclear factor kappa B (NF-kB), mitogen activated protein kinase (MAPK) (Falck-Hansen et al., 2013). Depending upon the specific TLR various types of adaptor molecules can be recruited (Luo et al., 2019). For example, TLR1, TLR2, and TLR6 utilize MyD88 and TIRAP (TIR-containing adaptor protein) (Horng et al., 2002; Jenkins & Mansell, 2010), while the TLR5, TLR7, TLR9, and TLR11 recruit MyD88. TLR3 only utilizes the TRIF adaptor, and TLR4 can employ four adaptor molecules such as MyD88, TIRAP, TRAM, and TRIF) (Häcker et al., 2006; Oganesyan et al., 2006).

Activation of TLR4 resulted in activation of MyD88-dependent pathways after encounter with bacterial LPS or some viral envelope proteins. This leads to initial phase activation of NF-kB and the TRIF-dependent pathway, which finally resulted in late-phase activation of NF-kB (Satoh & Akira, 2016; Leitner et al., 2019). Consecutively, IKK complex causes phosphorylation of IkB (inhibitor of kB) that resulted in polyubiquitination and breakdown through 26S proteasome, finally leading to NF-kB nuclear translocation. This canonical pathway ultimately resulted in induction of transcription of inflammatory cytokines, such as TNF-α and IL-6 (Sheedy & O'Neill, 2005; Carty et al., 2006). The non-canonical pathway is initiated in the form of TRIF-dependent signaling. Initially, IRF3 (interferon regulatory factor 3) is localized in the cytoplasm in its inactive form. However, upon stimulation by interaction of their TLR and ligands, IRF3 is phosphorylated at a specific location by TBK1 and IKKi. This resulted in the formation of a homodimer of IRF3 and transfer in to the nucleus. This leads to the formation of IRF3, NF-kB, and AP-1 complex which induces the transcription of IFN gene, specifically the IFN-B (Colonna, 2007; Brown et al., 2011; Oosenbrug et al., 2017).

3.3 TLRs IN CANCER PROGRESSION

Inflammatory and autoimmune illnesses, as well as cancer, are linked to TLRs and NF-kB. TLRs are primarily responsible for normal tissue homeostasis, which includes cell proliferation and death regulation. However, recent studies suggested the prominent role of TLRs and NF-kB are involved in inflammatory and autoimmune diseases, and also in cancer (Kawai & Akira, 2007; Brown et al., 2011; Narayanankutty et al., 2020). Usually, TLRs are mainly responsible for normal tissue homeostasis, including the regulation of cell proliferation and death. However, recent research has revealed that TLRs play an important role in cancer progression and development by supporting the tumor environment by influencing the inflammatory response, apoptosis, and angiogenesis processes (Huang et al., 2018; Angrini et al., 2020; McCall et al., 2020). There are three ways in which TLR-mediated inflammatory response can stimulate process of carcinogenesis: via inducing the anti-apoptotic effect of NF-κB, oxidative stress-induced DNA damage and inducing the tissue repair process (Medzhitov, 2001; Kowalczyk et al., 2013; Di Gioia & Zanoni, 2015). Several studies established that abnormal expression of TLRs have been observed in tumor tissues samples with various subtypes of TLRs, including colorectal cancer, prostate cancer, gastric cancer, pancreatic cancer, ovarian cancer, lung cancer, liver cancer, and breast cancer (Gambara et al., 2013; Li et al., 2014; Zhang et al., 2015; Shi et al., 2016; Dajon et al., 2017; Vlad et al., 2018; Liu et al., 2019).

In tumor cells, TLR-ligand interaction causes the production of cytokine and chemokine engaged in tumor invasion, inhibition of apoptosis, chemoresistance, and enhanced metastasis (Huang et al., 2008). Out of all the TLRs, TLR4 expression has been reported in various tumor cells, and is related to immunological escape by secreting immunosuppressive cytokines and preventing apoptosis (Basith et al., 2012) (Table 3.2). A previous study by Huang et al. (2005) revealed that LPS-induced TLR4 activation resulted in proinflammatory cytokines production (IL-6, IL-12, nitric oxide) that may induce tumor cell resistance and immune evasion by tumor cells. Another study demonstrated the mechanism of regulation of LPS-induced tumor cell growth by TLR4 that shows increased expression of TNF level, which resulted in the increased expression of NF-kB-mediated antiapoptotic molecules such as Bcl-XL, cIAP1, cIAP2 (Luo et al., 2004). A study conducted in murine model has also been demonstrated the association of LPS-induced TLR4 activation with tumor metastasis. In addition, NF-kB stimulation causes a rise in matrix metalloproteinase 2 (MMP2), and inducible nitric oxide synthase levels (iNOS) (Wang et al., 2003).

TABLE 3.2 TLRs in Different Tumor Subtypes

Tumor Samples	TLRs Expression
Breast cancer	TLR2, TLR3, TLR4, TLR9
Colorectal cancer	TLR2, TLR3, TLR4, TLR5, TLR9
Gastric cancer	TLR2, TLR4, TLR5, TLR9
Liver cancer	TLR2, TLR3, TLR4, TLR6, TLR9
Lung cancer	TLR2, TLR3, TLR4, TLR9
Ovarian cancer	TLR2, TLR3, TLR4, TLR5
Pancreatic cancer	TLR2, TLR4, TLR9
Prostate cancer	TLR4, TLR9

The involvement of TLR4 has been confirmed in almost all types of carcinomas, including liver, colon, esophageal, skin, prostate, and gynecological cancers (Dickinson et al., 2018; Jiang et al., 2018; Kang et al., 2018; Ou et al., 2018; Kohtz et al., 2019; Koliaraki et al., 2019). TLR4 activation in human colon cancer cells stimulates the production of immunosuppressive cytokines and induces apoptosis resistance through TNF-α and TRAIL (TNF-related apoptosis-inducing ligand) (Tang & Zhu, 2012). Subsequently, LPS-induced TLR4 activation in several murine cancer cells resulted in immune evasion via the secretion of IL-6, IL-12, and iNOS (Huang et al., 2005). In human neuroblastoma cells, TLR4 is not expressed at the cell surface and present in intracellular locations; thus, these cells are insensitive to LPS effects (Hassan et al., 2006). In human head and neck tumors, TLR4-mediated cancer progression was associated with an increase levels in IL-8, IL-6, VEGF, and macrophage colony-stimulating factor (Szczepanski et al., 2009). These results suggested that there are specific sequential and spatial TLR regulations in the different phases of cancer progression and development. The role of TLR4 is profoundly discussed in gynecological tumors and may serve as a crucial target for the development of potential and novel anticancer agents.

3.4 ROLE OF TLRs IN CERVICAL CANCER

The cervical cancer comprises approximately ~8% of total cancer mortalities detected in women (Bentivegna et al., 2016; Pan et al., 2021). The correlation between HPV infection and cervical cancer development includes an inflammatory component along with infection. Persistent cervical inflammation may result in cervical cancer development and TLRs play a dominant role in the generation of inflammatory response (DeCarlo et al., 2012; Husseinzadeh & Davenport, 2014). That is why, the activation and distribution of TLR4 and other TLRs were mainly examined in the normal cervix, invasive cervical cancer, and in HPV-related cervical cancer cells (Wang et al., 2014; Aggarwal et al., 2015). Recent studies suggested the overexpression of TLR2, TLR4, TLR5, and TLR9 were found in premalignant lesions and cervical cancer samples compared to normal samples (Figure 3.1). These studies also established that abnormal expression of TLR4, TLR5, and TLR9 is correlated with HPV infection and cervical cancer development. It has also been observed that expression of TLR4 established a relationship with the lesion grade, as higher expression was seen in cervical cancer than intraepithelial neoplasia and normal tissues. Moreover, HPV16 infection also induces TLR4 expression which established the correlation between HPV 16 and TLR4 (Hasimu et al., 2011; Li et al., 2013). Few studies also reported the role of bacterial infection in the stimulation of cancer progression in HPV-related cervical epithelium. A study performed by Werner et al. revealed the involvement of two pathogens viz. *Escherichia coli* and *Pseudomonas aeruginosa* in HeLa cells and reported increased TLR4 and integrin β6 expression that could be an important mechanism of cervical cancer development (Werner et al., 2012). A recent study explored the involvement of five single nucleotide polymorphism of TLR4 gene with disease progression in 130 cervicitis patients (Chauhan et al., 2019). These researchers also reported that TLR genes could also be used as an important marker for early diagnosis of cervical cancer in high-risk HPV (HPV 16 and 18) infected cancer patients in Western India.

A study was conducted in Chinese Han population to determine the probability of cervical cancer and their correlation with TLR gene polymorphisms and HPV infection, and found that polymorphisms in minor alleles TLR4-rs7873784, TLR2-rs3775290, and TLR9-rs352140 were associated with increased chances of cervical cancer (Jin et al., 2017). A recent study also explored the predominant role of HPV 16 in cervical squamous cell carcinoma associated with decreased levels of TLR4 and Th1 cytokines as well as increased expression of cancer-related genes (Guleria et al., 2019). Tables 3.3 and 3.4 summarizes the polymorphism associated with the major TLRs and cervical cancer progression.

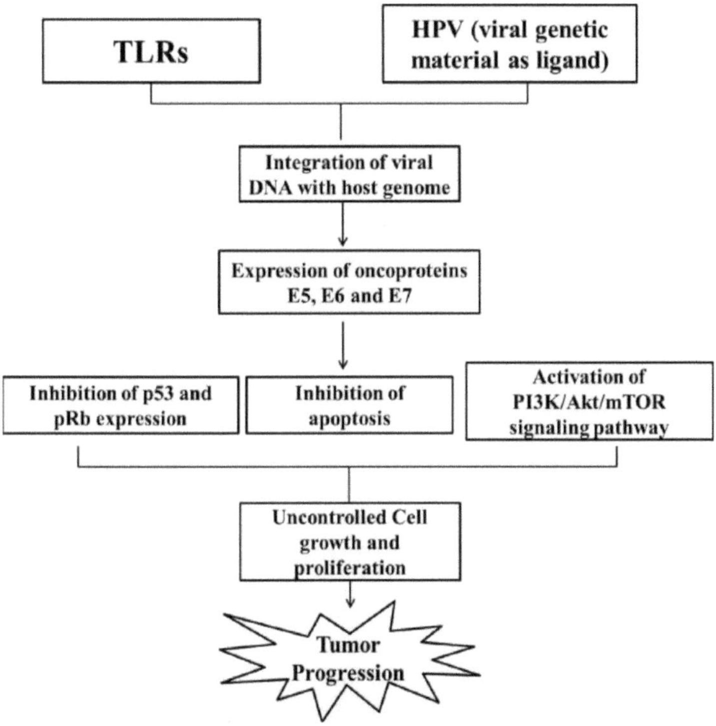

FIGURE 3.1 Possible mechanism behind the TLR-mediated cervical cancer progression and development via inhibition of tumor suppressor genes (p53, pRb), apoptosis resistance, and activation of PI3K/Akt/mTOR signaling pathway.

Li et al. studied HPV-positive cervical cancer samples in 43 patients and compared them to healthy HPV-positive and control patients to illustrate the role of HPV in TLR/nitric oxide (NO) signaling. The cervical canal of HPV-positive cervical cancer patients had a higher NO concentration (≈68.63) than healthy HPV-positive patients (≈21.71) and healthy controls (≈10.38). In addition, HPV-positive cervical cancer tissue had a high level of iNOS in the nucleus and cytoplasm. They looked at the activation of the TLR4/NO pathway in cervical cancer cell lines (Caski, HeLa, and C33a cells) to see if there was a link between NO levels and TLR signaling. At both the mRNA and protein levels, TLR4, NF-kB, and iNOS were greater in HPV-positive HeLa and CaSki cells than in HPV-negative C33A cells (Li et al., 2017).

TABLE 3.3 Meta-Analysis from Association between Polymorphisms in TLR2, TLR3, and TLR4 Genes and the Risk of Cervical Cancer According to Genetic Model

Poly	Comparisons	Test of Association			Model	Test of Heterogeneity			Egger Test	
		OR (95% CI)	Z	p-Value		$\chi 2$	p-Value	I^2 (%)	Z	P
TLR2 del¡196–174 (rs111200466)					Allele					
	Del vs. Ins	1.24 (0.93–1.66)	1.45	0.15	F	1.38	0.24	27	NA	NA
					Codominant Model					
	Del/Del vs. Ins/Ins	1.65 (0.28–9.64)	0.56	0.58	R	2.62	0.11	62	NA	NA
	Ins/Del vs. Ins/Ins	1.42 (0.97–2.08)	1.81	0.07	F	–	0.85	0	NA	NA
					Dominant Model					
	Ins/Del+Del/Del vs. Ins/Ins	1.34 (0.95–1.89)	1.66	0.10	F	–	0.57	0	NA	NA
					Recessive Model					
	Del/Del vs. Ins/ Ins+Ins/Del	1.52 (0.26–8.79)	0.47	0.64	R	–	0.11	62	NA	NA
TLR3 þ1377C>T (rs3775290)					Allele					
	T vs. C	1.18 (0.74–1.86)	0.70	0.49	R	16.83	0.0002	88	5.6978	<0.0001
					Codominant Model					
	T/T vs. C/C	1.45 (0.62–3.39)	0.86	0.39	R	8.87	0.01	77	1.5596	0.1189
	C/T vs. C/C	1.13 (0.64–2.00)	0.42	0.67	R	14.91	0.0006	87	3.5558	0.0004
					Dominant Model					
	C/T+T/T vs. C/C	1.17 (0.65–2.12)	0.52	0.60	R	17.59	0.0002	89	5.5882	<0.0001
					Recessive Model					
	T/T vs. C/C+C/T	1.44 (0.80–2.60)	1.22	0.22	R	4.60	0.10	56	1.1507	0.2498

TABLE 3.3 *(Continued)*

Poly	Comparisons	Test of Association			Model	Test of Heterogeneity			Egger Test	
		OR (95% CI)	Z	p-Value		χ2	p-Value	I^2 (%)	Z	P
TLR4 þ1196C>T Thr399Ile (rs4986791)					Allele					
	T vs. C	1.34 (1.12–1.62)	3.12	0.002	F	0.04	0.85	0	7.6363	<0.0001
					Codominant Model					
	T/T vs. C/C	1.82 (1.15–2.87)	2.57	0.01	F	0.01	0.91	0	2.0422	0.0411
	C/T vs. C/C	1.28 (1.01–1.62)	2.03	0.04	F	0.05	0.83	0	8.0258	<0.0001
					Dominant Model					
	C/T+T/T vs. C/C	1.35 (1.08–1.69)	2.64	0.008	F	0.02	0.89	0	10.0681	<0.0001
					Recessive Model					
	T/T vs. C/C+C/T	1.67 (1.07–2.61)	2.26	0.02	F	0.02	0.88	0	1.6604	0.0968
TLR4 þ896A>G Asp299Gly (rs4986790)					Allele					
	G vs. A	1.18 (0.71–1.95)	0.63	0.53	R	6.02	0.05	67	–0.6060	0.5445
					Codominant Model					
	G/G vs. A/A	1.97 (0.84–4.63)	1.55	0.12	F	0.21	0.90	0	0.2292	0.8187
	A/G vs. A/A	0.89 (0.31–2.58)	0.21	0.83	R	16.01	0.0003	88	–0.8842	0.3766
					Dominant Model					
	A/G+G/G vs. A/A	1.08 (0.50–2.36)	0.20	0.84	R	10.89	0.004	82	–1.0560	0.2910
					Recessive Model					
	G/G vs. A/A+A/G	2.08 (0.88–4.89)	1.67	0.09	F	0.33	0.85	0	–0.2137	0.8308

TABLE 3.3 *(Continued)*

Poly	Comparisons	Test of Association			Model	Test of Heterogeneity			Egger Test	
		OR (95% CI)	Z	p-Value		χ2	p-Value	I^2 (%)	Z	P
TLR4 þ7263G>C (rs11536889)					**Allele**					
	C vs. G	1.08 (0.75–1.55)	0.41	0.68	R	8.45	0.01	76	3.2563	0.0011
					Codominant Model					
	C/C vs. G/G	1.13 (0.54–2.36)	0.34	0.74	R	2.77	0.10	64	NA	NA
	G/C vs. G/G	1.21 (0.95–1.53)	1.56	0.12	F	0.72	0.40	0	3.7104	0.0002
					Dominant Model					
	G/C+C/C vs. G/G	1.22 (0.97–1.52)	1.73	0.08	F	0.05	0.82	0	3.2301	0.0012
					Recessive Model					
	C/C vs. G/G+G/C	1.11 (0.50–2.46)	0.26	0.79	R	16.10	0.0003	88	–0.2583	0.7962

Note: Poly.: Polymorphism; R: Random effects model; F: Fixed effects model; NA: Not available; OR: Odds ratio; Statistically significant p values ($p < 0.05$).

Source: Reproduced with permission from Moura et al. (2022); Copyright © Elsevier (2022).

TABLE 3.4 Meta-Analysis from Association between Polymorphisms in TLR4 and TLR9 Genes and the Risk of Cervical Cancer According to Genetic Model

Poly	Comparisons	Test of Association			Model	Test of Heterogeneity			Egger Test	
		OR (95% CI)	Z	p-Value		χ2	p-Value	I^2 (%)	Z	P
TLR4-2604A>G (rs10759931)				**Allele**						
	G vs. A	1.28 (1.00–1.65)	1.95	0.05	F	0.16	0.69	0	NA	NA
				Codominant Model						
	G/G vs. A/A	1.50 (0.92–2.45)	1.64	0.10	F	0.24	0.62	0	NA	NA
	A/G vs. A/A	1.07 (0.68–1.69)	0.29	0.77	F	0.90	0.34	0	NA	NA
				Dominant Model						
	A/G+G/G vs. A/A	1.24 (0.81–1.89)	1.01	0.31 F 0.67 0.41 0 NA NA	F	0.67	0.41	0	NA	NA
				Recessive Model						
	G/G vs. A/A+A/G	1.48 (1.02–2.17)	2.05	0.04	F	0.02	0.90	0	NA	NA
TLR4 þ7764C>T (rs1927911)				**Allele**						
	T vs. C	1.71 (1.31–2.24)	3.90	<0.0001	F	0.01	0.94	0	NA	NA
				Codominant Model						
	T/T vs. C/C	2.57 (1.21–5.45)	2.46	0.01	F	0.05	0.82	0	NA	NA
	C/T vs. C/C	2.20 (1.52–3.19)	4.17	<0.0001	F	0.02	0.89	0	NA	NA
				Dominant Model						
	C/T+T/T vs. C/C	2.24 (1.56–3.21)	4.39	<0.0001	F	0.02	0.88	0	NA	NA
				Recessive Model						
	T/T vs. C/C+C/T	1.71 (0.83–3.52)	1.45	0.15	F	0.03	0.87	0	NA	NA

TABLE 3.4 *(Continued)*

Poly	Comparisons	Test of Association			Model	Test of Heterogeneity			Egger Test	
		OR (95% CI)	Z	p-Value		$\chi 2$	p-Value	I^2 (%)	Z	P
TRL9-1486T>C (rs187084)		**Allele**								
	C vs. T	1.22 (1.09–1.37)	3.53	0.0004	F	5.01	0.17	40	2.9240	0.0035
		Codominant Model								
	C/C vs. T/T	1.38 (1.09–1.74)	2.71	0.007	F	3.99	0.26	25	1.4403	0.1498
	T/C vs. T/T	1.58 (1.12–2.23)	2.62	0.009	R	7.35	0.06	59	1.8262	0.0678
		Dominant Model								
	T/C+C/C vs. T/T	1.54 (1.13–2.08)	2.77	0.006	R	6.75	0.08	56	1.7492	0.0803
		Recessive Model								
	A/A vs. G/G+G/A	1.56 (1.13–2.15)	2.73	0.006	R	15.50	0.02	61	1.1647	0.2441
TLR9 þ2848G>A (rs352140)		**Allele**								
	A vs. G	1.42 (1.11–1.84)	2.73	0.006	R	31.13	<0.0001	81	1.3645	0.1724
		Codominant Model								
	A/A vs. G/G	1.74 (1.18–2.58)	2.78	0.005	R	18.01	0.006	67	0.1381	0.8901
	G/A vs. G/G	1.30 (0.96–1.76)	1.71	0.09	R	17.13	0.009	65	0.9538	0.3402
		Dominant Model								
	G/A+A/A vs. G/G	1.47 (1.07–2.01)	2.39	0.02	R	21.75	0.001	72	0.7173	0.4732
		Recessive Model								
	A/A vs. G/G+G/A	1.56 (1.13–2.15)	2.73	0.006	R	15.50	0.02	61	1.1647	0.2441

TABLE 3.4 *(Continued)*

Poly	Comparisons	Test of Association			Model	Test of Heterogeneity			Egger Test	
		OR (95% CI)	Z	p-Value		χ2	p-Value	I^2 (%)	Z	P
TLR9-1237T>C (rs5743836)	**Allele**									
	C vs. T	1.13 (0.40–3.23)	0.23	0.82	R	10.11	0.001	90	NA	NA
	Codominant Model									
	C/C vs. T/T	2.88 (1.41–5.86)	2.91	0.004	F	0.99	0.32	0	NA	NA
	T/C vs. T/T	0.86 (0.36–2.03)	0.35	0.73	R	4.31	0.04	77	NA	NA
	Dominant Model									
	T/C+C/C vs. T/T	1.02 (0.34–3.01)	0.03	0.98	R	7.83	0.005	87	NA	NA
	Recessive Model									
	C/C vs. T/T+T/C	2.70 (1.35–5.38)	2.82	0.005	F	0.61	0.44	0	NA	NA

Source: Reproduced with permission from Moura et al. (2022); Copyright © Elsevier (2022).

TLR4 has been linked to a variety of immune responses in cervical cancer patients. de Matos et al. identified a substantial correlation between TLR4 and TNF-α/TNFβ-expression in both premalignant lesions and cervical cancer after examining 35 specimens with cervical intraepithelial neoplasia and 10 specimens with cervical squamous cell carcinoma. There's also a correlation that IgG-expressing cervical cancer cells are engaged in TLR4 signaling modulation (de Matos et al., 2017). Wang et al. discovered a significant reduction in LPS-related proinflammatory cytokines when IgG was reduced, and showed that IgG knockdown repressed NF-kB and MAPK, affecting nuclear translocation of NF-kB and the activity of its response element. IgG was recruited to TLR4 in the cytoplasm of cells in response to LPS stimulation, and when IgG was silenced, TLR4 expression was downregulated; while total TLR4 was present in increased amount in control shRNA HeLa cells, IGHG1-silenced HeLa cells downregulated TLR4 levels as well as inflammatory molecules (TNF-α, IL-6, IL-1) at both the mRNA and protein levels (Wang et al., 2014).

Cervical cancer vaccines based on novel virus-like particles have been developed. In wild-type animals, CD4+ T-cells and TLR4 receptor-deficient animals, and mice defective in CD8+ T cells, a recombinant protein comprising immunogenic multi-epitopes of HPV-16 E6 and E7 demonstrated anticancer effects; however, no protective action was detected in mice deficient in CD8+ T cells (de Oliveira et al., 2015). Clinical aspects of HPV-related illnesses are connected to cellular immunity to E7. In the therapy of cervical cancer, Mansilla et al. combined HPVE7 with a fusion protein containing extra domain A (EDA) from fibronectin (a TLR4 ligand). EDA-HPVE7-immunized animals have anticancer CD8+ T cell responses, indicating that the vaccine complex (EDA-HPVE7) was successfully acquired by dendritic cells and stimulated *in vitro* maturation with additional IL-12 production (Mansilla et al., 2012). In TLR4 mutant mice, the immunogenicity of HPV 16 L1 capsomeres was also observed that suggested an intriguing potential for vaccine development against cervical cancer (Schädlich et al., 2009).

Altogether, identification of new targets that disrupt the TLR signaling pathway (mainly TLR4) could help to reduce the impact of inflammation and immunology on tumor formation and progression (Figure 3.2). There is mounting evidence that novel TLR/TLR4 antagonists or TLR/TLR4 gene silencers may play a significant role in the inhibition of tumor development and aggressiveness.

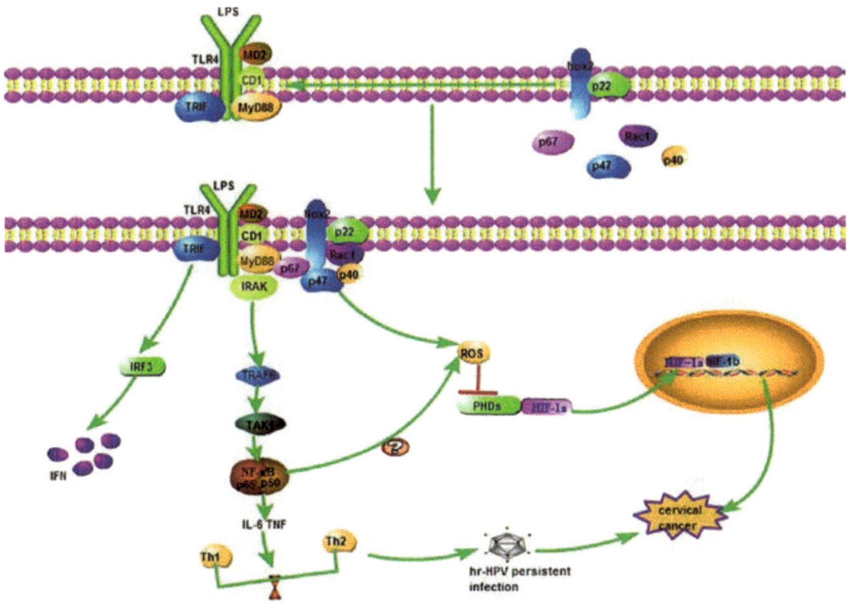

FIGURE 3.2 The possible mechanism of TLR4 being correlated with cervical cancer. The combination of TLR4 and its ligand (LPS) can trigger lipid rafts flowing which results in the change of lipid raft space conformation. This conformational change provides a condition for the aggregation of NADPH oxidase subunits on lipid rafts, which activates the redox reaction of lipid rafts to produce ROS and inhibits the degradation of HIF-1α, leading to the high expression of HIF-1α.

Source: Adapted from Yang et al. (2017); https://creativecommons.org/licenses/by/4.0/

3.5 TLR AGONISTS AND HPV VACCINES AS ADJUVANT THERAPY IN CERVICAL CANCER

HPV vaccine development is an important accomplishment for cervical cancer therapies since HPV is a primary cause of cervical cancer. Although, it still encounters certain drawbacks in clinical practice. Present research focused on improving the efficacy of the HPV vaccine via eliminating HPV infected tumor cells through stimulation of immune response. However, a therapeutic vaccine was less effective as having severe side effects and problems in identifying tumor specific antigens (E6 and E7) (Paavonen et al., 2009; Luchner et al., 2021). Some therapeutic vaccines against HPV-mediated cervical cancer, such as Gardasil, Cervarix shows very low response rate (2.6%) in a clinical study performed with 440 cancer patients. The reason behind the low response of prophylactic vaccines observed in cancer patients was lack of potent adjuvants that could overcome the immunosuppressive role of tumor cells (Rosenberg et al., 2004; Paavonen et al., 2009). The molecules or compounds that can trigger TLRs might be used as adjuvants for vaccine development. Ongoing research and development for the investigation of novel vaccine adjuvants are predominantly concentrated on various TLR ligands. Clinical studies have been performed by targeting TLR pathways to enhance the immunogenic properties of DNA vaccines and stimulate the T cell-mediated immune response in preventing viral infection (Hedayat et al., 2011). Research findings revealed that concomitant stimulation of numerous TLR signaling pathways by cancer vaccines resulted in enhanced immunogenic responses. TLR signaling mediated immune response generation mechanism not only associated with HPV vaccine, but also found in other types of vaccines, such as measles, rubella, and hepatitis (Dabbagh & Lewis, 2003). Moreover, several experimental findings revealed the significant role of TLR signaling pathways in different types of infectious diseases and explored the therapeutic benefits of new agonists and antagonist ligands against TLRs (Rosenberg et al., 2004). Presently, international regulatory agencies approved only three TLR agonists for cancer therapeutics viz. MPL (monophosphoryl lipid A), BCG (Bacillus Calmette-Guérin), and imiquimod (Hemmi et al., 2002; Hoffman et al., 2005; Mata-Haro et al., 2007). A clinical trial study involving the Cervarix/Gardasil vaccine with adjuvant aluminum-MPL demonstrated that MPL adjuvants could improve the efficacy of both vaccines. However, results of antibody titers show that increased neutralization antibodies were observed in Cervarix plus adjuvant in comparison with Gardasil plus adjuvant (Einstein et al., 2009). Recent studies of some clinical trials on vaccine adjuvants suggested that MPLs are safe and have enhanced immunogenic properties (Neidhart et al., 2004). Furthermore, numerous preclinical and clinical studies are in progress to investigate the potential of several TLR agonists (for example, TMX-101: TLR7 agonist) and vaccine adjuvants (CpG ODNs), which could help in the development of novel immunotherapeutic agents for cervical cancer.

KEYWORDS

- **Cervarix plus adjuvant**
- **cervical cancer**
- **Gardasil plus adjuvant**
- **immunotherapeutic agents**
- **signaling pathways**
- **vaccine adjuvants**

REFERENCES

Aggarwal, R., Misra, S., Guleria, C., et al., (2015). Characterization of toll-like receptor transcriptome in squamous cell carcinoma of cervix: A case-control study. *Gynecologic Oncology, 138*(2), 358–362.

Angrini, M., Varthaman, A., & Cremer, I., (2020). Toll-like receptors (TLRs) in the tumor microenvironment (TME): A dragon-like weapon in a non-fantasy game of thrones. *Advances in Experimental Medicine and Biology, 1263*, 145–173.

Basith, S., Manavalan, B., Yoo, T. H., Kim, S. G., & Choi, S., (2012). Roles of toll-like receptors in cancer: A double-edged sword for defense and offense. *Arch Pharm Res., 35*(8), 1297–1316.

Bentivegna, E., Gouy, S., Maulard, A., Chargari, C., Leary, A., & Morice, P., (2016). Oncological outcomes after fertility-sparing surgery for cervical cancer: A systematic review. *The Lancet. Oncology, 17*(6), e240–e253.

Brown, J., Wang, H., Hajishengallis, G. N., & Martin, M., (2011). TLR-signaling networks: An integration of adaptor molecules, kinases, and crosstalk. *Journal of Dental Research, 90*(4), 417–427.

Calich, V. L., Pina, A., Felonato, M., Bernardino, S., Costa, T. A., & Loures, F. V., (2008). Toll-like receptors and fungal infections: The role of TLR2, TLR4 and MyD88 in paracoccidioidomycosis. *FEMS Immunology and Medical Microbiology, 53*(1), 1–7.

Carty, M., Goodbody, R., Schröder, M., Stack, J., Moynagh, P. N., & Bowie, A. G., (2006). The human adaptor SARM negatively regulates adaptor protein TRIF-dependent toll-like receptor signaling. *Nature Immunology, 7*(10), 1074–1081.

Chauhan, A., Pandey, N., Desai, A., et al., (2019). Association of TLR4 and TLR9 gene polymorphisms and haplotypes with cervicitis susceptibility. *PLoS One, 14*(7), e0220330.

Colonna, M., (2007). TLR pathways and IFN-regulatory factors: To each its own. *European Journal of Immunology, 37*(2), 306–309.

Dabbagh, K., & Lewis, D. B., (2003). Toll-like receptors and T-helper-1/T-helper-2 responses. *Current Opinion in Infectious Diseases, 16*(3), 199–204.

Dajon, M., Iribarren, K., & Cremer, I., (2017). Toll-like receptor stimulation in cancer: A pro– and anti-tumor double-edged sword. *Immunobiology, 222*(1), 89–100.

De Matos, L. G., Cândido, E. B., Vidigal, P. V., Bordoni, P. H., Lamaita, R. M., Carneiro, M. M., & Da Silva-Filho, A. L., (2017). Association between toll-like receptor and tumor necrosis factor immunological pathways in uterine cervical neoplasms. *Tumori, 103*(1), 81–86.

De Oliveira, L. M., Morale, M. G., Chaves, A. A., et al., (2015). Design, immune responses and anti-tumor potential of an HPV16 E6E7 multi-epitope vaccine. *PLoS One, 10*(9), e0138686.

DeCarlo, C. A., Rosa, B., Jackson, R., Niccoli, S., Escott, N. G., & Zehbe, I., (2012). Toll-like receptor transcriptome in the HPV-positive cervical cancer microenvironment. *Clinical and Developmental Immunology, 2012*, 785825.

Di Gioia, M., & Zanoni, I., (2015). Toll-like receptor co-receptors as master regulators of the immune response. *Molecular Immunology, 63*(2), 143–152.

Dickinson, S. E., & Wondrak, G. T., (2018). TLR4-directed molecular strategies targeting skin photodamage and carcinogenesis. *Current Medicinal Chemistry, 25*(40), 5487–5502.

Einstein, M. H., Baron, M., Levin, M. J., et al., (2009). Comparison of the immunogenicity and safety of cervarix and gardasil human papillomavirus (HPV) cervical cancer vaccines in healthy women aged 18–45 years. *Human Vaccines, 5*(10), 705–719.

Falck-Hansen, M., Kassiteridi, C., & Monaco, C., (2013). Toll-like receptors in atherosclerosis. *International Journal of Molecular Sciences, 14*(7), 14008–14023.

Gambara, G., De Cesaris, P., De Nunzio, C., Ziparo, E., Tubaro, A., Filippini, A., & Riccioli, A., (2013). Toll-like receptors in prostate infection and cancer between bench and bedside. *Journal of Cellular and Molecular Medicine, 17*(6), 713–722.

Guleria, C., Suri, V., Kapoor, R., Minz, R. W., & Aggarwal, R., (2019). Human papillomavirus 16 infection alters the toll-like receptors and downstream signaling cascade: A plausible early event in cervical squamous cell carcinoma development. *Gynecologic Oncology, 155*(1), 151–160.

Häcker, H., Redecke, V., Blagoev, B., et al., (2006). Specificity in toll-like receptor signaling through distinct effector functions of TRAF3 and TRAF6. *Nature, 439*(7073), 204–207.

Hasimu, A., Ge, L., Li, Q. Z., Zhang, R. P., & Guo, X., (2011). Expressions of toll-like receptors 3, 4, 7, and 9 in cervical lesions and their correlation with HPV16 infection in Uighur women. *Chinese Journal of Cancer, 30*(5), 344–350.

Hassan, F., Islam, S., Tumurkhuu, G., et al., (2006). Intracellular expression of toll-like receptor 4 in neuroblastoma cells and their unresponsiveness to lipopolysaccharide. *BMC Cancer, 6*, 281.

Hedayat, M., Netea, M. G., & Rezaei, N., (2011). Targeting of toll-like receptors: A decade of progress in combating infectious diseases. *The Lancet Infectious Diseases, 11*(9), 702–712.

Hemmi, H., Kaisho, T., Takeuchi, O., et al., (2002). Small anti-viral compounds activate immune cells via the TLR7 MyD88-dependent signaling pathway. *Nature Immunology, 3*(2), 196–200.

Hoffman, E. S., Smith, R. E., & Renaud, R. C., (2005). From the analyst's couch: TLR-targeted therapeutics. *Nature Reviews Drug Discovery, 4*(11), 879–880.

Horng, T., Barton, G. M., Flavell, R. A., & Medzhitov, R., (2002). The adaptor molecule TIRAP provides signaling specificity for toll-like receptors. *Nature, 420*(6913), 329–333.
Huang, B., Zhao, J., Li, H., et al., (2005). Toll-like receptors on tumor cells facilitate evasion of immune surveillance. *Cancer Research, 65*(12), 5009–5014.
Huang, B., Zhao, J., Unkeless, J. C., Feng, Z. H., & Xiong, H., (2008). TLR signaling by tumor and immune cells: A double-edged sword. *Oncogene, 27*(2), 218–224.
Huang, L., Xu, H., & Peng, G., (2018). TLR-mediated metabolic reprogramming in the tumor microenvironment: Potential novel strategies for cancer immunotherapy. *Cellular and Molecular Immunology, 15*(5), 428–437.
Husseinzadeh, N., & Davenport, S. M., (2014). Role of toll-like receptors in cervical, endometrial and ovarian cancers: A review. *Gynecologic Oncology, 135*(2), 359–363.
Jenkins, K. A., & Mansell, A., (2010). TIR-containing adaptors in toll-like receptor signaling. *Cytokine, 49*(3), 237–244.
Jiang, Y., Zhou, J., Luo, P., et al., (2018). Prosaposin promotes the proliferation and tumorigenesis of glioma through toll-like receptor 4 (TLR4)-mediated NF-κB signaling pathway. *eBioMedicine, 37*, 78–90.
Jin, Y., Qiu, S., Shao, N., & Zheng, J., (2017). Association of toll-like receptor gene polymorphisms and its interaction with HPV infection in determining the susceptibility of cervical cancer in Chinese Han population. *Mammalian Genome, 28*(5, 6), 213–219.
Kang, Y., Su, G., Sun, J., & Zhang, Y., (2018). Activation of the TLR4/MyD88 signaling pathway contributes to the development of human hepatocellular carcinoma via upregulation of IL-23 and IL-17A. *Oncology Letters, 15*(6), 9647–9654.
Kawai, T., & Akira, S., (2007). Signaling to NF-kappaB by toll-like receptors. *Trends in Molecular Medicine, 13*(11), 460–469.
Kawai, T., & Akira, S., (2007). TLR signaling. *Seminars in Immunology, 19*(1), 24–32.
Kohtz, P. D., Halpern, A. L., Eldeiry, M. A., et al., (2019). Toll-like receptor-4 is a mediator of proliferation in esophageal adenocarcinoma. *The Annals of Thoracic Surgery, 107*(1), 233–241.
Koliaraki, V., Chalkidi, N., Henriques, A., et al., (2019). Innate sensing through mesenchymal TLR4/MyD88 signals promotes spontaneous intestinal tumorigenesis. *Cell Reports, 26*(3), 536–545.
Kowalczyk, E., Siednienko, J., & Matuszyk, J., (2013). Regulation of the inflammatory response mediated by toll-like receptors. *Advances in Hygiene and Experimental Medicine, 67*, 201–213.
Leitner, G. R., Wenzel, T. J., Marshall, N., Gates, E. J., & Klegeris, A., (2019). Targeting toll-like receptor 4 to modulate neuroinflammation in central nervous system disorders. *Expert Opinion on Therapeutic Targets, 23*(10), 865–882.
Li, J., Rao, H., Jin, C., & Liu, J., (2017). Involvement of the toll-like receptor/nitric oxide signaling pathway in the pathogenesis of cervical cancer caused by high-risk human papillomavirus infection. *BioMed Research International, 2017*, 7830262.
Li, Q., Ayshamgul, H., Jiang, Y., Liu, Y., & Li, G., (2013). Expression of toll-like receptor 4 in cervical cell lines and cervical epithelial lesions and its relationship with HPV16 infection. *Journal of Central South University (Medical Edition), 38*(11), 1110–1116.
Li, T. T., Ogino, S., & Qian, Z. R., (2014). Toll-like receptor signaling in colorectal cancer: Carcinogenesis to cancer therapy. *World Journal of Gastroenterology, 20*(47), 17699–17708.

Lim, K. H., & Staudt, L. M., (2013). Toll-like receptor signaling. *Cold Spring Harbor Perspectives in Biology, 5*(1), a011247.

Liu, C., Han, C., & Liu, J., (2019). The role of toll-like receptors in oncotherapy. *Oncology Research, 27*(8), 965–978.

Luchner, M., Reinke, S., & Milicic, A., (2021). TLR agonists as vaccine adjuvants targeting cancer and infectious diseases. *Pharmaceutics, 13*(2), 142.

Luo, J. L., Maeda, S., Hsu, L. C., Yagita, H., & Karin, M., (2004). Inhibition of NF-kappaB in cancer cells converts inflammation-induced tumor growth mediated by TNFalpha to TRAIL-mediated tumor regression. *Cancer Cell, 6*(3), 297–305.

Luo, L., Lucas, R. M., Liu, L., & Stow, J. L., (2019). Signaling, sorting and scaffolding adaptors for toll-like receptors. *Journal of Cell Science, 133*(5), jcs239194.

Mansilla, C., Berraondo, P., Durantez, M., et al., (2012). Eradication of large tumors expressing human papillomavirus E7 protein by therapeutic vaccination with E7 fused to the extra domain A from fibronectin. *International Journal of Cancer, 131*(3), 641–651.

Mata-Haro, V., Cekic, C., Martin, M., Chilton, P. M., Casella, C. R., & Mitchell, T. C., (2007). The vaccine adjuvant monophosphoryl lipid A as a TRIF-biased agonist of TLR4. *Science, 316*(5831), 1628–1632.

McCall, K. D., Muccioli, M., & Benencia, F., (2020). Toll-like receptors signaling in the tumor microenvironment. *Advances in Experimental Medicine and Biology, 1223*, 81–97.

Medzhitov, R., (2001). Toll-like receptors and innate immunity. *Nature Reviews Immunology, 1*(2), 135–145.

Moura, E. L., Santos, I. F. D., Freitas, P. P., et al., (2022). Polymorphisms in toll-like receptors genes changes the host's immune response and is associated with cervical cancer. *Immunobiology, 227*(2), 152187. doi: 10.1016/j.imbio.2022.152187.

Mukherjee, S., Huda, S., & Sinha, B. S. P., (2019). Toll-like receptor polymorphism in host immune response to infectious diseases: A review. *Scandinavian Journal of Immunology, 90*(1), e12771.

Narayanankutty, A., Sasidharan, A., & Job, J. T., (2020). Targeting toll like receptors in cancer: Role of TLR natural and synthetic modulators. *Current Pharmaceutical Design, 26*(39), 5040–5053.

Neidhart, J., Allen, K. O., Barlow, D. L., Carpenter, M., Shaw, D. R., Triozzi, P. L., & Conry, R. M., (2004). Immunization of colorectal cancer patients with recombinant baculovirus-derived KSA (Ep-CAM) formulated with monophosphoryl lipid A in liposomal emulsion, with and without granulocyte-macrophage colony-stimulating factor. *Vaccine, 22*(5, 6), 773–780.

O'Neill, L. A., & Bowie, A. G., (2007). The family of five: TIR-domain-containing adaptors in toll-like receptor signaling. *Nature Reviews Immunology, 7*(5), 353–364.

O'Neill, L. A., Dunne, A., Edjeback, M., Gray, P., Jefferies, C., & Wietek, C., (2003). Mal and MyD88: Adapter proteins involved in signal transduction by toll-like receptors. *Journal of Endotoxin Research, 9*(1), 55–59.

Oganesyan, G., Saha, S. K., Guo, B., He, J. Q., Shahangian, A., Zarnegar, B., Perry, A., & Cheng, G., (2006). Critical role of TRAF3 in the toll-like receptor-dependent and –independent antiviral response. *Nature, 439*(7073), 208–211.

Oosenbrug, T., Van De, G. M. J., Ressing, M. E., & Van, K. S. I., (2017). Chemical tools for studying TLR signaling dynamics. *Cell Chemical Biology, 24*(7), 801–812.

Ou, T., Lilly, M., & Jiang, W., (2018). The pathologic role of toll-like receptor 4 in prostate cancer. *Frontiers in Immunology, 9*, 1188.

Paavonen, J., Naud, P., Salmerón, J., et al., (2009). Efficacy of human papillomavirus (HPV)-16/18 AS04-adjuvanted vaccine against cervical infection and precancer caused by oncogenic HPV types (PATRICIA): Final analysis of a double-blind, randomized study in young women. *Lancet, 374*(9686), 301–314.

Pan, S., Jiang, W., Xie, S., Zhu, H., & Zhu, X., (2021). Clinicopathological features and survival of adolescent and young adults with cervical cancer. *Cancer Control, 28*, 10732748211051558.

Rosenberg, S. A., Yang, J. C., & Restifo, N. P., (2004). Cancer immunotherapy: Moving beyond current vaccines. *Nature Medicine, 10*(9), 909–915.

Satoh, T., & Akira, S., (2016). Toll-like receptor signaling and its inducible proteins. *Microbiology Spectrum, 4*(6), 10.1128/microbiolspec.MCHD-0040-2016.

Schädlich, L., Senger, T., Kirschning, C. J., Müller, M., & Gissmann, L., (2009). Refining HPV 16 L1 purification from *E. coli*: Reducing endotoxin contaminations and their impact on immunogenicity. *Vaccine, 27*(10), 1511–1522.

Sheedy, F. J., & O'Neill, L. A., (2007). The troll in toll: Mal and tram as bridges for TLR2 and TLR4 signaling. *Journal of Leukocyte Biology, 82*(2), 196–203.

Shi, M., Chen, X., Ye, K., Yao, Y., & Li, Y., (2016). Application potential of toll-like receptors in cancer immunotherapy: Systematic review. *Medicine, 95*(25), e3951.

Szczepanski, M. J., Czystowska, M., Szajnik, M., et al., (2009). Triggering of toll-like receptor 4 expressed on human head and neck squamous cell carcinoma promotes tumor development and protects the tumor from immune attack. *Cancer Research, 69*(7), 3105–3113.

Takeda, K., & Akira, S., (2005). Toll-like receptors in innate immunity. *International Immunology, 17*(1), 1–14.

Tang, X., & Zhu, Y., (2012). TLR4 signaling promotes immune escape of human colon cancer cells by inducing immunosuppressive cytokines and apoptosis resistance. *Oncology Research, 20*(1), 15–24.

Vijay, K., (2018). Toll-like receptors in immunity and inflammatory diseases: Past, present, and future. *International Immunopharmacology, 59*, 391–412.

Vlad, C., Dina, C., Kubelac, P., Vlad, D., Pop, B., & Achimas, C. P., (2018). Expression of toll-like receptors in ovarian cancer. *Journal of B.U.ON, 23*(6), 1725–1731.

Wang, J. H., Manning, B. J., Wu, Q. D., Blankson, S., Bouchier-Hayes, D., & Redmond, H. P., (2003). Endotoxin/lipopolysaccharide activates NF-kappa B and enhances tumor cell adhesion and invasion through a beta 1 integrin-dependent mechanism. *Journal of Immunology, 170*(2), 795–804.

Wang, Y., Weng, Y., Shi, Y., Xia, X., Wang, S., & Duan, H., (2014). Expression and functional analysis of toll-like receptor 4 in human cervical carcinoma. *The Journal of Membrane Biology, 247*(7), 591–599.

Watters, T. M., Kenny, E. F., & O'Neill, L. A., (2007). Structure, function, and regulation of the toll/IL-1 receptor adaptor proteins. *Immunology and Cell Biology, 85*(6), 411–419.

Werner, J., Decarlo, C. A., Escott, N., Zehbe, I., & Ulanova, M., (2012). Expression of integrins and toll-like receptors in cervical cancer: Effect of infectious agents. *Innate Immunity, 18*(1), 55–69.

Yang, X., Cheng, Y., & Li, C., (2017). The role of TLRs in cervical cancer with HPV infection: A review. *Sig. Transduct. Target Ther., 2*, 17055. https://doi.org/10.1038/sigtrans.2017.55.

Zhang, C., Ben, A., Reville, J., Calabrese, V., Villa, N. N., Bandyopadhyay, M., & Dasgupta, S., (2015). Immunotherapeutic impact of toll-like receptor agonists in breast cancer. *Anti-Cancer Agents in Medicinal Chemistry, 15*(9), 1134–1140.

CHAPTER 4

PI3K-Akt-mTOR Signaling Pathways

4.1 PHOSPHATIDYLINOSITOL-3-KINASE (PI3K)/Akt/ MAMMALIAN TARGET OF RAPAMYCIN (mTOR) SIGNALING

PI3K is a set of lipid kinases associated with the plasma membrane, which consists of three subunits with regulatory and catalytic functions (Whitman et al., 1985; Foukas & Okkenhaug, 2003). The main three subunits are p85 (regulatory), p55 (regulatory), and p110 (catalytic). During normal conditions, the catalytic p110 subunit is sequestered by p85 regulatory subunit dimerization (Geering et al., 2007; Vanhaesebroeck et al., 2010). PI3K/Akt/mTOR signaling pathway gets activated by interaction of external signals such as growth factors, cytokines, and hormones with the receptor. After activation, PI3K catalyzes the phosphorylation of PIP2 (phosphatidylinositol-4,5-bis-phosphate) to PIP3 (phosphatidylinositol-3,4,5-triphosphate). Subsequent accumulation of PIP3 resulted in activation of a signaling protein Akt (a serine–threonine kinase) (Krasilnikov, 2000; Ersahin et al., 2015). A tumor suppressor PTEN (Phosphatase and tensin homolog) regulates this pathway by dephosphorylation of PIP3 and subsequent Akt deactivation which prevents activation of downstream target proteins. In contrast to PTEN's inhibitory effect, PIP3 causes Akt phosphorylation, which activates mTOR further (Fresno Vara et al., 2004; Dibble & Cantley, 2015). Following mTOR activation, two downstream effector molecules, S6k-1 (ribosomal protein S6 kinase-1) and 4E-BP1, were phosphorylated and activated (eukaryotic translation initiation factor 4E binding protein 1). Activated S6k-1 and 4E-BP1 lead to increased target protein translation that are responsible for cell growth, proliferation, apoptosis, and survival (Chappell et al., 2011; Guenthe et al., 2013; Asati

Cervical Cancer: Signaling Pathways, Molecular Mechanisms, Natural Products, and Therapeutic Approaches. Pratibha Pandey, Fahad Khan, Saher Islam, and Devarajan Thangadurai, (Eds.)

et al., 2016). Altogether, the PI3K/Akt/mTOR signaling pathway crosstalk with diverse complex signaling pathways which correlates the cellular response to numerous stimuli, thereby influencing critical processes involved in cancer progression.

4.2 THE PI3K/Akt/mTOR PATHWAY AND CANCER

Phosphatidylinositol-3-kinase (PI3K)/Akt/mammalian target of rapamycin (mTOR) signaling cascade is an important intracellular signaling pathway which controls cell proliferation, survival, metabolic pathway and process of angiogenesis (Kaplan et al., 1987; Katso et al., 2001; Engelman et al., 2006). Abnormal activation/hyperactivation of this pathway can lead to the cancer progression and resistance towards antitumor therapies (Martini et al., 2014). The two most studied non-coding RNAs which are mainly responsible for the regulation of gene expression are miRNA (microRNA) and long non-coding RNA (lncRNA). Crosstalk of these two ncRNA and PI3K/Akt/mTOR pathway form a basis in the process of carcinogenesis (Benetatos et al., 2017; Klingenberg et al., 2017). The PI3K/Akt/mTOR signaling has been found to be deregulated approximately in all type of human carcinoma, such as colorectal cancer, prostate cancer, breast cancer, and other malignancies (Figure 4.1). This notion highlights the significance of targeting this signaling pathway as a possible therapeutic option in the treatment of various types of cancer (Hennessy et al., 2005; Pópulo et al., 2012; Alzahrani, 2019). Suppression of PI3K and their intermediate signaling molecules can lead to both decreased cell growth and augmented apoptosis (Yuan & Cantley, 2008). Firstly, immunohistochemical studies detected the antibody mediated abnormal activation of Akt in different types of cancers, such as lung cancer, multiple myeloma (MM), breast cancer, head and neck cancer, brain cancer, gastric cancer, endometrial cancer, renal cell carcinoma, prostate cancer, ovarian cancer, and colon cancer (Alkan & Izban, 2002; Choe et al., 2003; Dai et al., 2005; Chen et al., 2014; Kim et al., 2017; Deng et al., 2019; Ippen et al., 2019; Lian et al., 2019; Narayanankutty et al., 2019; Braglia et al., 2020; Liu et al., 2020; Miricescu et al., 2020, 2021; Wang et al., 2020; Ye et al., 2020; Liu et al., 2021; Moura et al., 2021). Immunohistochemical investigation has also been employed to reveal the prognostic implication of

Akt activation. Several studies demonstrating the Akt phosphorylation at S473 amino acid residue has been correlated with poor prognosis in numerous carcinoma, including pancreas, skin, breast, liver, prostate, endometrium, stomach, blood, and brain (Ermoian et al., 2002; Perez-Tenorio & Stal, 2002; Kreisberg et al., 2004; Min et al., 2004; Dai et al., 2005; Nakanishi et al., 2005; Murakami et al., 2007; Zaczek et al., 2020; Kisling et al., 2021; Mehra et al., 2021). Tsurutani et al. extended this research by targeting two amino acid residues of Akt phosphorylation (S473 and T308) using antibodies in non-small cell lung cancer (NSCLC) and also illustrate that targeting both these sites could be a strong predictor of poor prognosis in NSCLC (Tsurutani et al., 2006). Furthermore, low frequency of Akt isoforms amplification has also been observed in some tumors (Bellacosa et al., 1995; Cheng et al., 1996; Ruggeri et al., 1998). Another frequently observed genetic modification in PI3K/Akt/mTOR signaling pathway associated with human cancer progression is down-regulation of tumor suppressor PTEN gene which inhibits signaling pathway activation. Numerous research findings have revealed an association of loss of function of PTEN with several types of human cancers, including bladder, brain, endometrial, breast, and prostate cancers (Cairns et al., 1998; Lin et al., 1998; Escudero et al., 2011; Rodríguez-Lin, 2014; Osei-Amponsa et al., 2020; He et al., 2021). Loss of function of PTEN is mainly associated with genetic mutations/deletions; however, in some tumor types, epigenetic silencing may occur, such as lung cancer (Forgacs et al., 1998; Kim et al., 1998; Kohno et al., 1998). Altogether, these experimental data have established the fact that suppression of PTEN is an important mechanism linked with the instigation of the PI3K/Akt/mTOR pathway as well as poor prognostic factor in human tumors. There are several PI3K inhibitors that have been used to target PI3K/Akt/mTOR signaling pathway such as PI3K/mTOR inhibitors, isoform-selective PI3K inhibitors, and pan-PI3K inhibitors. The safety and effectiveness of these targeting therapeutic methods have been explored in various research experimental findings, including preclinical and clinical studies, which clearly indicate the efficacy of PI3K inhibitors against several tumors. One of the PI3K inhibitor, idelalisib is the first FDA (United States Food and Drug Administration) approved drug that proved the efficacy in cancer treatment.

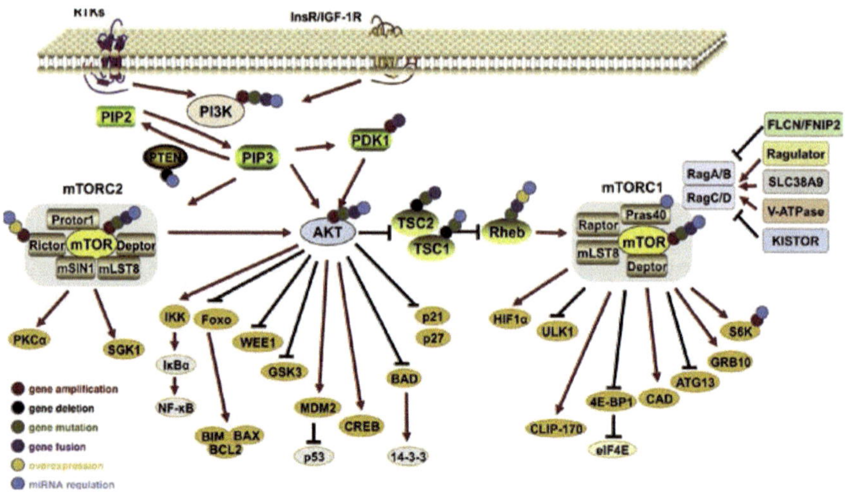

FIGURE 4.1 Summary of changes of the PI3K/Akt/mTOR signaling pathway at DNA and RNA levels. Upon stimulation by growth factors or cytokines, activated RTKs (receptor tyrosine kinases) recruit PI3K to plasma membrane where PI3K catalyzes PI(4,5)P2 to generate PI(3,4,5)P3. PI(3,4,5)P3 activates Akt through PDK1 and mTORC2 and activation of Akt potentiates cell cycle progression, cell proliferation, apoptosis, glucose metabolism, cell survival, actin organization, transcription, cell motility and motion through phosphorylating downstream substrates including TSC2 to alleviate TSC2 suppression on Rheb, leading to mTORC1 activation on lysosome. mTORC1 activation is also controlled by amino acids through distinct amino acid sensors, regulator, V-ATPase, and more importantly, Rags that recruit mTORC1 to lysosome. Activated mTORC1 promotes protein translation, potentiates nucleotide synthesis, suppresses autophagy and proteasomal degradation. Regulatory mechanisms for key signaling components are labeled with indicated colored dots.

Abbreviations: RTKs: receptor tyrosine kinase; PI3K: phosphatidylinositol 3-kinase; PIP2: phosphatidylinositol 4,5-bisphosphate; PIP3: phosphatidylinositol 3,4,5-triphosphate; PTEN: phosphatase and tensin homolog; PDK1: 3-phosphoinositide-dependent kinase 1; mTOR: mechanistic target of rapamycin; TSC1: tuberous sclerosis 1; TSC2: tuberous sclerosis 2; 4E-BP: eIF4E-binding protein; GRB10: growth factor receptor-bound protein 10; IGF-1R: insulin-like growth factor 1 receptor; mLST8: mammalian lethal with SEC 13 8; RICTOR: rapamycin-insensitive companion of mTOR; S6K: ribosomal S6 kinase; FLCN: folliculin; ULK1: UNC-51-like kinase 1; RAPTOR: regulatory-associated protein of mTOR; RICTOR: rapamycin-insensitive companion of mTOR.

Source: Reproduced with permission from Le et al. (2021); Copyright © Elsevier (2021).

4.3 THE PI3K/Akt/mTOR PATHWAY AND CERVICAL CANCER

The phosphatidylinositol 3-kinase/protein kinase B/mammalian target of rapamycin (PI3K/Akt/mTOR) pathway is frequently disrupted in cervical cancer, indicating that it may be a potential therapeutic target in the therapy and management of this disease. This route has the potential to be exploited as a novel and powerful biomarker in the assessment of cervical cancer risk. The PI3K/Akt/mTOR pathway involves in the regulation of several cellular and molecular activities, which plays an important role in tumor progression and metastasis. Several research have revealed that stimulation of PI3K/Akt/mTOR signaling is crucially involved in a variety of human cancers such as ovary, breast, gliomas, and endometrium cancers. Furthermore, in cervical cancer, activation of the PI3K/Akt/mTOR pathway is linked to an inadequate response (Schwarz et al., 2012). The critical significance of the PI3K/Akt/mTOR signaling pathway in cervical cancer progression has been demonstrated through genomic expression analyses. The PIK3CA gene has been shown to have genomic expression and stimulating mutations in 23–36% of cervical cancer samples (McIntire et al., 2013). The highest mutation rate was found in cervical cancer specimens especially, in the PIK3CA gene, according to high-throughput genotyping research analysis of 80 samples of cervical tumor targeted for 139 cancer genes and 1,250 mutations (31.3%) (Wright et al., 2013). In another study, investigation of 675 cervical tumor samples revealed enhanced expression of PIK3CA and other PI3K/Akt signaling pathway genes in squamous cell carcinoma (31%) and adenocarcinoma (24%) (Lou et al., 2015). McIntire et al. (2013) have presented a better prognosis in patients having mutation in PIK3CA in early stage of cervical cancer. Other research findings have also indicated higher expression and constitutive activation of the mTOR pathway in cervical cancer (Feng et al., 2016). Liao et al. (2014) reported over expressed Akt, PI3K, and MDM2 and down expression of p53 in cervical cancer. Active HPV infection has been linked to the development of both malignant and benign neoplasms in the cervix by interfering with multiple host cell biological pathways (Shiraz et al., 2020). HPVs interact with four upstream pathways, namely Notch receptor, Ras, growth factor receptor, and PI3KCA genes, for inducing host cell survival and proliferation, which leads to carcinogenesis via alteration and activation of PI3K pathway downstream compounds, in addition to p53 and pRb suppression (Keysar et al., 2013). Altogether, aberrantly activated pathway offers the basis behind the association of PI3K/mTOR/Akt inhibitors and pathway in cervical cancer for being utilized as diagnostic and prognostic uses.

4.4 PI3K/Akt/mTOR PATHWAY AS PROGNOSTIC BIOMARKER IN CERVICAL CANCER

PI3K was found to be overexpressed in cervical cancer cells in numerous *in vitro* experiments, and treatment with PI3K inhibitors decreased cell growth and proliferation (Figure 4.2). Others have calculated the predictive value of PI3K over-regulation in cervical cancer patients receiving chemotherapy (cisplatin) (Faried et al., 2006, 2008). p-mTOR expression level has been a potent prognostic biomarker (independent) in the cervix. Research findings from cervical cancer cells have demonstrated PI3K pathway activation leading to unrestrained positive feedback triggered by PTEN ubiquitination (Lee et al., 2015). Using cell line generated xenografts, researchers investigated downstream mTOR inhibition and discovered robust *in vivo* efficacy. HPV controls the Akt/mTOR signaling pathway through regulating E2F (Banister et al., 2017). Another study found that oncogenic HPV E6 activates the mTOR pathway in cervical cancer cell lines, which is consistent with these findings (Callejas-Valera et al., 2016). The PI3K/Akt/mTOR pathway is connected to the overexpression of the tumor suppressor p16INK4a by HPVs. Elevated expression of p16INK4a is common in CC, where HPVs have a high risk of inactivating the pRb protein (Paolini et al., 2011). S6K phosphorylation has been associated with HPV16 infection in cervical cancer (Zhou et al., 2007). According to immunohistochemical analysis of 140 CC specimens, both p-S6K and p-S6 were significantly more frequent in HPV16 (+) CC samples than in HPV16 (–) samples. The oncoprotein HPV16 E6 activates S6K via Akt signaling, increasing S6K phosphorylation and keeping the mTORC1 and mTORC2 signaling pathways active. HPV E7 has been related to an increase in Akt activity, which is dependent on E7's ability to inactivate the pRb protein family. AKT activity was elevated and pRb was diminished when HPV (+) cervical advanced squamous intraepithelial lesions were compared to normal cervical tissue. Thus, pRb expression is negatively related with Akt activation in HPV (+) cervical advanced squamous intraepithelial lesions (Menges et al., 2006). E7 promotes Akt by phosphorylating it, which causes BAD to phosphorylate (a downstream target of Akt). Akt phosphorylation is linked to the activation of the Notch1 signaling system, which regulates the PI3K pathway (Wu et al., 2013). The serine/threonine phosphatase Protein Phosphatase 2 (PP2A) has been discovered to dephosphorylate Akt by establishing a complex with the structural components of p-Akt. The activity of Akt in preventing cell apoptosis is reduced when it is dephosphorylated (Li et al., 2003). E7 binds to the PP2A subunits and prevents them from interacting with p-Akt, keeping the Akt signal active. Inhibition of the PI3K pathway may have a crucial role in the clinic, according to this preclinical research (Pim et al., 2005). Inhibitors of PI3K/Akt/mTOR as a therapeutic target for cervical cancer are frequently treated with a combination of platinum-based chemotherapy and radiation; nevertheless, some tumors acquire chemotherapeutic resistance, resulting in treatment failure. A variety of natural medicines derived from plants have been shown to inhibit cell proliferation, induce apoptosis, restore metastasis, and reduce angiogenesis in CC by regulating the PI3K/Akt/mTOR signaling pathway. It has been hypothesized that these substances could be used to cure cancer. The effects of natural substances in CC cell lines have been studied *in vitro* in several research. In 52% of CC patients, tissue microarray analysis demonstrated that p-mTOR is expressed in the cytoplasm and on the membrane of tumor cells (Faried et al., 2006). According to Lee and colleagues, pre-treatment of CC cell lines with the PI3K/Akt inhibitor LY294002 increased radiation sensitivity *in vitro* (Lee et al., 2006). Furthermore, in Caski and HeLa cells, LY294002 significantly reduced the viability loss caused by cisplatin, showing a role for the PI3K/Akt pathway in Cisplatin-resistant CC cells (Shu et al., 2015). Rapamycin and other rapalogs inhibit mTOR1, preventing S6 kinase1, 4E-BP1, and other proteins from being phosphorylated, resulting in cell cycle arrest and reduced angiogenesis (Diaz-Padilla et al., 2012). In a recent study, AKT1 activity was reduced in CC cell lines treated with LY294002. According to the researchers, LY294002 treatment triggered G1 cycle arrest in cervix cancer-derived cells (Prasad et al., 2015).

Many targeted therapeutic techniques have been proposed as a result of the distinctions between HPV-inactive and HPV-active cancers. Gefitinib, an EGF-receptor inhibitor, is more effective in treating HPV-active cervical malignancies than dasatinib in treating HPV-inactive tumors, for example (Zheng et al., 2019). Somatic gene alterations upstream of AKT are more common in HPV-inactive malignancies, suggesting that dual PI3K/mTOR inhibitors may be more effective in these individuals (Guo et al., 2015). Genetic differences in the PI3K/Akt pathway have been associated with sensitivity to platinum-based neoadjuvant chemotherapy in individuals with cervical squamous cervical carcinoma (CSCC). HeLa cells have also been shown to be significantly reduced in viability when

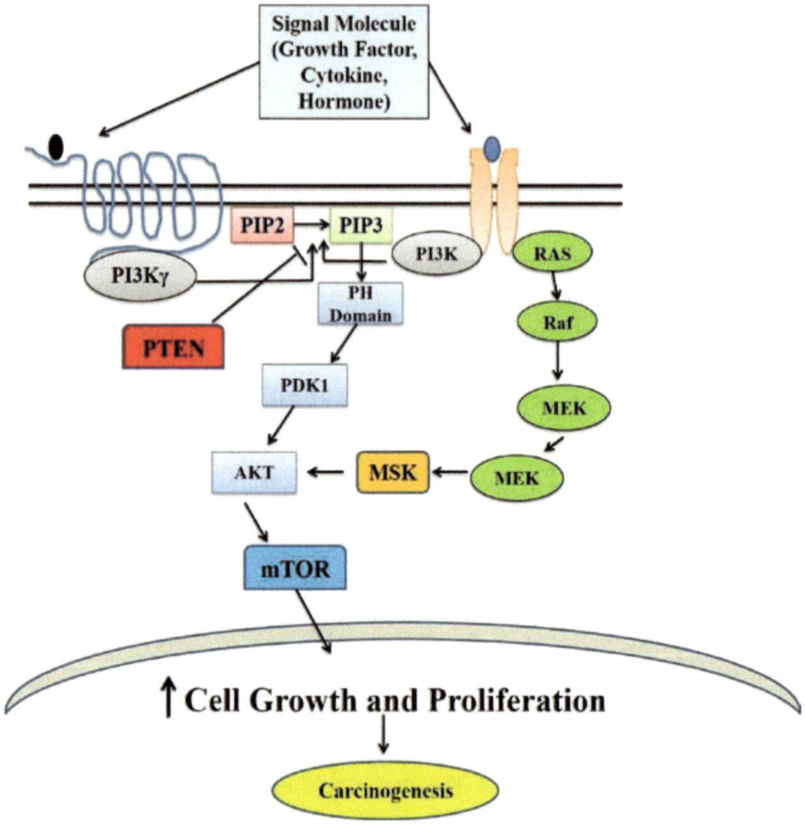

FIGURE 4.2 PI3K/Akt/mTOR pathway and cancer.

treated with a combination of PI3K inhibitors and NaBT. Inhibiting PI3K promotes NaBT-mediated apoptosis in human CC cells by activating caspase-3 and -9 and cleaving poly(ADP-ribose) polymerase (Park et al., 2006). In multiple studies, mTOR activation has been seen in at least 60% of HPV-related cancer patients, showing that mTOR activation plays a key role in HPV-induced carcinogenesis. The preclinical efficacy of mTOR inhibitors such as RAD001 and rapamycin when paired with standard-of-care cisplatin/radiation therapy has been investigated in HPV (+) cervical cancer squamous cell carcinomas (CCSCC) tumor xenografts and mouse models (Coppock et al., 2013). Both inhibitors reduce mTOR activity in immune-compromised animals, lowering tumor burden and enhancing survival (Molinolo et al., 2012). A substantial incidence of PIK3CA mutations has been found in CC, adding to the suggestion that mTOR inhibitors may play a role in this disease (Lamsisi et al., 2021). Table 4.1 summarizes all the potential inhibitors against PI3K/Akt/mTOR oncogenic signaling pathway components evaluated in clinical trials for the efficient management of several human cancers. These research findings support the use of PI3K/Akt/mTOR inhibitors as a molecular targeted therapy for HPV-related cancers in medicinal aspects.

TABLE 4.1 Inhibitors Targeting the PI3K/Akt/mTOR Oncogenic Signaling Pathway Components Evaluated in Clinical Trials to Treat Human Cancer

Inhibitors/Natural Products	Target	Disease	Phase	References
Idelalisib/CAL-101	p110δ	B-cell malignancies	Approved	Tripathy et al. (2020)
AMG319	p110δ	HNSCC	II	Cushing et al. (2015)
Duvelisib (Copiktra)	p110δ	CLL or SLL	III	Patel et al. (2019)
Copanlisib (BAY 80-6946)	pan-class I PI3K	Follicular lymphoma	Approved	Kumar et al. (2020)
Alpelisib (BYL719)	p110δ	Diverse cancers	Approved	Markham (2019)
LY294002	pan-PI3K class I	Pancreatic cancer	–	Fujiwara et al. (2008)
Buparlisib (BKM120)	pan-class I PI3K	Breast cancer	II, III	Martin et al. (2017)
Pictilisib	pan-class I PI3K	Breast cancer	II	Krop et al. (2016)
Pilaralisib	pan-class I PI3K	Breast, endometrial cancers	II	Matulonis et al. (2015); Tolaney et al. (2015)
AZD6482	p110β	Glioblastoma	I	Xu et al. (2019)
GSK2636771	p110β	Diverse cancers	II	Mateo et al. (2017)
AZD8186	p110β	Solid tumors	I	Barlaam et al. (2015)
IPI-549	p110γ	Melanoma, pancreatic cancer	I	Zhang et al. (2019)
GDC-0032 (Taselisib)	p1100α, p110δ, and p110γ	Lung, breast cancer	I, II	Dickler et al. (2018); Baird et al. (2019); Langer et al. (2019)
GDC-0077	p110α	PIK3CA-mutant HR+/HER2-locally advanced or metastatic breast cancer	III	ClinicalTrial.gov
Ipatasertib (GDC-0068)	pan-Akt	Breast, prostate cancer	II, III	de Bono et al. (2019); Ippen et al. (2019)
AZD5363	pan-Akt	Gastric, prostate cancer	I, II	Li et al. (2013); Kolinsky et al. (2020)

TABLE 4.1 *(Continued)*

Inhibitors/Natural Products	Target	Disease	Phase	References
Afuresertib (GSK2110183)	Akt1 and Akt2	Ovarian cancer	I	Blagden et al. (2019)
MK2206	pan-Akt	NSCLC	II	Lopez-Chavez et al. (2015)
Temsirolimus (CCI-779)	mTORC1	Renal cell carcinoma	Approved	Hudes et al. (2007)
Everolimus (RAD001)	mTORC1	Renal cancer, HR+ breast cancer	Approved	Hasskarl (2018)
Sirolimus	mTORC1	Solid tumors	II	Yanik et al. (2015)
Ridaforolimus	mTORC1	Soft-tissue sarcoma	III	Demetri et al. (2017)
CC-223	mTORC1/C2	Lymphoma	II	Wolin et al. (2019)
Vistusertib (AZD2014)	mTORC1/C2	NSCLC, ovarian cancer	II	Basu et al. (2018)
AZD8055	mTORC1/2	Advanced solid tumors and lymphoma	I	Naing et al. (2012)
Dactolisib (BEZ235)	dual PI3K/mTOR	Advanced solid tumors	I, II	Wise-Draper et al. (2017)
Voxtalisib (SAR245409, XL765)	Class-I PI3Ks, mTORC1, and mTORC2	Solid tumors	I	Janne et al. (2014)
Apitolisib (GDC0980)	pan-PI3K and mTORC1/mTORC2	Advanced solid tumors	I	Dolly et al. (2016)
PQR309	pan-PI3K and mTORC1/mTORC2	Solid tumors	I	Wicki et al. (2018)

Source: Slightly modified with permission from Le et al. (2021); Copyright © Elsevier (2021).

KEYWORDS

- **cervical cancer squamous cell carcinomas**
- **human cancers**
- **lipid kinases**
- **mammalian target of rapamycin**
- **phosphatidylinositol-3-kinase**
- **plasma membrane**

REFERENCES

Alkan, S., & Izban, K. F., (2002). Immunohistochemical localization of phosphorylated AKT in multiple myeloma. *Blood, 99*(6), 2278–2279.

Alzahrani, A. S., (2019). PI3K/Akt/mTOR inhibitors in cancer: At the bench and bedside. *Seminars in Cancer Biology, 59*, 125–132.

Asati, V., Mahapatra, D. K., & Bharti, S. K., (2016). PI3K/Akt/mTOR and Ras/Raf/MEK/ERK signaling pathways inhibitors as anticancer agents: Structural and pharmacological perspectives. *European Journal of Medicinal Chemistry, 109*, 314–341.

Baird, R. D., Van, R. A. G. J., Oliveira, M., et al., (2019). POSEIDON trial phase 1b results: Safety, efficacy and circulating tumor DNA response of the beta isoform-sparing PI3K inhibitor taselisib (GDC-0032) combined with tamoxifen in hormone receptor positive metastatic breast cancer patients. *Clin. Cancer Res., 25*(22), 6598–6605.

Banister, C. E., Liu, C., Pirisi, L., Creek, K. E., & Buckhaults, P. J., (2017). Identification and characterization of HPV-independent cervical cancers. *Oncotarget, 8*(8), 13375–13386.

Barlaam, B., Cosulich, S., Degorce, S., et al., (2015). Discovery of (R)-8-(1-(3,5-difluorophenylamino)ethyl)-N,N-dimethyl-2-morpholino-4-oxo-4H-chrom ene-6-carboxamide (AZD8186): A potent and selective inhibitor of PI3Kbeta and PI3Kdelta for the treatment of PTEN-deficient cancers. *J. Med. Chem., 58*(2), 943–962.

Basu, B., Krebs, M. G., Sundar, R., et al., (2018). Vistusertib (dual m-TORC1/2 inhibitor) in combination with paclitaxel in patients with high-grade serous ovarian and squamous non-small-cell lung cancer. *Ann. Oncol., 29*(9), 1918–1925.

Bellacosa, A., De Feo, D., Godwin, A. K., et al., (1995). Molecular alterations of the AKT2 oncogene in ovarian and breast carcinomas. *International Journal of Cancer, 64*(4), 280–285.

Benetatos, L., Voulgaris, E., & Vartholomatos, G., (2017). The crosstalk between long non-coding RNAs and PI3K in cancer. *Medical Oncology, 34*(3), 39.

Blagden, S. P., Hamilton, A. L., Mileshkin, L., et al., (2019). Phase IB dose escalation and expansion study of AKT inhibitor afuresertib with carboplatin and paclitaxel in recurrent platinum-resistant ovarian cancer. *Clin. Cancer Res., 25*(5), 472–1478.

Braglia, L., Zavatti, M., Vinceti, M., Martelli, A. M., & Marmiroli, S., (2020). Deregulated PTEN/PI3K/AKT/mTOR signaling in prostate cancer: Still a potential druggable target? *Biochimica et Biophysica Acta Molecular Cell Research, 1867*(9), 118731.

Cairns, P., Evron, E., Okami, K., et al., (1998). Point mutation and homozygous deletion of PTEN/MMAC1 in primary bladder cancers. *Oncogene, 16*(24), 3215–3218.

Callejas-Valera, J. L., Iglesias-Bartolome, R., Amornphimoltham, P., et al., (2016). mTOR inhibition prevents rapid-onset of carcinogen-induced malignancies in a novel inducible HPV-16 E6/E7 mouse model. *Carcinogenesis, 37*(10), 1014–1025.

Chappell, W. H., Steelman, L. S., Long, J. M., et al., (2011). Ras/Raf/MEK/ERK and PI3K/PTEN/Akt/mTOR inhibitors: Rationale and importance to inhibiting these pathways in human health. *Oncotarget, 2*(3), 135–164.

Chen, J., Zhao, K. N., Li, R., Shao, R., & Chen, C., (2014). Activation of PI3K/Akt/mTOR pathway and dual inhibitors of PI3K and mTOR in endometrial cancer. *Current Medicinal Chemistry, 21*(26), 3070–3080.

Cheng, J. Q., Ruggeri, B., Klein, W. M., Sonoda, G., Altomare, D. A., Watson, D. K., & Testa, J. R., (1996). Amplification of AKT2 in human pancreatic cells and inhibition of AKT2 expression and tumorigenicity by antisense RNA. *Proceedings of the National Academy of Sciences of the United States of America, 93*(8), 3636–3641.

Choe, G., Horvath, S., Cloughesy, T. F., et al., (2003). Analysis of the phosphatidylinositol 3'-kinase signaling pathway in glioblastoma patients *in vivo*. *Cancer Research, 63*(11), 2742–2746.

Coppock, J. D., Wieking, B. G., Molinolo, A. A., Gutkind, J. S., Miskimins, W. K., & Lee, J. H., (2013). Improved clearance during treatment of HPV-positive head and neck cancer through mTOR inhibition. *Neoplasia, 15*(6), 620–630.

Cushing, T. D., Hao, X., Shin, Y., et al., (2015). Discovery and *in vivo* evaluation of (S)-N-(1-(7-fluoro-2-(pyridin-2-yl)quinolin-3-yl)ethyl)-9H-purin-6-amine (AMG319) and related PI3Kdelta inhibitors for inflammation and autoimmune disease. *J. Med. Chem., 58*(1), 480–511.

Dai, D. L., Martinka, M., & Li, G., (2005). Prognostic significance of activated Akt expression in melanoma: A clinicopathologic study of 292 cases. *Journal of Clinical Oncology, 23*(7), 1473–1482.

De Bono, J. S., De Giorgi, U., Rodrigues, D. N., et al., (2019). Randomized phase II study evaluating Akt blockade with ipatasertib, in combination with abiraterone, in patients with metastatic prostate cancer with and without PTEN loss. *Clin. Cancer Res., 25*(3), 928–936.

Demetri, G. D., Chawla, S. P., Ray-Coquard, I., et al., (2017). A phase Ib study of the dual PI3K/ mTOR inhibitor dactolisib (BEZ235) combined with everolimus in patients with advanced solid malignancies. *Target. Oncol., 12*(3), 323–332.

Deng, J., Bai, X., Feng, X., Ni, J., Beretov, J., Graham, P., & Li, Y., (2019). Inhibition of PI3K/Akt/mTOR signaling pathway alleviates ovarian cancer chemoresistance through reversing epithelial-mesenchymal transition and decreasing cancer stem cell marker expression. *BMC Cancer, 19*(1), 618.

Diaz-Padilla, I., Duran, I., Clarke, B. A., & Oza, A. M., (2012). Biologic rationale and clinical activity of mTOR inhibitors in gynecological cancer. *Cancer Treatment Reviews, 38*(6), 767–775.

Dibble, C. C., & Cantley, L. C., (2015). Regulation of mTORC1 by PI3K signaling. *Trends in Cell Biology, 25*(9), 545–555.

Dickler, M. N., Saura, C., Richards, D. A., et al., (2018). Phase II study of taselisib (GDC-0032) in combination with fulvestrant in patients with HER2-Negative, hormone receptor-positive advanced breast cancer. *Clin. Cancer Res., 24*(18), 4380–4387.

Dolly, S. O., Wagner, A. J., Bendell, J. C., et al., (2016). Phase I study of apitolisib (GDC-0980), dual phosphatidylinositol-3-Kinase and mammalian target of rapamycin kinase inhibitor, in patients with advanced solid tumors. *Clin. Cancer Res., 22*(12), 2874–2884.

Engelman, J. A., Luo, J., & Cantley, L. C., (2006). The evolution of phosphatidylinositol 3-kinases as regulators of growth and metabolism. *Nature Reviews Genetics, 7*(8), 606–619.

Ermoian, R. P., Furniss, C. S., Lamborn, K. R., et al., (2002). Dysregulation of PTEN and protein kinase B is associated with glioma histology and patient survival. *Clinical Cancer Research, 8*(5), 1100–1106.

Ersahin, T., Tuncbag, N., & Cetin-Atalay, R., (2015). The PI3K/AKT/mTOR interactive pathway. *Molecular BioSystems, 11*(7), 1946–1954.

Faried, L. S., Faried, A., Kanuma, T., et al., (2006). Predictive and prognostic role of activated mammalian target of rapamycin in cervical cancer treated with cisplatin-based neoadjuvant chemotherapy. *Oncology Reports, 16*(1), 57–63.

Faried, L. S., Faried, A., Kanuma, T., et al., (2008). Expression of an activated mammalian target of rapamycin in adenocarcinoma of the cervix: A potential biomarker and molecular target therapy. *Molecular Carcinogenesis, 47*(6), 446–457.

Feng, T., Zheng, L., Liu, F., et al., (2016). Growth factor progranulin promotes tumorigenesis of cervical cancer via PI3K/Akt/mTOR signaling pathway. *Oncotarget, 7*(36), 58381–58395.

Forgacs, E., Biesterveld, E. J., Sekido, Y., et al., (1998). Mutation analysis of the PTEN/MMAC1 gene in lung cancer. *Oncogene, 17*(12), 1557–1565.

Foukas, L. C., & Okkenhaug, K., (2003). Gene-targeting reveals physiological roles and complex regulation of the phosphoinositide 3-kinases. *Archives of Biochemistry and Biophysics, 414*(1), 13–18.

Fresno, V. J. A., Casado, E., De Castro, J., Cejas, P., Belda-Iniesta, C., & González-Barón, M., (2004). PI3K/Akt signaling pathway and cancer. *Cancer Treatment Reviews, 30*(2), 193–204.

Fujiwara, M., Izuishi, K., Sano, T., Hossain, M. A., Kimura, S., Masaki, T., & Suzuki, Y., (2008). Modulating effect of the PI3-kinase inhibitor LY294002 on cisplatin in human pancreatic cancer cells. *J. Exp. Clin. Cancer Res., 27,* 76.

Geering, B., Cutillas, P. R., Nock, G., Gharbi, S. I., & Vanhaesebroeck, B., (2007). Class IA phosphoinositide 3-kinases are obligate p85-p110 heterodimers. *Proceedings of the National Academy of Sciences of the United States of America, 104*(19), 7809–7814.

Guenther, M. K., Graab, U., & Fulda, S., (2013). Synthetic lethal interaction between PI3K/Akt/mTOR and Ras/MEK/ERK pathway inhibition in rhabdomyosarcoma. *Cancer Letters, 337*(2), 200–209.

Guo, L., Wu, H., Zhu, J., Zhang, C., Ma, J., Lan, J., & Xie, X., (2015). Genetic variations in the PI3K/AKT pathway predict platinum-based neoadjuvant chemotherapeutic sensitivity in squamous cervical cancer. *Life Sciences, 143*, 217–224.

Hasskarl, J., (2018). Everolimus, recent results in cancer research, Fortschritte der krebsforschung. *Progres Dans les Recherches sur le Cancer, 211*(2018), 101–123.

He, T., Zhang, X., Hao, J., & Ding, S., (2021). Phosphatase and tensin homolog in non-neoplastic digestive disease: More than just tumor suppressor. *Frontiers in Physiology, 12*, 684529.

Hennessy, B. T., Smith, D. L., Ram, P. T., Lu, Y., & Mills, G. B., (2005). Exploiting the PI3K/AKT pathway for cancer drug discovery. *Nature Reviews Drug Discovery, 4*(12), 988–1004.

Hudes, G., Carducci, M., Tomczak, P., et al., (2007). Temsirolimus, interferon alfa, or both for advanced renal-cell carcinoma. *N. Engl. J. Med., 356*(22), 2271–2281.

Ippen, F. M., Alvarez-Breckenridge, C. A., Kuter, B. M., et al., (2019). The dual PI3K/mTOR pathway inhibitor GDC-0084 achieves antitumor activity in PIK3CA-mutant breast cancer brain metastases. *Clinical Cancer Research, 25*(11), 3374–3383.

Ippen, F. M., Grosch, J. K., Subramanian, M., et al., (2019). Targeting the PI3K/Akt/mTOR pathway with the pan-Akt inhibitor GDC-0068 in PIK3CA-mutant breast cancer brain metastases. *Neurooncology, 21*(11), 1401–1411.

Janne, P. A., Cohen, R. B., Laird, A. D., et al., (2014). Phase I safety and pharmacokinetic study of the PI3K/mTOR inhibitor SAR245409 (XL765) in combination with erlotinib in patients with advanced solid tumors. *J. Thorac. Oncol., 9*(3), 316–323.

Kaplan, D. R., Whitman, M., Schaffhausen, B., Pallas, D. C., White, M., Cantley, L., & Roberts, T. M., (1987). Common elements in growth factor stimulation and oncogenic transformation: 85 kd phosphoprotein and phosphatidylinositol kinase activity. *Cell, 50*(7), 1021–1029.

Katso, R., Okkenhaug, K., Ahmadi, K., White, S., Timms, J., & Waterfield, M. D., (2001). Cellular function of phosphoinositide 3-kinases: Implications for development, homeostasis, and cancer. *Annual Review of Cell and Developmental Biology, 17*, 615–675.

Keysar, S. B., Astling, D. P., Anderson, R. T., et al., (2013). A patient tumor transplant model of squamous cell cancer identifies PI3K inhibitors as candidate therapeutics in defined molecular bins. *Molecular Oncology, 7*(4), 776–790.

Kim, K. Y., Park, K. I., Kim, S. H., et al., (2017). Inhibition of autophagy promotes salinomycin-induced apoptosis via reactive oxygen species-mediated PI3K/AKT/mTOR and ERK/p38 MAPK-dependent signaling in human prostate cancer cells. *International Journal of Molecular Sciences, 18*(5), 1088.

Kim, S. K., Su, L. K., Oh, Y., Kemp, B. L., Hong, W. K., & Mao, L., (1998). Alterations of PTEN/MMAC1, a candidate tumor suppressor gene, and its homologue, PTH2, in small cell lung cancer cell lines. *Oncogene, 16*(1), 89–93.

Kisling, S. G., Natarajan, G., Pothuraju, R., Shah, A., Batra, S. K., & Kaur, S., (2021). Implications of prognosis-associated genes in pancreatic tumor metastasis: Lessons from global studies in bioinformatics. *Cancer Metastasis Reviews, 40*(3), 721–738.

Klingenberg, M., Matsuda, A., Diederichs, S., & Patel, T., (2017). Non-coding RNA in hepatocellular carcinoma: Mechanisms, biomarkers and therapeutic targets. *Journal of Hepatology, 67*(3), 603–618.

Kohno, T., Takahashi, M., Manda, R., & Yokota, J., (1998). Inactivation of the PTEN/MMAC1/TEP1 gene in human lung cancers. *Genes, Chromosomes and Cancer, 22*(2), 152–156.

Kolinsky, M. P., Rescigno, P., Bianchini, D., et al., (2020). A phase I dose-escalation study of enzalutamide in combination with the AKT inhibitor AZD5363 (capivasertib) in patients with metastatic castration-resistant prostate cancer. *Ann. Oncol., 31*(5), 619–625.

Krasilnikov, M. A., (2000). Phosphatidylinositol-3 kinase dependent pathways: The role in control of cell growth, survival, and malignant transformation. *Apoptosis, 3*, 10–12.

Kreisberg, J. I., Malik, S. N., Prihoda, T. J., Bedolla, R. G., Troyer, D. A., Kreisberg, S., & Ghosh, P. M., (2004). Phosphorylation of Akt (Ser473) is an excellent predictor of poor clinical outcome in prostate cancer. *Cancer Research, 64*(15), 5232–5236.

Krop, I. E., Mayer, I. A., Ganju, V., et al., (2016). Pictilisib for oestrogen receptor-positive, aromatase inhibitor-resistant, advanced or metastatic breast cancer (FERGI): A randomized, double-blind, placebo-controlled, phase 2 trial. *The Lancet, Oncology, 17*(6), 811–821.

Kumar, A., Bhatia, R., Chawla, P., Anghore, D., Saini, V., & Rawal, R. K., (2020). Copanlisib: Novel PI3K inhibitor for the treatment of lymphoma, anticancer agents. *Med. Chem., 20*(10), 1158–1172.

Lamsisi, M., Wakrim, L., Bouziyane, A., et al., (2021). The biological significance of long noncoding RNAs dysregulation and their mechanism of regulating signaling pathways in cervical cancer. *International Journal of Molecular and Cellular Medicine, 10*(2), 75–101.

Langer, C. J., Redman, M. W., Wade, III. J. L., et al., (2019). SWOG S1400B (NCT02785913), a phase II study of GDC-0032 (Taselisib) for previously treated PI3K-positive patients with stage IV squamous cell lung cancer (Lung-MAP sub-study). *J. Thorac. Oncol., 14*(10), 1839–1846.

Le, Y., Jessica, W., & Pengda, L., (2021). Attacking the PI3K/Akt/mTOR signaling pathway for targeted therapeutic treatment in human cancer. *Seminars in Cancer Biology*. https://doi.org/10.1016/j.semcancer.2021.06.019.

Lee, E. R., Kim, J. Y., Kang, Y. J., et al., (2006). Interplay between PI3K/Akt and MAPK signaling pathways in DNA-damaging drug-induced apoptosis. *Biochimica et Biophysica Acta, 1763*(9), 958–968.

Lee, M. S., Jeong, M. H., Lee, H. W., et al., (2015). PI3K/AKT activation induces PTEN ubiquitination and destabilization accelerating tumourigenesis. *Nature Communications, 6*, 7769.

Li, J., Davies, B. R., Han, S., et al., (2013). The AKT inhibitor AZD5363 is selectively active in PI3KCA mutant gastric cancer and sensitizes a patient-derived gastric cancer xenograft model with PTEN loss to taxotere. *J. Transl. Med., 11*, 241.

Li, L., Ren, C. H., Tahir, S. A., Ren, C., & Thompson, T. C., (2003). Caveolin-1 maintains activated Akt in prostate cancer cells through scaffolding domain binding site interactions with and inhibition of serine/threonine protein phosphatases PP1 and PP2A. *Mol Cell Biol., 23*(24), 9389–9404. doi: 10.1128/MCB.23.24.9389-9404.2003.

Lian, G., Chen, S., Ouyang, M., Li, F., Chen, L., & Yang, J., (2019). Colon cancer cell secretes EGF to promote M2 polarization of TAM through EGFR/PI3K/AKT/mTOR pathway. *Technology in Cancer Research and Treatment, 18*, 1533033819849068.

Liao, S., Xiao, S., Zhu, G., et al., (2014). CD38 is highly expressed and affects the PI3K/Akt signaling pathway in cervical cancer. *Oncology Reports, 32*(6), 2703–2709.

Lin, M. F., (2014). Cellular prostatic acid phosphatase, a PTEN-functional homologue in prostate epithelia, functions as a prostate-specific tumor suppressor. *Biochimica et Biophysica Acta, 1846*(1), 88–98.

Lin, W. M., Forgacs, E., Warshal, D. P., Yeh, I. T., Martin, J. S., Ashfaq, R., & Muller, C. Y., (1998). Loss of heterozygosity and mutational analysis of the PTEN/MMAC1 gene in synchronous endometrial and ovarian carcinomas. *Clinical Cancer Research, 4*(11), 2577–2583.

Liu, X., Xiao, M., Zhang, L., et al., (2021). The m6A methyltransferase METTL14 inhibits the proliferation, migration, and invasion of gastric cancer by regulating the PI3K/AKT/mTOR signaling pathway. *Journal of Clinical Laboratory Analysis, 35*(3), e23655.

Liu, Z., Hong, Z., & Qu, P., (2020). Proteomic analysis of human endometrial tissues reveals the roles of PI3K/AKT/mTOR pathway and tumor angiogenesis molecules in the pathogenesis of endometrial cancer. *BioMed Research International, 2020*, 5273969.

Lopez-Chavez, A., Thomas, A., Rajan, A., et al., (2015). Molecular profiling and targeted therapy for advanced thoracic malignancies: A biomarker-derived, multiarm, multihistology phase II basket trial. *J. Clin. Oncol., 33*(9), 1000–1007.

Lou, H., Villagran, G., Boland, J. F., et al., (2015). Genome analysis of Latin American cervical cancer: Frequent activation of the PIK3CA pathway. *Clinical Cancer Research, 21*(23), 5360–5370.

Markham, A., (2019). Alpelisib: First global approval. *Drugs, 79*(11), 1249–1253.

Martin, M., Chan, A., Dirix, L., et al., (2017). A randomized adaptive phase II/III study of buparlisib, a pan-class I PI3K inhibitor, combined with paclitaxel for the treatment of HER2– advanced breast cancer (BELLE-4). *Ann. Oncol., 28*(2), 313–320.

Martini, M., De Santis, M. C., Braccini, L., Gulluni, F., & Hirsch, E., (2014). PI3K/AKT signaling pathway and cancer: An updated review. *Annals of Medicine, 46*(6), 372–383.

Mateo, J., Ganji, G., Lemech, C., et al., (2017). A first-time-in-Human study of GSK2636771, a phosphoinositide 3 kinase beta-selective inhibitor, in patients with advanced solid tumors. *Clin. Cancer Res., 23*(19), 5981–5992.

Matulonis, U., Vergote, I., Backes, F., et al., (2015). Phase II study of the PI3K inhibitor pilaralisib (SAR245408; XL147) in patients with advanced or recurrent endometrial carcinoma. *Gynecol. Oncol., 136*(2), 246–253.

McIntyre, J. B., Wu, J. S., Craighead, P. S., et al., (2013). PIK3CA mutational status and overall survival in patients with cervical cancer treated with radical chemoradiotherapy. *Gynecologic Oncology, 128*(3), 409–414.

Mehra, S., Deshpande, N., & Nagathihalli, N., (2021). Targeting PI3K pathway in pancreatic ductal adenocarcinoma: Rationale and progress. *Cancers, 13*(17), 4434.

Menges, C. W., Baglia, L. A., Lapoint, R., & McCance, D. J., (2006). Human papillomavirus type 16 E7 up-regulates AKT activity through the retinoblastoma protein. *Cancer Research, 66*(11), 5555–5559.

Miricescu, D., Balan, D. G., Tulin, A., et al., (2021). PI3K/AKT/mTOR signaling pathway involvement in renal cell carcinoma pathogenesis. *Experimental and Therapeutic Medicine, 21*(5), 540.

Miricescu, D., Totan, A., Stanescu-Spinu, I. I., Badoiu, S. C., Stefani, C., & Greabu, M., (2020). PI3K/AKT/mTOR signaling pathway in breast cancer: From molecular landscape to clinical aspects. *International Journal of Molecular Sciences, 22*(1), 173.

Molinolo, A. A., Marsh, C., El Dinali, M., et al., (2012). mTOR as a molecular target in HPV-associated oral and cervical squamous carcinomas. *Clinical Cancer Research, 18*(9), 2558–2568.

Moura, A. C., Assad, D. X., Amorim, D. S. J., et al., (2021). Worldwide prevalence of PI3K-AKT-mTOR pathway mutations in head and neck cancer: A systematic review and meta-analysis. *Critical Reviews in Oncology/Hematology, 160*, 103284.

Murakami, D., Tsujitani, S., Osaki, T., Saito, H., Katano, K., Tatebe, S., & Ikeguchi, M., (2007). Expression of phosphorylated Akt (pAkt) in gastric carcinoma predicts prognosis and efficacy of chemotherapy. *Gastric Cancer, 10*(1), 45–51.

Naing, A., Aghajanian, C., Raymond, E., et al., (2012). Safety, tolerability, pharmacokinetics and pharmacodynamics of AZD8055 in advanced solid tumors and lymphoma. *Br. J. Cancer, 107*(7), 1093–1099.

Nakanishi, K., Sakamoto, M., Yamasaki, S., Todo, S., & Hirohashi, S., (2005). Akt phosphorylation is a risk factor for early disease recurrence and poor prognosis in hepatocellular carcinoma. *Cancer, 103*(2), 307–312.

Narayanankutty, A., (2019). PI3K/Akt/mTOR pathway as a therapeutic target for colorectal cancer: A review of preclinical and clinical evidence. *Current Drug Targets, 20*(12), 1217–1226.

Osei-Amponsa, V., Buckwalter, J. M., Shuman, L., et al., (2020). Hypermethylation of FOXA1 and allelic loss of PTEN drive squamous differentiation and promote heterogeneity in bladder cancer. *Oncogene, 39*(6), 1302–1317.

Paolini, F., Carbone, A., Benevolo, M., et al., (2011). Human papillomaviruses, p16INK4a and Akt expression in basal cell carcinoma. *Journal of Experimental and Clinical Cancer Research, 30*(1), 108.

Park, J. K., Cho, C. H., Ramachandran, S., Shin, S. J., Kwon, S. H., Kwon, S. Y., & Cha, S. D., (2006). Augmentation of sodium butyrate-induced apoptosis by phosphatidylinositol 3-kinase inhibition in the human cervical cancer cell line. *Cancer Research and Treatment, 38*(2), 112–117.

Patel, K., Danilov, A. V., & Pagel, J. M., (2019). Duvelisib for CLL/SLL and follicular non-Hodgkin lymphoma. *Blood, 134*(19), 1573–1577.

Pérez-Tenorio, G., Stål, O., & Southeast Sweden Breast Cancer Group, (2002). Activation of AKT/PKB in breast cancer predicts a worse outcome among endocrine treated patients. *British Journal of Cancer, 86*(4), 540–545.

Pim, D., Massimi, P., Dilworth, S. M., & Banks, L., (2005). Activation of the protein kinase B pathway by the HPV-16 E7 oncoprotein occurs through a mechanism involving interaction with PP2A. *Oncogene, 24*(53), 7830–7838.

Pópulo, H., Lopes, J. M., & Soares, P., (2012). The mTOR signaling pathway in human cancer. *International Journal of Molecular Sciences, 13*(2), 1886–1918.

Prasad, S. B., Yadav, S. S., Das, M., et al., (2015). PI3K/AKT pathway-mediated regulation of p27 (Kip1) is associated with cell cycle arrest and apoptosis in cervical cancer. *Cellular Oncology, 38*(3), 215–225.

Rodríguez-Escudero, I., Oliver, M. D., Andrés-Pons, A., Molina, M., Cid, V. J., & Pulido, R., (2011). A comprehensive functional analysis of PTEN mutations: Implications in tumor- and autism-related syndromes. *Human Molecular Genetics, 20*(21), 4132–4142.

Ruggeri, B. A., Huang, L., Wood, M., Cheng, J. Q., & Testa, J. R., (1998). Amplification and overexpression of the AKT2 oncogene in a subset of human pancreatic ductal adenocarcinomas. *Molecular Carcinogenesis, 21*(2), 81–86.

Schwarz, J. K., Payton, J. E., Rashmi, R., et al., (2012). Pathway-specific analysis of gene expression data identifies the PI3K/Akt pathway as a novel therapeutic target in cervical cancer. *Clinical Cancer Research, 18*(5), 1464–1471.

Shiraz, A., Crawford, R., Egawa, N., Griffin, H., & Doorbar, J., (2020). The early detection of cervical cancer. The current and changing landscape of cervical disease detection. *Cytopathology, 31*(4), 258–270.

Shu, X. R., Wu, J., Sun, H., Chi, L. Q., & Wang, J. H., (2015). PAK4 confers the malignance of cervical cancers and contributes to the cisplatin-resistance in cervical cancer cells via PI3K/AKT pathway. *Diagnostic Pathology, 10*, 177.

Surviladze, Z., Sterk, R. T., DeHaro, S. A., & Ozbun, M. A., (2013). Cellular entry of human papillomavirus type 16 involves activation of the phosphatidylinositol 3-kinase/Akt/mTOR pathway and inhibition of autophagy. *Journal of Virology, 87*(5), 2508–2517.

Tolaney, S., Burris, H., Gartner, E., et al., (2015). Phase I/II study of pilaralisib (SAR245408) in combination with trastuzumab or trastuzumab plus paclitaxel in trastuzumab-refractory HER2-positive metastatic breast cancer. *Breast Cancer Res. Treat., 149*(1), 151–161.

Tripathy, H. K., Manju, N. S. V., Dittakavi, S., Zakkula, A., & Mullangi, R., (2020). DBS assay with LC-MS/MS for the determination of idelalisib, a selective PI3K-delta inhibitor in mice blood and its application to a pharmacokinetic study. *Drug Res., 71*(1), 36–42. doi:10.1055/a-1252-2476.

Tsurutani, J., Fukuoka, J., Tsurutani, H., et al., (2006). Evaluation of two phosphorylation sites improves the prognostic significance of Akt activation in non-small-cell lung cancer tumors. *Journal of Clinical Oncology, 24*(2), 306–314.

Vanhaesebroeck, B., Guillermet-Guibert, J., Graupera, M., & Bilanges, B., (2010). The emerging mechanisms of isoform specific PI3K signaling. *Nature Reviews Molecular Cell Biology, 11*(5), 329–341.

Wang, J., Jiang, C., Li, N., et al., (2020). The circEPSTI1/mir-942-5p/LTBP2 axis regulates the progression of OSCC in the background of OSF via EMT and the PI3K/Akt/mTOR pathway. *Cell Death and Disease, 11*(8), 682.

Whitman, M., Kaplan, D. R., Schaffhausen, B., Cantley, L., & Roberts, T. M., (1985). Association of phosphatidylinositol kinase activity with polyoma middle-T competent for transformation. *Nature, 315*(6016), 239–242.

Wicki, A., Brown, N., Xyrafas, A., et al., (2018). First-in human, phase 1, dose-escalation pharmacokinetic and pharmacodynamic study of the oral dual PI3K and mTORC1/2 inhibitor PQR309 in patients with advanced solid tumors (SAKK 67/ 13). *Eur. J. Cancer* 96, 6–16.

Wise-Draper, T. M., Moorthy, G., Salkeni, M. A., et al., (2017). A phase Ib study of the dual PI3K/ mTOR inhibitor dactolisib (BEZ235) combined with everolimus in patients with advanced solid malignancies. *Target. Oncol., 12*(3), 323–332.

Wolin, E., Mita, A., Mahipal, A., et al., (2019). A phase 2 study of an oral mTORC1/ mTORC2 kinase inhibitor (CC-223) for non-pancreatic neuroendocrine tumors with or without carcinoid symptoms. *PLoS One, 14*(9), e0221994.

Wright, A. A., Howitt, B. E., Myers, A. P., et al., (2013). Oncogenic mutations in cervical cancer: Genomic differences between adenocarcinomas and squamous cell carcinomas of the cervix. *Cancer, 119*(21), 3776–3783.

Wu, J., Ji, Z., Liu, H., et al., (2013). Arsenic trioxide depletes cancer stem-like cells and inhibits repopulation of neurosphere derived from glioblastoma by downregulation of notch pathway. *Toxicol. Lett., 220*(1), 61–69. doi: 10.1016/j.toxlet.2013.03.019.

Xu, P. F., Yang, J. A., Liu, J. H., et al., (2019). PI3Kbeta inhibitor AZD6482 exerts antiproliferative activity and induces apoptosis in human glioblastoma cells. *Oncol. Rep., 41*(1), 125–132.

Yanik, E. L., Siddiqui, K., & Engels, E. A., (2015). Sirolimus effects on cancer incidence after kidney transplantation: A meta-analysis. *Cancer Med., 4*(9), 1448–1459.

Ye, X., Ruan, J. W., Huang, H., Huang, W. P., Zhang, Y., & Zhang, F., (2020). PI3K-Akt-mTOR inhibition by GNE-477 inhibits renal cell carcinoma cell growth *in vitro* and *in vivo*. *Aging, 12*(10), 9489–9499.

Yuan, T. L., & Cantley, L. C., (2008). PI3K pathway alterations in cancer: Variations on a theme. *Oncogene, 27*(41), 5497–5510.

Zaczek, A., Jóźwiak, P., Ciesielski, P., et al., (2020). Relationship between polycomb-group protein BMI-1 and phosphatases regulating AKT phosphorylation level in endometrial cancer. *Journal of Cellular and Molecular Medicine, 24*(2), 1300–1310.

Zhang, X., Shen, L., Liu, Q., Hou, L., & Huang, L., (2019). Inhibiting PI3 kinase-gamma in both myeloid and plasma cells remodel the suppressive tumor microenvironment in desmoplastic tumors. *J. Control. Release, 309*, 173–180.

Zheng, J., Yu, J., Yang, M., & Tang, L., (2019). Gefitinib suppresses cervical cancer progression by inhibiting cell cycle progression and epithelial-mesenchymal transition. *Experimental and Therapeutic Medicine, 18*(3), 1823–1830.

Zhou, Y., Pan, Y., Zhang, S., Shi, X., Ning, T., & Ke, Y., (2007). Increased phosphorylation of p70 S6 kinase is associated with HPV16 infection in cervical cancer and esophageal cancer. *British Journal of Cancer, 97*(2), 218–222.

CHAPTER 5

Notch Signaling Pathway

5.1 NOTCH SIGNALING

Notch signaling is mainly involved in cell fate determination and regulation of many cellular processes like cell proliferation, differentiation, survival, and apoptosis (Kopan & Ilagan, 2009; Wang et al., 2011; Kovall et al., 2017). Notch genes code for heterodimeric, single-pass trans-membrane receptors that are involved in cell-to-cell communication between neighboring cells. Mature Notch receptors processed after proteolytic cleavage by furin-like protease enzyme from large single polypeptide precursors into (Blaumueller et al., 1997; Logeat et al., 1998) heterodimers consisting of an extracellular subunit and a transmembrane subunit (NTM) associated with non-covalent interactions. The mammalian family of Notch receptors comprises four different kinds of receptors including Notch1, Notch2, Notch3, Notch4 and contains multiple EGF-like repeats on their extracellular domain (Fleming, 1998; Klueg & Muskavitch, 1999). These four receptors different from each other on the basis of intracellular domain length and EGF-like repeat (Egan et al., 1998; Kortschak et al., 2001). There are five members of cell membrane-associated Notch ligand were known which belongs to the Delta or Jagged families, including Jagged1/2 and Delta-like 1, -3 and -4 (Dll1/3/4) (Handford et al., 2018; Hozumi, 2020) (Figure 5.1).

Cervical Cancer: Signaling Pathways, Molecular Mechanisms, Natural Products, and Therapeutic Approaches. Pratibha Pandey, Fahad Khan, Saher Islam, and Devarajan Thangadurai, (Eds.)

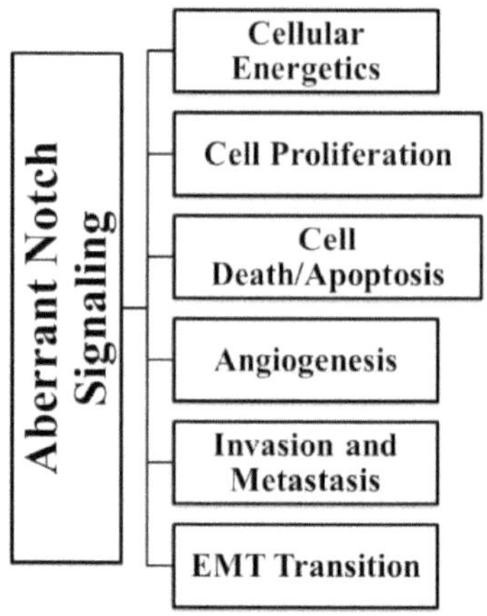

FIGURE 5.1 Modulatory effect of Notch signaling pathway on key events that promotes carcinogenesis process.

Activation of Notch receptors is mediated by association of cell membrane associated Notch ligand which resulted in initiation of Notch signaling. The relative affinity of particular receptors for various ligands is regulated by glycosylation of extracellular domain which is catalyzed by associated glycosyltransferases (Fortini, 2002, 2009, 2012). The ligand-receptor interaction caused a conformational change in the Notch receptor, which resulted in two consecutive proteolytic cleavages.

The first cleavage is catalyzed by TNF-alpha converting enzyme (TACE), a member of the ADAM (A disintegrin and metalloprotease) group of metalloproteases within the Notch extracellular domain (Mumm & Kopan, 2000). Subsequently, receptor underwent second cleavage mediated by a presenilin-1-dependent γ-secretase within the trans-membrane sequence, releasing the Notch intracellular domain (NICD). NICD then translocate to the nucleus where it primarily effect gene expression by associating to a transcriptional factor known as CBF1 (Rbp-Jk) (Bray, 2006; Bray & Gomez-Lamarca, 2018). This association resulted in dissociation of CBF-1 from a co-repressor complex which transforms its role from transcriptional repressor into an activator. The target genes of Notch involves helix–loop–helix inhibitory transcription factors of the hairy enhancer of split (HES) family, NF-kB family and PPAR family transcription factors which mainly regulates cellular differentiation and mediators of cell cycle, including $p21^{cip1/waf1}$ and cyclin D1 (Zhang et al., 2018).

5.2 NOTCH SIGNALING IN CANCER

During the past several years, numerous research reports suggested the dysregulation of a Notch signaling pathway in various malignancies and could be a potential target for therapeutic implications (Jang et al., 2000; Zhdanovskaya et al., 2021). The first evidence of Notch signaling and human carcinoma association was revealed by 9: 7 chromosomal translocations in approximately 10% of T-cell lymphoblastic leukemia which resulted in generation of a truncated human Notch-1 lacking extracellular subunit (Ellisen et al., 1991). These truncated forms of all four Notch isoforms have shown transforming ability in *in-vitro* and *in-vivo* system both (Pear et al., 1996; Capobianco et al., 1997; Bellavia et al., 2000; Felli et al., 2005). In humans, aberrant expression level of Notch ligands, receptors, and associated targets is detected in an increasing number of solid tumors, such as cervical, head and neck, lung and breast carcinomas, endometrial, and renal (Daniel et al., 1997; Dang et al., 2000; Leethanakul et al., 2000; Rae et al., 2000; Suzuki et al., 2000; Hendrix et al., 2002; Bocchetta et al., 2003; Crabtree et al., 2016), as well as in hematological cancers like Hodgkin lymphomas, subsets of acute myeloid leukemias and B-cell chronic lymphoid leukemia (BCLL) (Hubmann et al., 2002; Jundt et al., 2002, 2004). SV40 and HPV16 viral oncoproteins also involved in increased expression of Notch-1, resulted in SV40-mediated (Bocchetta et al., 2003; Weijzen et al., 2003) and HPV16-mediated transformation (Rangarajan et al., 2001), while EBNA2, an EBV oncoprotein imitates active Notch-1 or -2 (Hsieh et al., 1996; Crow & Albig, 2020). Repression of Notch activity by antisense retrovirus or drug-mediated regulation of gamma secretase activity have remarkable antineoplastic effects in transformed cells (Notch expressing) *in vitro* and in xenograft models (Weijzen et al., 2002, 2003; Bocchetta et al., 2003; Liu et al., 2006). Thus, existing reports suggested that, in those carcinomas that express intracellular forms of Notch receptors, inhibition of Notch signaling may be a potential therapeutic strategy (Figure 5.2). Some reports also suggested that role of Notch-1 may serve as a onco-suppressor rather than an oncogene like in case of murine epidermis, presenilin-1-deficient mice (Xia et al., 2001; Nicolas et al., 2003). This may be associated to the growth suppressive, p21-mediated effects of Notch-1 in keratinocytes (Okuyama et al., 2004). In the case of Malignant Melanomas, cells are sensitive to Notch suppression which clearly indicates the oncogenic role of Notch signaling (Müller, 2012). Overall, these evidences suggested that inhibition of Notch signaling could be a viable approach for the treatment of various solid and hematopoietic malignancies (Figure 5.3).

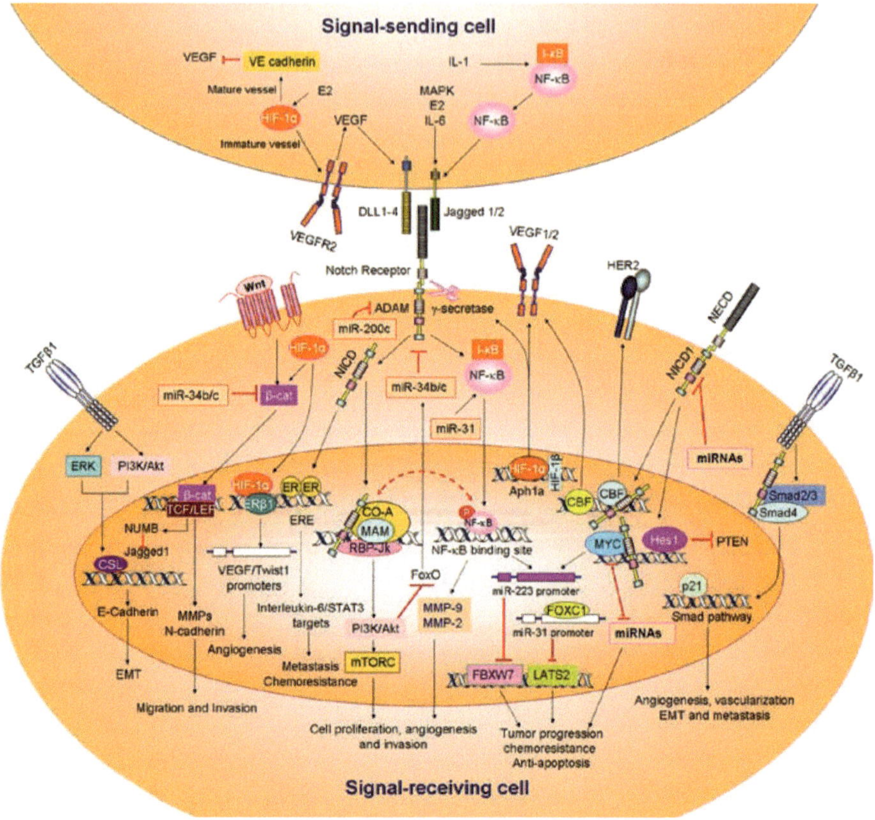

FIGURE 5.2 Role of Notch signaling in driving hallmarks of tumor progression. The scientific illustration summarizes the role of Notch signaling via its receptor-ligand interactions in the transmembrane region in driving tumorigenesis via regulating cell proliferation, angiogenesis, tumor migration and invasion, metastasis. The key players in the process of Notch mediated oncogenic progression is through hypoxia inducible factor 1 alpha (HIF-1α), β-catenin (CTNNB1), mammalian target of rapamycin (mTORC), matrix metalloproteinases (MMPs), p21, and microRNAs (miRNAs).

Source: Reproduced with permission from Aggarwal et al. (2021); Copyright © Elsevier (2021).

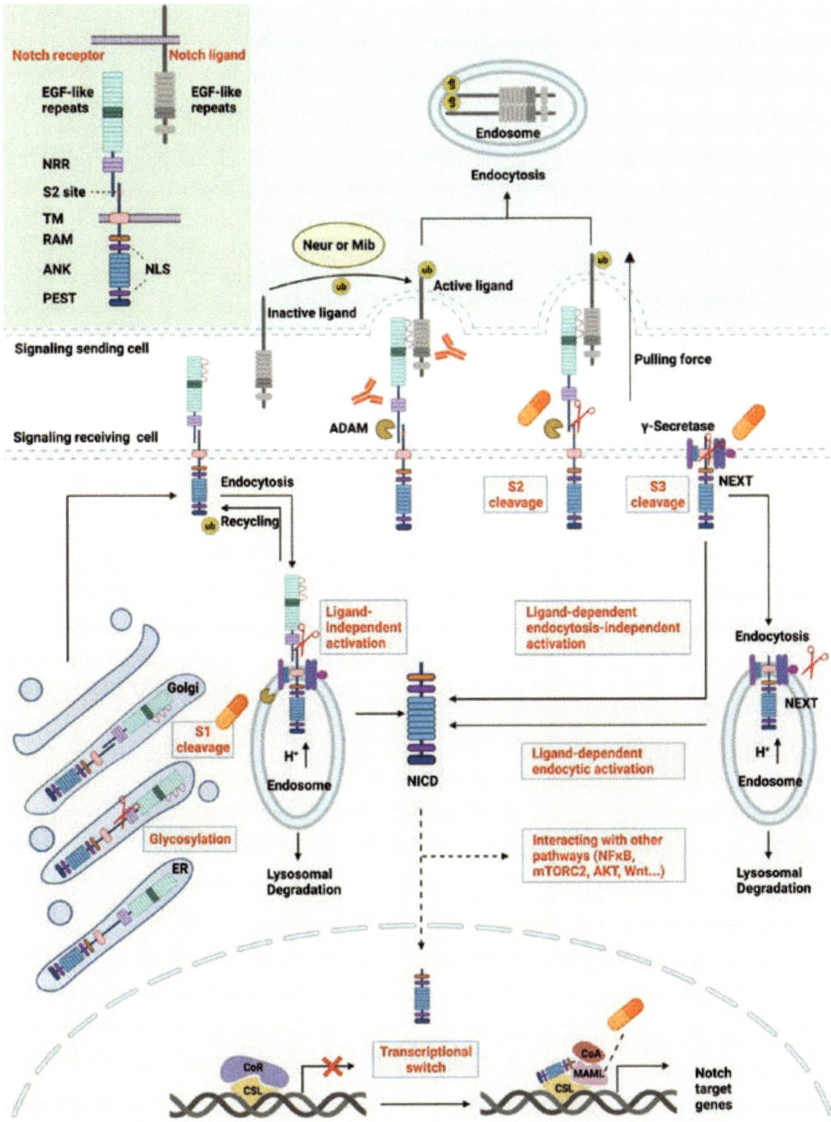

FIGURE 5.3 Overview of the Notch signaling pathway and therapeutic targets. In signal-receiving cells, Notch receptors are first generated in the ER and then trafficked to the Golgi apparatus. During trafficking, notch receptors are glycosylated at the EGF-like repeat domain (red curves). Then, in the Golgi apparatus, notch receptors are cleaved into heterodimers (S1 cleavage) and transported to the cell membrane. With the help of ubiquitin ligases, some of the notch receptors on the cell membrane are endocytosed into endosomes. Endosomes contain an acidic environment with ADAMs and γ-secretase. The

notch receptors in endosomes can be recycled to the cell membrane, cleaved into NICD, or transported into lysosomes for degradation. In signal-sending cells, notch ligands are distributed on the cell membrane and can bind to notch receptors on signal-receiving cells. However, the ligands are inactive before ubiquitylation by Neur or Mib. After ubiquitylation, ligands can be endocytosed, thus producing a pulling force for the binding receptors. Without the pulling force, the S2 site (red marks) of notch receptors is hidden by the NRR domain, and thus, the notch receptors are resistant to cleavage by ADAMs. With the pulling force, the NRR domain is extended, therefore exposing the S2 site for cleavage. ADAMs and the pulling force are both necessary for S2 cleavage. After S2 cleavage, the remaining part of the notch receptor is called NEXT. NEXT can be further cleaved on the cell membrane by γ-secretase or endocytosed into endosomes. In the former mode, NICD is released on the cell membrane. In the latter mode, NEXT can be cleaved into NICD or transported into lysosomes for degradation. In total, there are three approaches to generate NICD, classified as ligand-independent activation, ligand-dependent endocytosis-independent activation, and ligand-dependent endocytic activation. NICD can be translocated into the nucleus or remain in the cytoplasm to crosstalk with other signaling pathways, such as NFκB, mTORC2, Akt, and Wnt. The classical model proposes that, in the absence of NICD, CSL binds with corepressors to inhibit the transcription of target genes. Once NICD enters the nucleus, it can bind with CSL and recruit MAMLs, releasing corepressors, recruiting coactivators, and thus promoting the transcription of notch target genes. There are two main approaches to inhibit notch signaling for therapy. One is designing inhibitors of the key components of the pathways, including the enzymes that participate in S1 cleavage, ADAMs, γ-secretase, and MAML. The other one is producing antibody-drug conjugates against notch receptors and ligands. The protein structures of notch ligands and receptors are shown in the top left corner.

Abbreviations: NICD: notch intracellular domain; ADAM: a disintegrin and metalloproteinase domain-containing protein; Neur: Neutralized; Mib: Mindbomb; NRR: negative regulatory region; NEXT: notch extracellular truncation; CSL: CBF-1/suppressor of hairless/Lag1; MAMLs: mastermind-like proteins; TM: transmembrane domain; RAM: RBPJ association module; ANK: ankyrin repeats; PEST: proline/glutamic acid/serine/threonine-rich motifs; NLS: nuclear localization sequence; CoR: corepressor; CoA: coactivator; ub: ubiquitin.

Source: Adapted from Zhou et al. (2022); https://creativecommons.org/licenses/by/4.0/.

5.3 ABERRANT NOTCH SIGNALING IN CERVICAL CANCER

Recent investigations suggested that hyper activated Notch signaling was associated with Notch receptors in T-cell acute lymphoblastic leukemia while FBXW7 negatively regulate Notch signaling. In the absence of any activating mutations as in case of T-ALL, it is required to explore different cytogenetic anomalies such as amplification, deletion that might be associated with the activation of the Notch pathway (Palomero & Ferrando, 2009).

The data obtained from cancer database namely The Cancer Genome Atlas (TCGA) (https://www.cancer.gov/tcga) have outlined the gene mutation in various genes including EP300, NFE2L2, FBXW7, TP53, PTEN, PIK3CA, and ERBB2 in primary cervical cancers (Ojesina et al., 2014; Cancer Genome Atlas Research Network, 2017). Out of these, deep deletion, truncating, and missense mutation in FBXW7 gene was reported in 15% of the primary squamous cell cervical cancer (Ojesina et al., 2014). This information directed researchers to further explore genetic variations in other Notch signaling components such as NOTCH 1-4, DLL1, 3, 4, JAG1-2, MYC, HES1, DELTEX1, NUMB, and ADAM17 in cervical cancer tissues. It is clearly known that different genetic lesions can be resulted in activation of the Notch pathway. These genetic lesions are mainly associated with Notch receptor mutations (NOTCH 1-4), overexpression of Notch ligands and down regulated mutations of E3 ligases. The meta-analysis data of TCGA revealed that significant abnormal expression of Notch pathway constituents was detected in more than 80% of primary cervical cancer. Additionally, in half of the primary cervical cancer tissue, some of these constituents were disturbed by genetic alterations like amplification, point mutations and deletion. Genetic alterations related with positive regulators amplification (including Notch receptor, ligand, Hes1, c-Myc) and negative regulators deletion (including FBW7, CBL components), may resulted in increased expression of the key players of Notch pathway (Lian et al., 2019; Khan et al., 2020). Furthermore, Hes1 overexpression by amplification was significantly observed in cervical cancer tissues. Altogether, these data suggested that genetic anomalies might be one of the possible reasons for modulated expression and activity of the key players of the Notch pathway, as observed in several primary cervical cancer tissues.

Genetic alterations of the Notch signaling pathway are identified and limited to only primary cervical cancer tissues, and the other regulatory processes are also involved in other cases of advanced cervical cancers. The other mechanism involved in the modulation of Notch signaling includes ligand-dependent Notch activation, regulation by long noncoding RNAs and HPV (Steinbuck & Winandy, 2018). One of the mechanisms involved in the progression of cervical cancer is aberrant activation of the Notch pathway by different ligands. Various reports suggested the overexpression of various ligand of Notch signaling, including Jagged1, Notch1 in an advanced stage of cervical carcinoma (Palmer & Deng, 2015).

Another regulatory mode of the Notch signaling pathway occurs through noncoding RNAs. One study of Pang et al. revealed that binding of miR34a to the 3′ UTR site of Notch1 and Jagged1 resulted in their decreased protein expression and thus inhibited cell migration in human cervical cancer HeLa cells (Pang et al., 2010). Furthermore, increased expression of a long noncoding RNA (HOTAIR) associated with up regulated expression of Hes1 and Notch1 at both gene and protein level which resulted in enhanced cell invasion and migration in SiHa and CaSki cervical cancer cell lines (Lee et al., 2016).

5.4 HPVs AND NOTCH SIGNALING PATHWAY

Notch signaling has been linked to the epithelial differentiation process, where hyper-activated Notch signaling leading to the basal cell differentiation (Fuchs, 2009). Given that the HPV life cycle is rely upon keratinocyte differentiation, it's worth wondering if HPV oncoproteins play a role in regulating the Notch pathway. The relationship between HPV proteins and Notch signaling in this case is dependent on the HPV subtype. HPVs can be classified according to which epithelia they affect. Cutaneous HPVs are members of the genus beta of HPVs, which attack the skin. Mucosal HPVs, on the other hand, belong to the genus alpha of HPVs and infect mucosal epithelium (such as the cervical epithelium) (Bzhalava et al., 2013). High-risk HPVs (e.g., HPV16, HPV18, and HPV31) are known to generate cancers, whereas low-risk HPVs (e.g., HPV5, HPV8) create benign lesions but do not cause carcinomas (Muñoz et al., 2003).

High-risk HPV E6 proteins (e.g., HPV16, HPV18) can form a trimeric complex with Ubiquitin ligase E6AP and bind to p53 that leads to the breakdown of p53 (Scheffner et al., 1990; Werness et al., 1990; Huibregtse et al., 1993; Ramachandran & Dörk, 2021). Notch1 is down regulated as a consequence of P53 breakdown, resulting in suppression of differentiation markers in keratinocytes (Yugawa et al., 2007). In organotypic raft experiments, immortalized human keratinocyte cell line (NIKS) having HPV16 demonstrated uncontrolled differentiation, and loss of NICD. HPV E6 proteins from low-risk HPVs (such as HPV11 and HPV6) associate with E6AP however unable to degrade P53 (Crook et al., 1991; Brimer & Vande Pol, 2014; Vande Pol, 2015).

Cutaneous HPV E6 proteins, on the other hand, do not bind E6AP but rather MAML1, a transcriptional coactivator in the Notch complex, inhibiting Notch activation (Tan et al., 2012; Brimer et al., 2017). Furthermore, suppression of Notch signaling has been associated to slow rate of keratinocyte differentiation and persistent proliferation of differentiating keratinocytes (Kazem et al., 2012; Meyers et al., 2013). Other research studies, on the other hand, suggest that HPV causes an increase in Notch signaling. HPV16 E6 has also been shown to associate with NFX-123, a host cellular molecule that upregulates Notch1 expression (Vliet-Gregg et al., 2013). Weijzen et al. also revealed that E6 and E7 both upregulate Notch1 expression and its activation (Weijzen et al., 2003). Furthermore, Pattabiraman et al. demonstrated that ectopic expression of the HPV31 genome into human foreskin keratinocytes (HFKs) led to an increase in the quantity of Notch1 activation (Pattabiraman et al., 2014).

In Keratinocyte models, the majority of the reports summarized here look at how HPV oncoproteins regulate the Notch pathway (Lathion et al., 2003). These research findings may provide a better understanding of elements of normal HPV replication in Keratinocytes. The modulation of Notch signaling by HPV oncoproteins in cervical malignancies, on the other hand, has received less attention. The control of Notch signaling by HPV oncoproteins in cervical cancer cell lines would be intriguing to investigate, as these proteins still play critical and different roles in an advanced stage of cervical cancer. A study performed by Wang et al. demonstrated that utilizing an oncolytic adenovirus to delete HPV16 E6 and E7 reduces invasiveness and increases radio sensitivity in SiHa cells *in vitro* and *in vivo* (Wang et al., 2010). Kennedy et al. previously demonstrated that CRISPR/Cas9-mediated deletion of HPV18 E6 and E7 induces cell death in HeLa cells (Kennedy et al., 2014). These findings show that the Notch pathway caused by HPV may play a distinct role in cervical cancer, which has to be investigated further.

5.5 KEY MOLECULES ASSOCIATED WITH CERVICAL CANCER PROGRESSION

Given that Notch can act as both a tumor suppressor and an oncogene, it's critical to look at Notch and its downstream players throughout the evolution of cervical cancer. The expression of these players has been studied in a variety of studies during cervical cancer initiation and progression. These studies likewise show a complex pattern: the majority of them show Notch up regulation with advancement, but a few also show Notch down regulation during cancer development (Li et al., 2017; Gupta et al., 2018).

The expression of Notch1 pathway components was shown to be higher when cervical cancer progressed from normal to advance grade cervical carcinoma via cervical intraepithelial neoplasia III (CINI-III) (Rong et al., 2017). In cervical malignancies, Campos-Parra et al. found that Notch pathway components were up regulated as compared to control tissues (Campos-Parra et al., 2016). In addition, Daniel et al. found that invasive cervical tumors have higher levels of intracellular Notch than high-grade lesions (Daniel et al., 1997). Furthermore, CIN sections have higher amounts of nuclear Notch1 than invasive cervical malignancies. Notch1 cytoplasmic localization was found in the majority of invasive cervical malignancies, and this pattern was linked to cervical cancer growth. Nuclear Notch1 in tumors has also been linked to inferior clinical outcomes when compared to tumors with cytoplasmic Notch1 (Vázquez-Ulloa et al., 2018).

Rong et al. found that splicing of Numb (a negative regulator of Notch) was disrupted in cervical cancer, in addition to Notch expression and localization (Rong et al., 2017). NUMB-L and NUMB-S splice variants with and without exon 12 (NUMB-L and NUMB-S, respectively) were detected, and the NUMB-L variant's expression was found to be higher in cervical cancer tissue samples. Overexpression of the NUMB-L variant form enhanced Hes1 and Hey1 expression as well as cell proliferation in HeLa cells, but overexpression of the NUMB-S variant reduced it. In several cell types, including baby rat kidney cells, baby mouse kidney cells, and rat embryo fibroblasts, oncogenic HPV16 cooperates with Ras to drive transformation (Matlashewski et al., 1987; Crook et al., 1988; Chesters & McCance, 1989). Activated intracellular Notch 1 and 2 have been demonstrated to complement the adenoviral E1A oncogene during transformation, similar to Ras (Capobianco et al., 1997).

Rangarajan et al. demonstrated that activated intracellular Notch1 can phenocopy Ras in transforming immortalized HaCaT keratinocytes, with HPV16 E6 and E7 (Yin et al., 2017; Huo et al., 2020). HPV16, for example, has been shown to collaborate with c-Myc to transform and immortalize cells (Crook et al., 1989). HPV16 E6 influences cell immortalization by activating the human telomerase reverse transcriptase (hTERT) promoter via a c-Myc-dependent mechanism (Figure 5.4) (Veldman et al., 2003). Furthermore, c-Myc has been discovered to be an important component in E6/E7-Notch mediated cellular transformation (Subramanyam & Krishna, 2006). Based on this, it was also revealed that activated Notch1 might work in tandem with HPV16 oncogenes in these cells to induce tumor formation in nude mice (Chakrabarti et al., 2004).

Recent research has revealed comparable results using more genetically tractable model organisms like *Drosophila*, in addition to complementation analyzes of HPV oncogenes with active Notch signaling (Padash Barmchi et al., 2016). The expression of E6+UBE3A in combination with activated/oncogenic versions of Ras or Notch, for example, can induce tumorigenesis in this system. These model systems provide a platform to better understand these molecular interactions and, perhaps, developing genetic/drug screening.

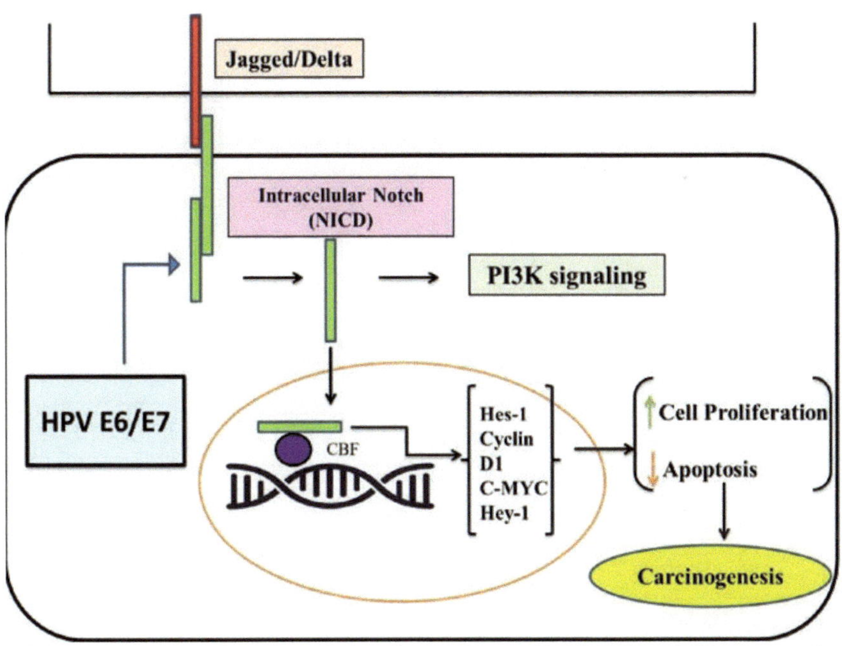

FIGURE 5.4 Association of notch signaling pathway with HPV E6 and E7 oncoproteins in cervical cancer pathogenesis.

TABLE 5.1 Drugs Targeting Notch Pathway in Clinical Trials

Notch Inhibitors	Class of Drug	Study Type	Study Detail	Clinical Trial Number
		Phase I Clinical Trial		
RO4929097 (R4733)	γ-secretase inhibitor	Phase I, non-randomized study	The study was aimed to evaluate the effect of the drug in refractory metastatic or advanced solid tumors.	NCT00532090
		Phase I interventional trial	The study was designed to evaluate the clinical efficiency of the drug against metastatic breast cancer where surgery cannot be performed.	NCT01071564
		Phase I interventional trial	The study was designed to evaluate the safe dose and any side effect against various solid tumors.	NCT01088763
		Phase I interventional trial	The study was designed to evaluate the safe dose and any side effect against various solid tumors.	NCT01096355
		Phase II interventional trial	The study was designed for clinical efficacy against metastatic colorectal cancer.	NCT01116687
		Phase I interventional trial	Evaluation of the combination of temozolomide and radiation with RO4929097 against malignant glioma.	NCT01119599
		Phase I interventional trial	Evaluation of the combination of cediranib with RO4929097 against solid tumors.	NCT01131234
		Phase I interventional trial	Evaluation of the combination of gemcitabine with RO4929097 against advanced solid tumors.	NCT01145456
		Phase I randomized trial	Evaluation of the combination of exemestane with RO4929097 among pre and postmenopausal patients of breast cancer.	NCT01149356
		Phase I interventional trial	Evaluation of the combination of capecitabine with RO4929097 among refractory solid tumors.	NCT01158274

TABLE 5.1 *(Continued)*

Notch Inhibitors	Class of Drug	Study Type	Study Detail	Clinical Trial Number
		Phase I, non-randomized	Evaluation of the combination of cetuximab with RO4929097 among colorectal cancer.	NCT01198535
		Phase I interventional trial	Evaluation of side effect and therapeutic combination of temsirolimus with RO4929097 among advanced solid tumors.	NCT01198184
		Phase I interventional trial	Evaluation of the combination of erlotinib with RO4929097 among stage IV non-small cell lung cancer patients.	NCT01193881
		Phase I interventional trial	The study was designed to evaluate the safe dose and any side effect against solid neoplasm.	NCT01192763
		Phase I randomized trial	The study was designed to evaluate the safe dose and any side effect of RO4929097 in combination with paclitaxel and carboplatin against stage II/III triple-negative breast cancer.	NCT01217411
		Phase I randomized trial	The study was designed to evaluate the safe dose and any side effect of RO4929097 in combination with bevacizumab against progressive/recurrent malignant glioma.	NCT01218620
		Phase I interventional trial	The study was designed to evaluate the safety of the combination of MK-0752 with docetaxel in breast cancer.	NCT01238133
		Phase I, non-randomized trial	The study was designed to evaluate the safety of PF-03084014 among patients with advanced cancer and leukemia.	NCT01189240

TABLE 5.1 *(Continued)*

Notch Inhibitors	Class of Drug	Study Type	Study Detail	Clinical Trial Number
MK-0752	–	Phase I, multi-center, non-randomized trial	The study was designed to evaluate the efficacy and tolerability of PF-03084014 in combination with docetaxel among patients with advanced breast cancer.	NCT00645333
Nirogacestat (PF-03084014)	γ-secretase inhibitor	Phase I non-randomized trial	The study was designed to evaluate the safety of PF-03084014 among patients with advanced cancer and leukemia.	NCT00878189
		Phase I non-open-label trial	The study was designed to evaluate the efficacy and tolerability of PF-03084014 in combination with docetaxel among patients with advanced breast cancer.	NCT01876251
LY3039478 (JSMD194)	γ-secretase inhibitor	Phase I, non-randomized trial	The study was designed to evaluate the safety of LY3039478 in Combination with other anticancer drugs among the patients of advanced/metastatic solid tumors.	NCT02784795
		Phase I interventional trial	The study was designed to evaluate the safe dose and any side effect of LY3039478 in combination with chimeric antigen receptor (CAR) T-cells against multiple myeloma.	NCT03502577
		Phase I, open-label, multicenter, nonrandomized	The drug was found to be safe and effective against breast cancer, cystic carcinoma, and leiomyosarcoma.	NCT01695005
AL101 (BMS-906024)	γ-secretase inhibitor	Phase I non-randomized trial	The study was designed to evaluate the safety as well as tolerability of metastatic breast cancer (advanced stage).	NCT01292655
		Phase I non-randomized trial	The study was designed to evaluate the safety as well as tolerability of AL101 in combination dexamethasone among the patients of T-cell acute lymphoblastic leukemia.	NCT01363817

TABLE 5.1 *(Continued)*

Notch Inhibitors	Class of Drug	Study Type	Study Detail	Clinical Trial Number
AL102 (BMS-986115)	γ-secretase inhibitor	Phase I non-randomized trial	The study was designed to evaluate the clinical efficacy and safety of AL102 among the patients of advanced cancer.	NCT01986218
MEDI0639	DLL-4 ligand-targeted antibodies	Phase 1 multicenter, open-label study	The study was designed to evaluate the clinical efficacy, safety, anticancer effect, and pharmacokinetic profile of AL102 among the patients of advanced cancer.	NCT01577745
Enoticumab (REGN421)	DLL-4 ligand-targeted antibodies	Phase I non-randomized trial	The study was designed to evaluate the clinical efficacy and safety of REGN421 among the patients of advanced cancer.	NCT00871559
CB-103	Notch transcription complex inhibitor	Phase I/II, non-randomized, open-label trial.	The study was designed to evaluate the clinical efficacy, tolerability, and safety of CB-103 among the patients of metastatic solid tumors as well as hematological malignancies.	NCT03422679
Brontictuzumab (OMP-52M51)	Notch receptor antibody	Phase I open-label trial.	Dose escalation study in refractory lymphoid carcinogenesis and evaluation of safety, efficacy, and pharmacokinetic profile.	NCT01703572
		Phase I open-label trial	Dose escalation study in Refractory solid tumors and evaluation of safety, efficacy, and pharmacokinetic profile.	NCT01778439
		Phase I double-blind randomized trial	The study was designed to explore the maximum tolerated dose of OMP-59R5 in combination with paclitaxel and gemcitabine among patients with pancreatic cancer (Stage IV).	NCT01647828

TABLE 5.1 *(Continued)*

Notch Inhibitors	Class of Drug	Study Type	Study Detail	Clinical Trial Number
Demcizumab	DLL-4 ligand-targeted antibodies	Phase I interventional trial	The study was designed to explore the safety and effective dose of gemcitabine in combination with demcizumab in pancreatic cancer.	NCT01189929
		Phase I non-randomized trial	The study was designed to explore the safety and effective dose of carboplatin and pemeterxed in combination with demcizumab among the patients of non-small cell lung cancer.	NCT01189968
		Phase I non-randomized trial	The study was designed to explore the effectiveness of paclitaxel in combination with demcizumab among the patients with ovarian, fallopian tube, or peritoneal cancer.	NCT01952249
		Phase I interventional trial	The study was designed to explore the safety and efficacy of pembrolizumab in combination with demcizumab among the patients of advanced/metastatic solid tumors.	NCT02722954
Phase II Clinical Trial				
Demcizumab	DLL-4 ligand-targeted antibodies	Phase 2 double-blind randomized trial	The study was designed to explore the efficacy and safety of combination with carboplatin and pemetrexed in combination with demcizumab among the patients of stage IV non-squamous non-small lung cancer.	NCT02259582
		Phase 2 double-blind randomized	The study was designed to explore the efficacy and safety of the combination of gemcitabine and Abraxane® with demcizumab among patients with pancreatic cancer.	NCT02289898
AL101 (BMS-906024)	γ-secretase inhibitor	Phase II open-label, multicenter study	The study was designed to explore the efficacy of AL101 among patients with adenoid cystic carcinoma.	NCT03691207

TABLE 5.1 *(Continued)*

Notch Inhibitors	Class of Drug	Study Type	Study Detail	Clinical Trial Number
Nirogacestat (PF-03084014)	γ-secretase inhibitor	Phase II open-label trial	The study was designed to explore the anticancer effect and tolerability of patients among the patients of advanced triple receptor-negative breast cancer.	NCT02299635
		Phase 2 open-label randomized trial	The study was designed to explore the maximum tolerated dose as well as the safety profile of nirogacestat in combination with gemcitabine and nab-paclitaxel among the patients with metastatic pancreas cancer.	NCT02109445
		Phase 2 open-label randomized trial	The study was designed to explore the efficacy of nirogacestat among patients with desmoid tumors.	NCT01981551
		Phase 2 open-label randomized trial	The study was designed to explore the efficacy, safety, and pharmacokinetic profile of nirogacestat among patients with desmoid tumors.	NCT04195399
RO4929097 (R4733)	γ-secretase inhibitor	Phase 2 open-label trial	The study was designed to explore the efficacy and the safety of RO4929097 among the patients of metastatic epithelial ovarian primary peritoneal cancer.	NCT01175343
		Phase 2 open-label trial	The study was designed to explore the efficacy and the safety of RO4929097 among the patients of advanced non-small cell lung cancer.	NCT01193868
		Phase 2 randomized trial	The study was designed to explore the efficacy of RO4929097 in combination with bicalutamide among patients with prostate cancer.	NCT01200810
		Phase 2 open-label randomized trial	The study was designed to explore the efficacy of chemotherapy and bevacizumab with or without RO4929097 among the patients of metastatic colorectal cancer.	NCT01270438

TABLE 5.1 *(Continued)*

Notch Inhibitors	Class of Drug	Study Type	Study Detail	Clinical Trial Number
		Phase 2 interventional trial	The study was designed to explore the efficacy of RO4929097 after autologous stem cell transplant among patients with multiple myeloma.	NCT01251172
		Phase II open-label trial	The study was designed to explore the efficacy of RO4929097 among the patients who were previously treated for metastatic pancreatic cancer.	NCT01232829
		Phase II non-randomized open-label trial	The study was designed to explore the anticancer, tolerability, and safety of RO4929097 among the patients of non-squamous non-small-cell lung cancer.	NCT01070927
		Phase II open-label trial	The study was designed to explore the anticancer effect (stage IV melanoma) of RO4929097.	NCT01120275
		Phase II non-randomized open-label trial	The study was designed to explore the clinical efficacy of RO4929097 among patients with recurrent or progressive glioblastoma.	NCT01122901
		Phase II open-label trial	The study was designed to explore the clinical efficacy of RO4929097 among patients with renal cell carcinoma.	NCT01141569
Phase III Clinical Trial				
Nirogacestat (PF-03084014)	γ-secretase inhibitor	Phase III double-blind randomized placebo-controlled trial	The study was designed to explore the clinical efficacy of nirogacestat against desmoid tumor.	NCT03785964

Source: Reproduced with permission from Aggarwal et al. (2021); Copyright © Elsevier (2021).

5.6 NOTCH SIGNALING IN CELL MIGRATION AND EMT

Akt signaling has been demonstrated to be critical in triggering Notch-mediated acceleration of cell migration and EMT in addition to other factors (Veeraraghavalu et al., 2005; Strickland & Vande Pol, 2016). HPV16 E7 is also known to directly stimulate Akt signaling in addition to working via the Notch pathway. By binding and sequestering PP2A, which otherwise dephosphorylates Akt, E7 has been shown to enhance the level of Akt phosphorylation (Pim et al., 2005). E7 has also been shown to improve cell migration in keratinocytes, which is also dependent on Akt (Charette & McCance, 2007). The ability of E7 to activate Akt signaling, which affects cell invasion through the regulation of MMP release, is directly influenced by its phosphorylation (Basukala et al., 2019).

Through RhoC, Notch1 signaling has also been identified to alter tumorigenic characteristics in cervical cancer cells. Both Notch1 receptor deletion and treatment with a Notch inhibitor (DAPT-gamma secretase inhibitor) reduced RhoC activity, which resulted in a reduction in cell motility and invasion in a cervical cancer cell line. Table 5.1 summarizes potent drugs targeting crucial elements of NOTCH signaling pathway evaluated in clinical trials. Finally, Notch1 and RhoC co-expression was detected in primary cervical carcinoma biopsies (Srivastava et al., 2010; Zubor et al., 2020).

5.7 CONCLUSION

In conclusion, we discussed the present state of knowledge about Notch signaling in cervical carcinoma, including its connections to HPV oncogenes, involvement in migration and metastasis, intratumoral heterogeneity, and mutations. These findings add to our understanding of Notch signaling in cervical cancer, while also highlighting the intricacy of the process, as well as various unknowns and future directions. Further knowledge could aid in re-evaluating and re-designing therapeutic techniques that target Notch components, as previous attempts to target Notch signaling in several abnormalities.

KEYWORDS

- **cervical cancer**
- **hematological malignancies**
- **heterogeneity**
- **Notch receptors**
- **Notch signaling**
- **proteolytic cleavage**

REFERENCES

Aggarwal, V., Tuli, H. S., Varol, M., et al., (2021). NOTCH signaling: Journey of an evolutionarily conserved pathway in driving tumor progression and its modulation as a therapeutic target. *Critical Reviews in Oncology/Hematology, 164*, 103403. https://doi.org/10.1016/j.critrevonc.2021.103403.

Basukala, O., Mittal, S., Massimi, P., Bestagno, M., & Banks, L., (2019). The HPV-18 E7 CKII phospho acceptor site is required for maintaining the transformed phenotype of cervical tumor-derived cells. *PLoS Pathogens, 15*(5), e1007769.

Bellavia, D., Campese, A. F., Alesse, E., et al., (2000). Constitutive activation of NF-kappaB and T-cell leukemia/lymphoma in notch3 transgenic mice. *The EMBO Journal, 19*(13), 3337–3348.

Blaumueller, C. M., Qi, H., Zagouras, P., & Artavanis-Tsakonas, S., (1997). Intracellular cleavage of notch leads to a heterodimeric receptor on the plasma membrane. *Cell, 90*(2), 281–291.

Bocchetta, M., Miele, L., Pass, H. I., & Carbone, M., (2003). Notch-1 induction, a novel activity of SV40 required for growth of SV40-transformed human mesothelial cells. *Oncogene, 22*(1), 81–89.

Bray, S. J., & Gomez-Lamarca, M., (2018). Notch after cleavage. *Current Opinion in Cell Biology, 51*, 103–109.

Bray, S. J., (2006). Notch signaling: A simple pathway becomes complex. *Nature Reviews Molecular Cell Biology, 7*(9), 678–689.

Brimer, N., & Vande, P. S. B., (2014). Papillomavirus E6 PDZ interactions can be replaced by repression of p53 to promote episomal human papillomavirus genome maintenance. *Journal of Virology, 88*(5), 3027–3030.

Brimer, N., Drews, C. M., & Vande, P. S. B., (2017). Association of papillomavirus E6 proteins with either MAML1 or E6AP clusters E6 proteins by structure, function, and evolutionary relatedness. *PLoS Pathogens, 13*(12), e1006781.

Bzhalava, D., Guan, P., Franceschi, S., Dillner, J., & Clifford, G., (2013). A systematic review of the prevalence of mucosal and cutaneous human papillomavirus types. *Virology, 445*(1, 2), 224–231.

Campos-Parra, A. D., Padua-Bracho, A., Pedroza-Torres, A., et al., (2016). Comprehensive transcriptome analysis identifies pathways with therapeutic potential in locally advanced cervical cancer. *Gynecologic Oncology, 143*(2), 406–413.

Cancer Genome Atlas Research Network, Albert Einstein College of Medicine, Analytical Biological Services, et al., (2017). Integrated genomic and molecular characterization of cervical cancer. *Nature, 543*(7645), 378–384.

Capobianco, A. J., Zagouras, P., Blaumueller, C. M., Artavanis-Tsakonas, S., & Bishop, J. M., (1997). Neoplastic transformation by truncated alleles of human NOTCH1/TAN1 and NOTCH2. *Molecular and Cellular Biology, 17*(11), 6265–6273.

Chakrabarti, O., Veeraraghavalu, K., Tergaonkar, V., Liu, Y., Androphy, E. J., Stanley, M. A., & Krishna, S., (2004). Human papillomavirus type 16 E6 amino acid 83 variants enhance E6-mediated MAPK signaling and differentially regulate tumorigenesis by notch signaling and oncogenic Ras. *Journal of Virology, 78*(11), 5934–5945.

Charette, S. T., & McCance, D. J., (2007). The E7 protein from human papillomavirus type 16 enhances keratinocyte migration in an Akt-dependent manner. *Oncogene, 26*(52), 7386–7390.

Chesters, P. M., & McCance, D. J., (1989). Human papillomavirus types 6 and 16 in cooperation with Ha-ras transform secondary rat embryo fibroblasts. *The Journal of General Virology, 70*(Pt 2), 353–365.

Crabtree, J. S., Singleton, C. S., & Miele, L., (2016). Notch signaling in neuroendocrine tumors. *Frontiers in Oncology, 6*, 94.

Crook, T., Almond, N., Murray, A., Stanley, M., & Crawford, L., (1989). Constitutive expression of c-myc oncogene confers hormone independence and enhanced growth-factor responsiveness on cells transformed by human papilloma virus type 16. *Proceedings of the National Academy of Sciences of the United States of America, 86*(15), 5713–5717.

Crook, T., Storey, A., Almond, N., Osborn, K., & Crawford, L., (1988). Human papillomavirus type 16 cooperates with activated ras and fos oncogenes in the hormone-dependent transformation of primary mouse cells. *Proceedings of the National Academy of Sciences of the United States of America, 85*(23), 8820–8824.

Crook, T., Tidy, J. A., & Vousden, K. H., (1991). Degradation of p53 can be targeted by HPV E6 sequences distinct from those required for p53 binding and trans-activation. *Cell, 67*(3), 547–556.

Crow, J. J., & Albig, A. R., (2020). Notch family members follow stringent requirements for intracellular domain dimerization at sequence-paired sites. *PLoS One, 15*(11), e0234101.

Dang, T. P., Gazdar, A. F., Virmani, A. K., et al., (2000). Chromosome 19 translocation, overexpression of Notch3, and human lung cancer. *Journal of the National Cancer Institute, 92*(16), 1355–1357.

Daniel, B., Rangarajan, A., Mukherjee, G., Vallikad, E., & Krishna, S., (1997). The link between integration and expression of human papillomavirus type 16 genomes and cellular changes in the evolution of cervical intraepithelial neoplastic lesions. *The Journal of General Virology, 78*(Pt 5), 1095–1101.

Egan, S. E., St-Pierre, B., & Leow, C. C., (1998). Notch receptors, partners and regulators: From conserved domains to powerful functions. *Protein Modules in Signal Transduction*, 273–324.

Ellisen, L. W., Bird, J., West, D. C., Soreng, A. L., Reynolds, T. C., Smith, S. D., & Sklar, J., (1991). TAN-1, the human homolog of the Drosophila notch gene, is broken by chromosomal translocations in T lymphoblastic neoplasms. *Cell, 66*(4), 649–661.

Felli, M. P., Vacca, A., Calce, A., et al., (2005). PKC theta mediates pre-TCR signaling and contributes to Notch3-induced T-cell leukemia. *Oncogene, 24*(6), 992–1000.

Fleming, R. J., (1998). Structural conservation of notch receptors and ligands. *Seminars in Cell and Developmental Biology, 9*(6), 599–607.

Fortini, M. E., (2002). Gamma-secretase-mediated proteolysis in cell-surface-receptor signaling. *Nature Reviews Molecular Cell Biology, 3*(9), 673–684.

Fortini, M. E., (2009). Notch signaling: The core pathway and its posttranslational regulation. *Developmental Cell, 16*(5), 633–647.

Fortini, M. E., (2012). Introduction-Notch in development and disease. *Seminars in Cell and Developmental Biology, 23*(4), 419–420.

Fuchs, E., (2009). Finding one's niche in the skin. *Cell Stem Cell, 4*(6), 499–502.

Gupta, S., Kumar, P., & Das, B. C., (2018). HPV: Molecular pathways and targets. *Current Problems in Cancer, 42*(2), 161–174.

Handford, P. A., Korona, B., Suckling, R., Redfield, C., & Lea, S. M., (2018). Structural insights into notch receptor-ligand interactions. *Advances in Experimental Medicine and Biology, 1066*, 33–46.

Hendrix, M. J., Seftor, R. E., Seftor, E. A., et al., (2002). Transendothelial function of human metastatic melanoma cells: Role of the microenvironment in cell-fate determination. *Cancer Research, 62*(3), 665–668.

Hozumi, K., (2020). Distinctive properties of the interactions between notch and notch ligands. *Development, Growth and Differentiation, 62*(1), 49–58.

Hsieh, J. J., Henkel, T., Salmon, P., Robey, E., Peterson, M. G., & Hayward, S. D., (1996). Truncated mammalian Notch1 activates CBF1/RBPJk-repressed genes by a mechanism resembling that of Epstein-Barr virus EBNA2. *Molecular and Cellular Biology, 16*(3), 952–959.

Hubmann, R., Schwarzmeier, J. D., Shehata, M., Hilgarth, M., Duechler, M., Dettke, M., & Berger, R., (2002). Notch2 is involved in the overexpression of CD23 in B-cell chronic lymphocytic leukemia. *Blood, 99*(10), 3742–3747.

Huibregtse, J. M., Scheffner, M., & Howley, P. M., (1993). Cloning and expression of the cDNA for E6-AP, a protein that mediates the interaction of the human papillomavirus E6 oncoprotein with p53. *Molecular and Cellular Biology, 13*(2), 775–784.

Huo, W., Zhai, S., Wang, Y., et al., (2020). Relevance research between the expression of p16INK4a, Notch1, and hTERC genes: The development of HPV16-positive cervical cancer. *Journal of Clinical Laboratory Analysis, 34*(5), e23207.

Jang, M. S., Zlobin, A., Kast, W. M., & Miele, L., (2000). Notch signaling as a target in multimodality cancer therapy. *Current Opinion in Molecular Therapeutics, 2*(1), 55–65.

Jundt, F., Anagnostopoulos, I., Förster, R., Mathas, S., Stein, H., & Dörken, B., (2002). Activated Notch1 signaling promotes tumor cell proliferation and survival in Hodgkin and anaplastic large cell lymphoma. *Blood, 99*(9), 3398–3403.

Jundt, F., Pröbsting, K. S., Anagnostopoulos, I., Muehlinghaus, G., Chatterjee, M., Mathas, S., Bargou, R. C., et al., (2004). Jagged1-induced notch signaling drives proliferation of multiple myeloma cells. *Blood, 103*(9), 3511–3515.

Kazem, S., Van, D. M. E., Struijk, L., De Gruijl, F. R., & Feltkamp, M. C., (2012). Human papillomavirus 8 E6 disrupts terminal skin differentiation and prevents pro-Caspase-14 cleavage. *Virus Research, 163*(2), 609–616.

Kennedy, E. M., Kornepati, A. V., Goldstein, M., et al., (2014). Inactivation of the human papillomavirus E6 or E7 gene in cervical carcinoma cells by using a bacterial CRISPR/Cas RNA-guided endonuclease. *Journal of Virology, 88*(20), 11965–11972.

Khan, F., Pandey, P., Jha, N. K., Khalid, M., & Ojha, S., (2021). Rutin mediated apoptotic cell death in Caski cervical cancer cells via Notch-1 and Hes-1 downregulation. *Life, 11*(8), 761.

Klueg, K. M., & Muskavitch, M. A., (1999). Ligand-receptor interactions and trans-endocytosis of delta, serrate and notch: Members of the notch signaling pathway in *Drosophila. Journal of Cell Science, 112*(Pt 19), 3289–3297.

Kopan, R., & Ilagan, M. X., (2009). The canonical notch signaling pathway: Unfolding the activation mechanism. *Cell, 137*(2), 216–233.

Kortschak, R. D., Tamme, R., & Lardelli, M., (2001). Evolutionary analysis of vertebrate notch genes. *Development, Genes and Evolution, 211*(7), 350–354.

Kovall, R. A., Gebelein, B., Sprinzak, D., & Kopan, R., (2017). The canonical notch signaling pathway: Structural and biochemical insights into shape, sugar, and force. *Developmental Cell, 41*(3), 228–241.

Lathion, S., Schaper, J., Beard, P., & Raj, K., (2003). Notch1 can contribute to viral-induced transformation of primary human keratinocytes. *Cancer Research, 63*(24), 8687–8694.

Lee, M., Kim, H. J., Kim, S. W., et al., (2016). The long non-coding RNA HOTAIR increases tumor growth and invasion in cervical cancer by targeting the notch pathway. *Oncotarget, 7*(28), 44558–44571.

Leethanakul, C., Patel, V., Gillespie, J., et al., (2000). Distinct pattern of expression of differentiation and growth-related genes in squamous cell carcinomas of the head and neck revealed by the use of laser capture microdissection and cDNA arrays. *Oncogene, 19*(28), 3220–3224.

Li, L., Tang, P., Li, S., Qin, X., Yang, H., Wu, C., & Liu, Y., (2017). Notch signaling pathway networks in cancer metastasis: A new target for cancer therapy. *Medical Oncology, 34*(10), 180.

Lian, H., Hui, Y., Xiaoping, T., Wei, T., Jiyi, X., & Xiaolan, Y., (2019). Baicalein suppresses the proliferation of human cervical cancer cells via notch 1/Hes signaling pathway. *Journal of Cancer Research and Therapeutics, 15*(6), 1216–1220.

Liu, Z. J., Xiao, M., Balint, K., et al., (2006). Notch1 signaling promotes primary melanoma progression by activating mitogen-activated protein kinase/phosphatidylinositol 3-kinase-Akt pathways and up-regulating N-cadherin expression. *Cancer Research, 66*(8), 4182–4190.

Logeat, F., Bessia, C., Brou, C., LeBail, O., Jarriault, S., Seidah, N. G., & Israël, A., (1998). The Notch1 receptor is cleaved constitutively by a furin-like convertase. *Proceedings of the National Academy of Sciences of the United States of America, 95*(14), 8108–8112.

Matlashewski, G., Schneider, J., Banks, L., Jones, N., Murray, A., & Crawford, L., (1987). Human papillomavirus type 16 DNA cooperates with activated ras in transforming primary cells. *The EMBO Journal, 6*(6), 1741–1746.

Meyers, J. M., Spangle, J. M., & Munger, K., (2013). The human papillomavirus type 8 E6 protein interferes with NOTCH activation during keratinocyte differentiation. *Journal of Virology, 87*(8), 4762–4767.

Müller, C. S., (2012). Notch signaling and malignant melanoma. *Advances in Experimental Medicine and Biology, 727*, 258–264.

Mumm, J. S., & Kopan, R., (2000). Notch signaling: From the outside in. *Developmental Biology, 228*(2), 151–165.

Muñoz, N., Bosch, F. X., De Sanjosé, S., et al., (2003). Epidemiologic classification of human papillomavirus types associated with cervical cancer. *The New England Journal of Medicine, 348*(6), 518–527.

Nicolas, M., Wolfer, A., Raj, K., et al., (2003). Notch1 functions as a tumor suppressor in mouse skin. *Nature Genetics, 33*(3), 416–421.

Ojesina, A. I., Lichtenstein, L., Freeman, S. S., et al., (2014). Landscape of genomic alterations in cervical carcinomas. *Nature, 506*(7488), 371–375.

Okuyama, R., LeFort, K., & Dotto, G. P., (2004). A dynamic model of keratinocyte stem cell renewal and differentiation: Role of the p21WAF1/Cip1 and Notch1 signaling pathways. *The Journal of Investigative Dermatology, 9*(3), 248–252.

Padash, B. M., Gilbert, M., Thomas, M., Banks, L., Zhang, B., & Auld, V. J., (2016). A Drosophila model of HPV E6-induced malignancy reveals essential roles for magi and the insulin receptor. *PLoS Pathogens, 12*(8), e1005789.

Palmer, W. H., & Deng, W. M., (2015). Ligand-independent mechanisms of notch activity. *Trends in Cell Biology, 25*(11), 697–707.

Palomero, T., & Ferrando, A., (2009). Therapeutic targeting of NOTCH1 signaling in T-cell acute lymphoblastic leukemia. *Clinical Lymphoma and Myeloma, 9*(S3), S205–S210.

Pang, R. T., Leung, C. O., Ye, T. M., et al., (2010). MicroRNA-34a suppresses invasion through downregulation of Notch1 and Jagged1 in cervical carcinoma and choriocarcinoma cells. *Carcinogenesis, 31*(6), 1037–1044.

Pattabiraman, C., Hong, S., Gunasekharan, V. K., et al., (2014). CD66+ cells in cervical precancers are partially differentiated progenitors with neoplastic traits. *Cancer Research, 74*(22), 6682–6692.

Pear, W. S., Aster, J. C., Scott, M. L., Hasserjian, R. P., Soffer, B., Sklar, J., & Baltimore, D., (1996). Exclusive development of T cell neoplasms in mice transplanted with bone marrow expressing activated notch alleles. *The Journal of Experimental Medicine, 183*(5), 2283–2291.

Pim, D., Massimi, P., Dilworth, S. M., & Banks, L., (2005). Activation of the protein kinase B pathway by the HPV-16 E7 oncoprotein occurs through a mechanism involving interaction with PP2A. *Oncogene, 24*(53), 7830–7838.

Rae, F. K., Stephenson, S. A., Nicol, D. L., & Clements, J. A., (2000). Novel association of a diverse range of genes with renal cell carcinoma as identified by differential display. *International Journal of Cancer, 88*(5), 726–732.

Ramachandran, D., & Dörk, T., (2021). Genomic risk factors for cervical cancer. *Cancers, 13*(20), 5137.

Rangarajan, A., Syal, R., Selvarajah, S., Chakrabarti, O., Sarin, A., & Krishna, S., (2001). Activated Notch1 signaling cooperates with papillomavirus oncogenes in transformation and generates resistance to apoptosis on matrix withdrawal through PKB/Akt. *Virology, 286*(1), 23–30.

Rong, C., Feng, Y., & Ye, Z., (2017). Notch is a critical regulator in cervical cancer by regulating numb splicing. *Oncology Letters, 13*(4), 2465–2470.

Scheffner, M., Werness, B. A., Huibregtse, J. M., Levine, A. J., & Howley, P. M., (1990). The E6 oncoprotein encoded by human papillomavirus types 16 and 18 promotes the degradation of p53. *Cell, 63*(6), 1129–1136.

Srivastava, S., Ramdass, B., Nagarajan, S., Rehman, M., Mukherjee, G., & Krishna, S., (2010). Notch1 regulates the functional contribution of RhoC to cervical carcinoma progression. *British Journal of Cancer, 102*(1), 196–205.

Steinbuck, M. P., & Winandy, S., (2018). A review of notch processing with new insights into ligand-independent notch signaling in T-cells. *Frontiers in Immunology, 9*, 1230.

Strickland, S. W., & Vande, P. S., (2016). The human papillomavirus 16 E7 oncoprotein attenuates AKT signaling to promote internal ribosome entry site-dependent translation and expression of c-MYC. *Journal of Virology, 90*(12), 5611–5621.

Subramanyam, D., & Krishna, S., (2006). c-Myc substitutes for Notch1-CBF1 functions in cooperative transformation with papillomavirus oncogenes. *Virology, 347*(1), 191–198.

Suzuki, T., Aoki, D., Susumu, N., Udagawa, Y., & Nozawa, S., (2000). Imbalanced expression of TAN-1 and human Notch4 in endometrial cancers. *International Journal of Oncology, 17*(6), 1131–1139.

Tan, M. J., White, E. A., Sowa, M. E., Harper, J. W., Aster, J. C., & Howley, P. M., (2012). Cutaneous β-human papillomavirus E6 proteins bind mastermind-like coactivators and repress notch signaling. *Proceedings of the National Academy of Sciences of the United States of America, 109*(23), E1473–E1480.

Vande, P. S., (2015). Papillomavirus E6 oncoproteins take common structural approaches to solve different biological problems. *PLoS Pathogens, 11*(10), e1005138.

Vázquez-Ulloa, E., Ramos-Cruz, A. C., Prada, D., et al., (2018). Loss of nuclear NOTCH1, but not its negative regulator NUMB, is an independent predictor of cervical malignancy. *Oncotarget, 9*(27), 18916–18928.

Veeraraghavalu, K., Subbaiah, V. K., Srivastava, S., Chakrabarti, O., Syal, R., & Krishna, S., (2005). Complementation of human papillomavirus type 16 E6 and E7 by Jagged1-specific Notch1-phosphatidylinositol 3-kinase signaling involves pleiotropic oncogenic functions independent of CBF1; Su(H); Lag-1 activation. *Journal of Virology, 79*(12), 7889–7898.

Veldman, T., Liu, X., Yuan, H., & Schlegel, R., (2003). Human papillomavirus E6 and Myc proteins associate *in vivo* and bind to and cooperatively activate the telomerase reverse transcriptase promoter. *Proceedings of the National Academy of Sciences of the United States of America, 100*(14), 8211–8216.

Vliet-Gregg, P. A., Hamilton, J. R., & Katzenellenbogen, R. A., (2013). NFX1-123 and human papillomavirus 16E6 increase notch expression in keratinocytes. *Journal of Virology, 87*(24), 13741–13750.

Wang, M. M., (2011). Notch signaling and notch signaling modifiers. *The International Journal of Biochemistry and Cell Biology, 43*(11), 1550–1562.

Wang, W., Sima, N., Kong, D., et al., (2010). Selective targeting of HPV-16 E6/E7 in cervical cancer cells with a potent oncolytic adenovirus and its enhanced effect with radiotherapy *in vitro* and *vivo*. *Cancer Letters, 291*(1), 67–75.

Weijzen, S., Rizzo, P., Braid, M., et al., (2002). Activation of Notch-1 signaling maintains the neoplastic phenotype in human Ras-transformed cells. *Nature Medicine, 8*(9), 979–986.

Weijzen, S., Zlobin, A., Braid, M., Miele, L., & Kast, W. M., (2003). HPV16 E6 and E7 oncoproteins regulate notch-1 expression and cooperate to induce transformation. *Journal of Cellular Physiology, 194*(3), 356–362.

Werness, B. A., Levine, A. J., & Howley, P. M., (1990). Association of human papillomavirus types 16 and 18 E6 proteins with p53. *Science, 248*(4951), 76–79.

Xia, X., Qian, S., Soriano, S., et al., (2001). Loss of presenilin 1 is associated with enhanced beta-catenin signaling and skin tumorigenesis. *Proceedings of the National Academy of Sciences of the United States of America, 98*(19), 10863–10868.

Yin, F., Wang, N., Wang, S., et al., (2017). HPV16 oncogenes E6 or/and E7 may influence the methylation status of RASSFIA gene promoter region in cervical cancer cell line HT-3. *Oncology Reports, 37*(4), 2324–2334.

Yousif, N. G., Sadiq, A. M., Yousif, M. G., Al-Mudhafar, R. H., Al-Baghdadi, J. J., & Hadi, N., (2015). Notch1 ligand signaling pathway activated in cervical cancer: Poor prognosis with high-level JAG1/Notch1. *Archives of Gynecology and Obstetrics, 292*(4), 899–904.

Yugawa, T., Handa, K., Narisawa-Saito, M., Ohno, S., Fujita, M., & Kiyono, T., (2007). Regulation of Notch1 gene expression by p53 in epithelial cells. *Molecular and Cellular Biology, 27*(10), 3732–3742.

Zhang, F., Zhang, J., Li, X., Li, B., Tao, K., & Yue, S., (2018). Notch signaling pathway regulates the cell cycle in proliferating hepatocytes involved in liver regeneration. *Journal of Gastroenterology and Hepatology, 33*(8), 1538–1547.

Zhdanovskaya, N., Firrincieli, M., Lazzari, S., et al., (2021). Targeting notch to maximize chemotherapeutic benefits: Rationale, advanced strategies, and future perspectives. *Cancers, 13*(20), 5106.

Zhou, B., Lin, W., Long, Y., et al., (2022). Notch signaling pathway: Architecture, disease, and therapeutics. *Signal Transduction and Targeted Therapy, 7*, 95. https://doi.org/10.1038/s41392-022-00934-y.

Zubor, P., Dankova, Z., Kolkova, Z., et al., (2020). Rho GTPases in gynecologic cancers: In-depth analysis toward the paradigm change from reactive to predictive, preventive, and personalized medical approach benefiting the patient and healthcare. *Cancers, 12*(5), 1292.

CHAPTER 6

Apoptotic Pathways in Cervical Cancer Management

6.1 APOPTOSIS IN CANCER

Cell death and survival must be balanced for the maintenance of tissue homeostasis, and any dysregulation in this balance can lead to carcinogenesis (Bunz, 2001; Kaczanowski, 2016; Xu et al., 2019; Kashyap et al., 2021). Cells have an intrinsic regulatory mechanism for controlling apoptosis associated tissue homeostasis (Godlewski & Kobylińska, 2016). Furthermore, any flaws in apoptosis-inducing pathways could lead to the growth of cancerous cells (Fulda, 2015; Kiraz et al., 2016; Pistritto et al., 2016). There are mainly two major alternative apoptotic initiation pathways viz. extrinsic and intrinsic apoptotic pathways. Extrinsic pathway (mediated via death receptors on cell surface) gets activated upon binding of death inducing ligands to death receptors and leading to activation of caspases (3, 6, 8, 10, and 7) activation (Solary et al., 2001; Fan et al., 2005; Kumar & Dorstyn, 2009). The intrinsic apoptosis process, which is controlled by mitochondria and is primarily regulated by Fas and TRAIL receptors expressed by many normal epithelial cells, is another apoptotic pathway (Sartorius et al., 2001). Pro caspase 9, which is activated downstream of mitochondrial pro-apoptotic events at the cytosolic death signaling protein complex (apoptosome) generated upon mitochondrial cytochrome c release, is part of the intrinsic apoptotic pathway. Procaspase-9 molecules dimerize primarily at the Apaf-1 scaffold, which is responsible for caspase-9 activation (Kim et al., 2015). Following the activation of initiator caspases, effector pro-caspases (7, 6, and 3)

Cervical Cancer: Signaling Pathways, Molecular Mechanisms, Natural Products, and Therapeutic Approaches. Pratibha Pandey, Fahad Khan, Saher Islam, and Devarajan Thangadurai, (Eds.)

are activated, resulting in the cleavage of particular protein substrates (Boatright & Salvesen, 2003; Wang et al., 2005). At various cellular levels, several proteins regulate these apoptotic events. FADD-like interleukin-1β converting enzyme-like protease (FLIPs) and FADD-like ICE (FLICE) are two inhibitory proteins that interfere with apoptosis initiation directly at the death receptor level (Gaur & Aggarwal, 2003). Another inhibitory protein IAPs (regulatory proteins) are mainly apoptosis protein inhibitors that inhibit caspases upon their binding. IAPs might also act as ubiquitin ligases that mainly promotes caspase (Straub, 2011; Kumar et al., 2020) (Figure 6.1 and Table 6.1).

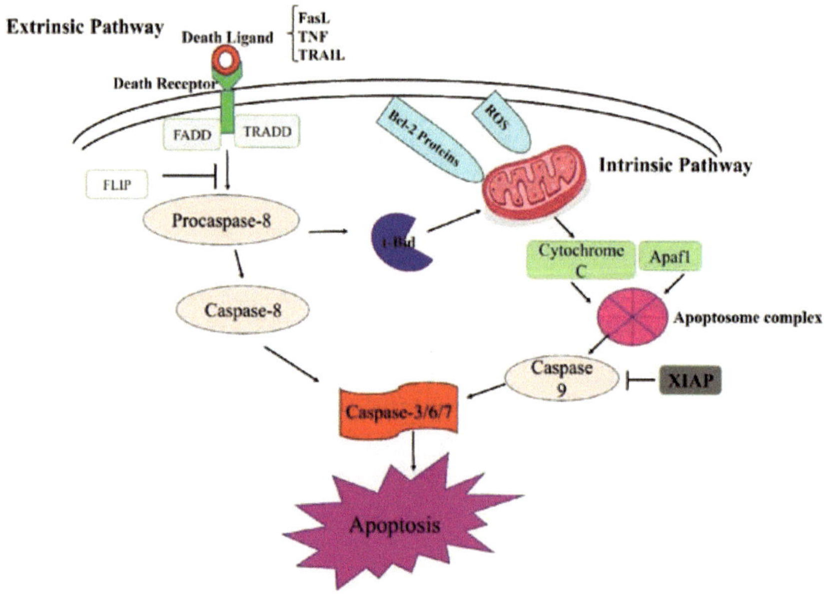

FIGURE 6.1 Outline of the extrinsic (mitochondrial-independent) and intrinsic (mitochondrial-dependent) apoptosis signaling cascade and their key regulatory mediators.

Most crucial feature in cancer progression is viral mediated apoptosis modulation supporting growth, immortalization, and cancer (Zhou et al., 2017). Overexpression of E6 protein leads to p53 degradation via ubiquitin proteasome pathways, and cervical cancer progression has been significantly linked to disruption of the apoptotic pathway (Li et al., 2005, 2019). In malignant cells, these apoptotic pathways are frequently reported to be dysregulated, resulting in uncontrolled cell growth and proliferation (Cai

TABLE 6.1 Clinical Trial Status of Bcl-2 Inhibitors

Drugs	Targets	Phase	Cancer types	Dose	ClinicalTrails.gov identifier
ABT-263 + Ruxolitinib	Bcl2, Bcl-xl, and Bcl-w	Phase II(R)	Myelofibrosis	ABT-263 QD at various doses + Ruxolitinib BID (≥10 mg)	NCT03222609
ABT-263		Phase II(C)	Chronic lymphocytic leukemia (CLL)	ABT-263 QD	NCT01557777
ABT-263 + Vistusertib		Phase I/II(R)	Relapsed small cell lung cancer and other solid tumors	ABT-263 orally QD and Vistusertib BID on days 1–28	NCT03366103
ABT-263 + Gemcitabine		Phase I(C)	Solid tumors	ABT-263 150 mg taken orally QD on Days 1–3 and Days 8–10 out of each 21-day cycle. ABT-263 325 mg taken orally QD on days 1–3, 8–10, 15–17 out of each 28-day cycle. Gemcitabine 1000 mg/m^2 administered on Day 1 and Day 8 intravenously of each 21-day cycle. Gemcitabine 1000 mg/m^2 administered on days 1, 8 and 15 intravenously of each 28-day cycle.	NCT00887757
ABT-263 + venetoclax + chemotherapy		Phase I(R)	Lymphoblastic lymphoma and acute lymphoblastic leukemia (ALL)	Venetoclax QD starting on Day 1 and ABT-263 QD starting on Day 3 weight-adjusted doses were administered orally + chemotherapy (peg-asparaginase, vincristine, dexamethasone) and tyrosine kinase inhibitor.	NCT03181126
ABT-263 + paclitaxel		Phase I(C)	Solid tumors	ABT-263 + paclitaxel Phase I(C) Solid tumors ABT-263 150 mg is administered orally QD on Days 1–3 + paclitaxel 175 mg/m^2 over 3 h administered intravenously on Day 1 of each 21-day cycle.	NCT00891605
Venetoclax	Bcl-2	Phase I(R)	Paediatric and young subjects with recurrent or refractory cancer.	Venetoclax is given orally QD with or without chemotherapy at various doses and dosing regimens.	NCT03236857

TABLE 6.1 (Continued)

Drugs	Targets	Phase	Cancer types	Dose	ClinicalTrails.gov identifier
Venetoclax		Phase III(A)	R/R CLL patients who have 17p deletion or TP53 mutation or who have previously undergone treatment with a B-cell receptor antagonist.	Venetoclax is given orally at a dose of 20 mg QD, starting with adose-titration stage, and increasing up to 400 mg QD.	NCT02756611
Venetoclax		Phase II(R)	Chronic lymphocytic leukemia (CLL) in presence of 17p deletion	Venetoclax is administered orally starting at a dose of 20 mg QD; dose escalation will proceed weekly in the following progression: 50, 100, 200, and 400 mg QD, as tolerated.	NCT02966756
Venetoclax + Standard chemotherapeutics		Phase I(R)	Acute lymphoblastic leukemia (ALL)	Venetoclax is given orally QD for 21 days in each cycle + Standard chemotherapy will be given every 28 days	NCT0331990
Azacitidine + Venetoclaxx		Phase II(R)	Old age patients with acute myeloid leukemia (AML)	Azacitidine is administered at dose of 75 mg/m^2 in days 1–7 of cycle; if no response repeat it in cycle 2 and 3 + Starting on day 2 of cycle 1, Venetoclax is given orally with increased dose upto 600 mg.	NCT03466294
Venetoclax + Ibrutinib		Phase II(R)	Chronic lymphocytic leukemia (CLL) or solid lymphocytic leukemia.	Venetoclax is administered at a dose of 20 mg QD; dose escalation will proceed weekly in the following progression: 50 mg QD, 100 mg QD, 200 mg QD, 400 mg QD, as tolerated + Ibrutinib is given orally up to 420 mg/day.	NCT02756897
Duvelisib + Ventoclax		Phase II(R)	Relapsed/refractory CLL or SLL	For the first seven days Duvelisib will be administered alone BID for the first seven days. On day 8 Venetoclax will be added orally QD.	NCT03534323

TABLE 6.1 (Continued)

Drugs	Targets	Phase	Cancer types	Dose	ClinicalTrails.gov identifier
Venetoclax + Alvocidib		Phase I(R)	Relapsed or refractory acute myeloid leukemia (AML)	Venetoclax given orally QD and Alvocidib is given as an intravenous infusion on days 1, 2, and 3 for all 28-day treatment cycles.	NCT03441555
Venetoclax + Dexamethasone		Phase I(R)	AL amyloidosis	Venetoclax administered at one of four escalating doses (100 mg/day, 200 mg/day, 400 mg/day, or 800 mg/day) orally on each day of the cycle + Dexamethasone administered at a dose of 20 mg orally on days 1, 8, 15, and 22 of each cycle.	NCT03000660
Oblimeresen + Cisplatin and 5-fluorouraci	Bcl-2	Phase I/II(T)	Gastric and esophageal cancer	In Phase I patients were given oblimersen I.V on days 1–7, fluorouracil I.V on days 4–8, and cisplatin I.V on day 4. Courses continue every 21 days in the absence of unacceptable toxicity or disease progression. Cohorts of 3–6 patients receive escalating doses of oblimersen until the maximum tolerated dose (MTD) is determined. An additional 12 patients are treated at the MTD. In Phase II Patients were treated as in phase I with oblimersen at the MTD.	NCT00064259
Oblimersen + Rituximab		Phase II(T)	Stage II, stage III, or stage IV follicular non-Hodgkin's lymphoma	In induction therapy, patients were administered with oblimeresen I.V on days 1–7 and 15–21 and rituximab I.V on days 3, 10, 17, and 24 in month 1. Then in extended induction therapy (months 3, 5, 7, and 9) Patients were administered with oblimersen I.V on days 22–28 and rituximab I.V on day 24 in months 3, 5, 7, and 9. Treatment continues for 9 months in the absence of unacceptable toxicity or disease progression.	NCT00301795

TABLE 6.1 (Continued)

Drugs	Targets	Phase	Cancer types	Dose	ClinicalTrails.gov identifier
Carboplatin and etoposide + Oblimersen		Phase I(C)	Aggressive small cell lung cancer stage	Patients were given oblimersen I.V on days 1–8, etoposide IV over 1 h on days 6–8 and carboplatin I.V over 30 min on day 6. Treatment was repeated for every three weeks for up to six times in the lack of disease advancement or intolerable toxicity.	NCT00017251
Fludarabine + cyclophosphamide with or without oblimersen		Phase III(C)	R/R CLL	In Arm 1 Patients were treated with oblimersen I.V on days 1–7 and fludarabine I.V over 20–30 min and cyclophosphamide I.V over 30–60 min on days 5–7. Patients were also given filgrastim S.C starting on 11 days and maintained until their blood levels improved. In Arm 2 Patients were treated with fludarabine I.V over 20–30 min followed by cyclophosphamide I.V over 30–60 min on days 1–3. Patients were also given filgrastim S.C starting on day 7 and ongoing until blood counts improved. Therapy across both arms repeated every 28 days for up to six sessions in the lack of unacceptable toxicity or disease progression.	NCT00024440
Oblimersen + Fludarabine and Rituximab		Phase I(C)	Chronic lymphocytic leukemia	4-week cycles; Cycle 1: oblimersen (1.5 mg/kg/d) by constant intravenous injection for 7 days, ending on Day 8; rituximab (125 mg/m^2) by intravenous injection on Day 4 and Day 6 (250 mg/m^2); fludarabine (25 mg/m^2) by constant intravenous injection for 3 days, beginning on Day 6. Successive cycles: oblimersen (3 mg/kg/d), finishing on Day 8; rituximab (375 mg/m^2) on Day 5; fludarabine (25 mg/m^2) for 3 days beginning on the same day as rituximab.	NCT00078234

TABLE 6.1 (Continued)

Drugs	Targets	Phase	Cancer types	Dose	ClinicalTrails.gov identifier
AT101 + erlotinib	Bcl-2, Bcl-xl, and Mcl-1	Phase II(T)	High grade non-small cell lung cancer (NSCLC)	Erlotinib 100 mg orally OQ was given to patients, and pulsed doses of AT-101 were given at a dose of 40 mg BID on days 1–3 of a 21-day cycle. If the initial combination doses are tolerated then, dose elevation of erlotinib upto 150 mg daily will be permitted.	NCT00988169
Obatoclax	Bcl-2, Bcl-w, Bclb, Bfl-1, Mcl-1 and Bcl-xl	Phase II(C)	Previously untreated acute myeloid leukemia	A 3-h IV infusion for 3 consecutive days or a 24-h infusion for 3 consecutive days every 2 weeks for up to 6 cycles.	NCT00684918
Obatoclax		Phase I(C)	Untreated chronic lymphocytic leukemia.	A 60-min or 3-h IV infusion every 2–3 weeks.	NCT00600964
Obatoclax+ Rituximab		Phase II(C)	Previously untreated follicular lymphoma	40 mg obatoclax mesaylate over 3 h q/weekly for 12 weeks, 4 weeks in combination with rituximab and another 8 weeks as a single-agent. About 60 mg obatoclax mesylate over 24 h, q/weekly for 12 weeks, 4 weeks combo with rituximab, another 8 weeks single agent obatoclax.	NCT00427856
Obatoclax + Fludarabine + Rituximab		Phase I(T)	Previously treated chronic lymphocytic leukemia	Patients receive obatoclax mesylate IV over 3 h on days 1 and 3, fludarabine IV over 20–30 min on days 1–5, and rituximab IV over 4 h on day 1 (days 1 and 3 of course 1 only). The treatment repeated every 28 days for up to six sessions in the lack of disease advancement or intolerable toxicity.	NCT00612612

TABLE 6.1 (Continued)

Drugs	Targets	Phase	Cancer types	Dose	ClinicalTrails.gov identifier
Obatoclax		Phase I(C)	Hematological malignancies	Patients receive obatoclax mesylate IV over 3 h on days 1 and 3, fludarabine IV over 20–30 min on days 1–5, and rituximab IV over 4 h on day 1 (days 1 and 3 of course 1 only). Treatment repeats every 28 days for up to 6 courses in the absence of disease progression or unacceptable toxicity.	NCT00438178
Obatoclax + Carboplatin and etoposide		Phase I/II(C)	Extensive-stage small cell lung cancer	In Phase IA Obatoclax for 3 h for 3 days with carboplatin/etoposide. In Phase IB Obatoclax for 24 h for 3 days with carboplatin/etoposide. In Phase IIA Obatoclax for 3 h for 3 days with carboplatin/etoposide. Phase II B Carboplatin + etoposide without further study-related care.	NCT00682981
S55746	Bcl-2	Phase I (ANR)	Chronic lymphocytic leukemia and B-cell non-Hodgkin lymphoma	Oral administration of drug S 55746 and dose increase from 50–1,500 mg. Treatment will be given in 21-day cycles to participants up until a stopping point is reached.	NCT02920697
BCL 201 + Idelalisib		Phase I(C)	Follicular lymphoma and mantle cell lymphoma	–	NCT02603445
APG-1252	Bcl-xl and Bcl-2	Phase I(R)	SCLC or advanced solid tumors	The starting dose for this study was 40 mg and 1 patient would be enrolled at this dose level. The dose escalation will convert to a standard 3 + 3 design following the occurrence of DLT or two ≥ Grade 2 adverse event or at doses 80 mg.	NCT03387332

Source: Reproduced with permission from Suvarna et al. (2019); Copyright © Elsevier (2019).

et al., 2013). In gynecological carcinomas, Fas down regulation has also been recognized as a frequent aberration (Nagat, 1996; Wu et al., 2012). In cervical cancer patients, TRAIL, FasL, and death receptors are widely expressed in the cytoplasm of tumor cells. Because TRAIL, DR4, and DR5 have been widely documented, and TRAIL expression has been found to be lacking in cervical cancer patients after radiotherapy (Zhou et al., 2006; Zucchi et al., 2009). In raft cultures of E5 expressing keratinocytes that were totally shielded against TRAIL and FasL induced cell death, HPV E5 protein damages FasL and TRAIL mediated apoptosis induction by downregulating Fas receptor and preventing DISC formation (Komposch et al., 2004). Similarly, E5 expressing human keratinocytes are protected against apoptosis when exposed to UV light for stress induction (Zhang et al., 2002).

6.2 APOPTOSIS PATHWAY IN CERVICAL CANCER

Apoptotic signaling pathways are connected with various therapeutic targets in cervical cancer. The fundamental mechanism of therapeutic techniques that have been developed or are being explored has been reported to be apoptosis induction (Liu et al., 2021). Several therapeutic techniques have successfully triggered apoptosis in cervical cancer cells, including the use of aspirin or luteolin alone or in combination with radiotherapy, or the use of TRAIL (apoptotic inducers) (Im & Jang, 2012; Hua et al., 2019). A broader spectrum of pro-apoptotic chemicals has been evaluated in cervical cancer cells in recent research studies (Figure 6.2).

In SiHa and CaSki cells, a Flavonoid derivate (N101-2 molecule) induced apoptosis by arresting cell cycle growth at the G1 phase, resulting in the activation of intrinsic pathways and inhibition of the PI3K/Akt signaling pathway (Kim et al., 2012). Likewise, silibilin treatment also resulted in dose dependent apoptosis induction in HeLa cells via activating both death receptor and mitochondrial mediated pathways (Zhang et al., 2012). Ganoderic acid derivatives have also displayed potent therapeutic potential in HeLa cervical cancer cells by apoptosis induction via reducing MMP (mitochondrial membrane potential) (Liu et al., 2015). Retinoids (Vitamin A related compound) has been reported to be a significant chemo preventive agent in HPV-associated cervical cancers. Studies conducted *in vitro* have demonstrated that retinoids exposure caused down-regulation

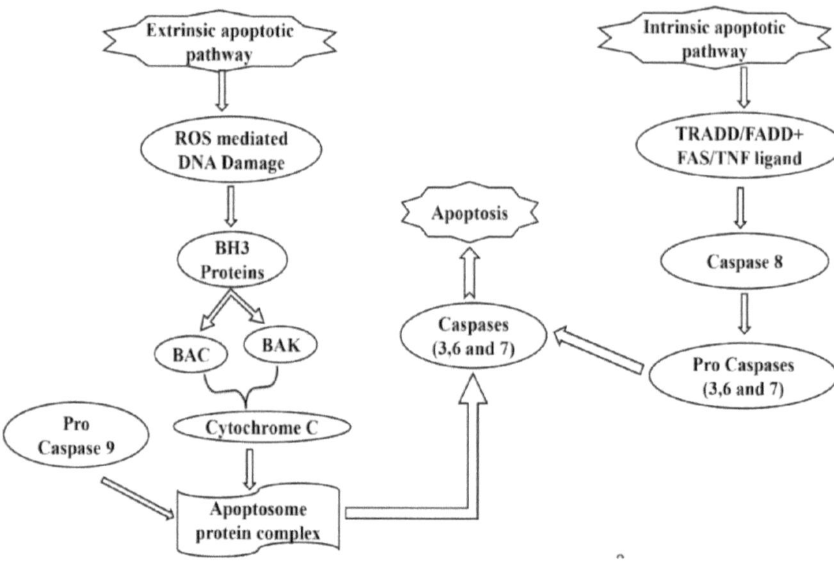

FIGURE 6.2 Apoptosis and cervical cancer.

of E6/E7 transcription level and up-regulation of p53 expression in HPV immortalized keratinocytes and cervical cancer cells along with deregulation of IGF and EGF cell signaling pathways, Fas induction and increased Fas or Fas ligand mediated apoptosis induction (Scribner & Benbrook, 2002; Abu et al., 2005; Helm et al., 2013). I3C has also displayed chemo preventive potential via apoptosis induction and anti-estrogenic potential in several preclinical studies (Jin et al., 1999; Grimminger et al., 2000; Chen et al., 2001). Studies have also reported a dramatic reduction in cancer incidences in transgenic mice fed with I3C supplemented diet (Qi et al., 2005).

On the other hand, DIM (3,3-diindolylmethane) polymer derived from I3C exhibited significant anti-proliferative and pro-apoptotic efficacies in cellular model via deregulating PI3K and MAPK signaling pathways when used as monodrug (Zhu et al., 2012).

Wen et al. has also reported apoptosis induction by arsenic trioxide treatment via reducing cell proliferation and specifically targeting HPV expressing cells in comparison to control cells. This reduction has been due to E6 down regulation and subsequent p53 release and caspase 3 levels leading to cell death (Wen et al., 2012). Cell death induction in tumor is undoubtedly an endpoint for cancer treatments related to cervical cancer and various registered protocols on www.clinicaltrails.gov aim to improve overall survival rate with low toxicity and a high apoptotic rate.

6.3 APOPTOSIS AND HPV

Pathogenic viruses utilize numerous strategies to deregulate apoptosis response during their infection to human. Loss of pro-apoptotic protein expression in several neoplasis may lead to delayed or dysregulated apoptosis, thereby promoting tumor growth (Zantl et al., 2007). Several studies have reported multiple variations in caspase (both effector and initiator) expression levels in HPV+ve cervical cancer cells (Hirchaud et al., 2013; Chiu et al., 2014; Wang et al., 2019). The viral genome is episomal during the initial stages of HPV-16 infection and comprises of increased E5 mRNA transcripts. Studies have proposed that death receptor mediated apoptotic inhibition in human keratinocytes are required for preventing apoptosis at the initial stage of viral infection, has been the key role of HR-HPV E5 protein. HPV16 E5 protein inhibits TRAIL and CD95L-mediated apoptosis in HaCaT cells via downregulating the CD95 receptor and its surface location, as well as modifying TRAIL-activated DISC formation (Lagunas-Martínez et al., 2010). E6 has also been shown to protect various cells (human and mouse species) and tissues from TNF-mediated cell death. In a p53-independent manner, E6 protects both U2OS and LM cells against TNF-mediated cell death. Because E6 binds to TNF-R1 C-terminal, limiting apoptotic signal transduction, TNF pathway suppression in the presence of E6 could be linked to TNF-R1 (intracellular death domain) failure to connect with TRADD (Duerksen-Hughes et al., 1999; Filippova et al., 2002). E6 could inhibit TNF mediated apoptotic induction via cIAP-2 (cellular inhibitor of apoptosis protein 2) stimulation, or through Bcl-2 over expression and Bak down regulation in U2OS and LM cells. E6 also protected U2OS cells from Fas-induced apoptosis by preventing caspase-3 and 8 activations through FADD binding and degradation. Accelerated FADD degradation and procaspase-8 were also found in a few cell lines harboring HPV-16 E6, impairing TRAIL-mediated apoptosis (Liu et al., 2005). Although both small and large HPV16 E6 isoforms bind to pro caspase 8, only the big isoform upregulates the enzyme's degradation. TNF-induced apoptosis is not always protected by E6 expression. It was also discovered that U2OS cells with low E6 expression levels are unaffected by TNF-mediated apoptosis, but U2OS cells with high E6 protein levels are sensitized (Filippova et al., 2004).

Due to pRb-E2F complex breakdown, E7 oncoproteins from HR HPVs are capable of immortalizing primary human keratinocytes by blocking differentiation and activating cell cycle progression, releasing active E2F and activating multiple genes essential for DNA synthesis. E7 oncoprotein is also a powerful inhibitor of $p27^{KIP1}$ and $p21^{CIP1}$ activities, allowing it to bypass the regular G1 checkpoint control. HPV-16 E7 oncoprotein induces pRb (anti-apoptotic) degradation via ubiquitin proteasome pathway thereby suggesting the positive correlation between E7 and apoptosis induction (Melillo et al., 1994; Chamulitrat et al., 2009). Cells expressing HPV-16 E7 oncoprotein have been pre-disposed to apoptosis induction (Thyrell et al., 2005). For example, increased HPV16 E7 expression induces apoptosis in the retina in transgenic mice, and p53 is required for apoptotic induction since mice with E7 expression produce retinal tumors rather than degeneration. In the lens of transgenic mice, HPV16 E7 expression promoted both p53 independent and p53 dependent apoptosis (Howes et al., 1994).

E7 has been shown to induce apoptosis in a variety of cell lines. For example, the conserved portions of E7 cause apoptosis in NIH3T3 (immortalized rodent fibroblasts) cells (CR1 and CR2) (Alunni-Fabbroni et al., 2000). Additionally, due to altered growth regulatory signals, simultaneous p21 and E7 protein expression promoted cell death (apoptosis) in U2OS cells. Cathepsin B activation has been linked to p21/E7-induced cell death (apoptosis mediator) (Kaznelson et al., 2004). HPV16 E7 protein has also increased both TNF-α induced apoptosis and spontaneous apoptotic induction in human keratinocytes (primary). Also, apoptosis induction via of E6 and E7 co-expression mediated apoptotic induction via TNF (Basile et al., 2001). Both TRAIL and TNFα along with cycloheximide (protein synthesis inhibitor) have been found to be positively associated with apoptotic induction in E7 expressing human keratinocytes. This is mostly due to E7-induced apoptosis and E7-E2F1 interaction. This interaction complex increased apoptosis by activating E2F1-mediated transcription (Cabeça et al., 2019). Cycloheximide therapy inhibited de novo c-FLIP (short-lived) protein synthesis and made cells more susceptible to ligand-induced apoptosis (Ogura et al., 2008). However, depending on the virus and cell type, E7 HPV oncoprotein may block apoptosis and lower sensitivity to cytokine-mediated senescence. In normal human fibroblasts, for example, HPV16 E7 oncoprotein has been shown to suppress TNF-mediated apoptosis and caspase-8 activation. Apoptosis induction was also inhibited in E7-expressing HaCaT cells after exposure to genotoxic stimuli, such as UVC or mitomycin C (alkylating agent) (Thompson et al., 2001).

In E7-expressing cancer cells, inhibiting HDAC (histone deacetylase) causes cell growth arrest and, subsequently, significant apoptotic induction. This might be associated with tumor suppressor gene activation and chromatin acetylation leading to pRb degradation and accidental intracellular E2F-1 accumulation leading to apoptosis induction. E2F-1 over expression induced either p53 independent or dependent apoptotic induction (Zheng et al., 2013; Wu et al., 2017).

KEYWORDS

- **apoptosis**
- **apoptotic induction**
- **cancer cells**
- **cell death**
- **histone deacetylase**
- **tumor suppressor gene activation**

REFERENCES

Abu, J., Batuwangala, M., Herbert, K., & Symonds, P., (2005). Retinoic acid and retinoid receptors: Potential chemopreventive and therapeutic role in cervical cancer. *The Lancet Oncology, 6*(9), 712–720.

Alunni-Fabbroni, M., Littlewood, T., Deleu, L., Caldeira, S., Giarrè, M., Dell' Orco, M., & Tommasino, M., (2000). Induction of S phase and apoptosis by the human papillomavirus type 16 E7 protein are separable events in immortalized rodent fibroblasts. *Oncogene, 19*(19), 2277–2285.

Basile, J. R., Zacny, V., & Münger, K., (2001). The cytokines tumor necrosis factor-alpha (TNF-alpha) and TNF-related apoptosis-inducing ligand differentially modulate proliferation and apoptotic pathways in human keratinocytes expressing the human papillomavirus-16 E7 oncoprotein. *The Journal of Biological Chemistry, 276*(25), 22522–22528.

Boatright, K. M., & Salvesen, G. S., (2003). Mechanisms of caspase activation. *Current Opinion in Cell Biology, 15*(6), 725–731.

Bunz, F., (2001). Cell death and cancer therapy. *Current Opinion in Pharmacology, 1*(4), 337–341.

Cabeça, T. K., De Mello, A. A., Andrette, R., et al., (2019). HPV-mediated resistance to TNF and TRAIL is characterized by global alterations in apoptosis regulatory factors, dysregulation of death receptors, and induction of ROS/RNS. *International Journal of Molecular Sciences, 20*(1), 198.

Cai, Q., Lv, L., Shao, Q., Li, X., & Dian, A., (2013). Human papillomavirus early proteins and apoptosis. *Archives of Gynecology and Obstetrics, 287*(3), 541–548.

Chamulitrat, W., Sattayakhom, A., Herold-Mende, C., & Stremmel, W., (2009). Human papillomavirus 16 E6/E7-immortalized human gingival keratinocytes with epithelial mesenchymal transition acquire increased expression of cIAP-1, Bclx and p27(Kip1). *Experimental Dermatology, 18*(12), 1067–1069.

Chen, D. Z., Qi, M., Auborn, K. J., & Carter, T. H., (2001). Indole-3-carbinol and diindolylmethane induce apoptosis of human cervical cancer cells and in murine HPV16-transgenic preneoplastic cervical epithelium. *The Journal of Nutrition, 131*(12), 3294–3302.

Chiu, T. H., Lan, K. Y., Yang, M. D., et al., (2013). Diallyl sulfide promotes cell-cycle arrest through the p53 expression and triggers induction of apoptosis via caspase- and mitochondria-dependent signaling pathways in human cervical cancer Ca Ski cells. *Nutrition and Cancer, 65*(3), 505–514.

Duerksen-Hughes, P. J., Yang, J., & Schwartz, S. B., (1999). HPV 16 E6 blocks TNF-mediated apoptosis in mouse fibroblast LM cells. *Virology, 264*(1), 55–65.

Fan, T. J., Han, L. H., Cong, R. S., & Liang, J., (2005). Caspase family proteases and apoptosis. *Acta Biochimica et Biophysica Sinica, 37*(11), 719–727.

Filippova, M., Parkhurst, L., & Duerksen-Hughes, P. J., (2004). The human papillomavirus 16 E6 protein binds to Fas-associated death domain and protects cells from Fas-triggered apoptosis. *The Journal of Biological Chemistry, 279*(24), 25729–25744.

Filippova, M., Song, H., Connolly, J. L., Dermody, T. S., & Duerksen-Hughes, P. J., (2002). The human papillomavirus 16 E6 protein binds to tumor necrosis factor (TNF) R1 and protects cells from TNF-induced apoptosis. *The Journal of Biological Chemistry, 277*(24), 21730–21739.

Fulda, S., (2015). Targeting extrinsic apoptosis in cancer: Challenges and opportunities. *Seminars in Cell and Developmental Biology, 39*, 20–25.

Gaur, U., & Aggarwal, B. B., (2003). Regulation of proliferation, survival and apoptosis by members of the TNF superfamily. *Biochemical Pharmacology, 66*(8), 1403–1408.

Godlewski, M., & Kobylińska, A., (2016). Programmed cell death – strategy for maintenance cellular organisms homeostasis. *Postepy. Hig. Med. Dosw., 70*(0), 1229–1244.

Grimminger, D., Howell, P., Mayeaux, E. J., Tucker, A., Turbat-Herrera, E. A., & Mathis, J. M., (2000). Placebo-controlled trial of indole-3-carbinol in the treatment of CIN. *Gynecologic Oncology, 78*(2), 123–129.

Helm, C. W., Lorenz, D. J., Meyer, N. J., Rising, W. W., & Wulff, J. L., (2013). Retinoids for preventing the progression of cervical intra-epithelial neoplasia. *The Cochrane Database of Systematic Reviews*, (6), CD003296.

Hirchaud, F., Hermetet, F., Ablise, M., Fauconnet, S., Vuitton, D. A., Prétet, J. L., & Mougin, C., (2013). Isoliquiritigenin induces caspase-dependent apoptosis via downregulation of HPV16 E6 expression in cervical cancer Ca Ski cells. *Planta Medica, 79*(17), 1628–1635.

Howes, K. A., Ransom, N., Papermaster, D. S., Lasudry, J. G., Albert, D. M., & Windle, J. J., (1994). Apoptosis or retinoblastoma: Alternative fates of photoreceptors expressing the HPV-16 E7 gene in the presence or absence of p53. *Genes and Development, 8*(11), 1300–1310.

Hua, H., Zhang, H., Kong, Q., Wang, J., & Jiang, Y., (2019). Complex roles of the old drug aspirin in cancer chemoprevention and therapy. *Medicinal Research Reviews, 39*(1), 114–145.

Im, S. R., & Jang, Y. J., (2012). Aspirin enhances TRAIL-induced apoptosis via regulation of ERK1/2 activation in human cervical cancer cells. *Biochemical and Biophysical Research Communications, 424*(1), 65–70.

Jin, L., Qi, M., Chen, D. Z., Anderson, A., Yang, G. Y., Arbeit, J. M., & Auborn, K. J., (1999). Indole-3-carbinol prevents cervical cancer in human papilloma virus type 16 (HPV16) transgenic mice. *Cancer Research, 59*(16), 3991–3997.

Kaczanowski, S., (2016). Apoptosis: Its origin, history, maintenance and the medical implications for cancer and aging. *Physical Biology, 13*(3), 031001.

Kashyap, D., Garg, V. K., & Goel, N., (2021). Intrinsic and extrinsic pathways of apoptosis: Role in cancer development and prognosis. *Advances in Protein Chemistry and Structural Biology, 125*, 73–120.

Kaznelson, D. W., Bruun, S., Monrad, A., Gjerløv, S., Birk, J., Röpke, C., & Norrild, B., (2004). Simultaneous human papilloma virus type 16 E7 and cdk inhibitor p21 expression induces apoptosis and cathepsin B activation. *Virology, 320*(2), 301–312.

Kim, B., Srivastava, S. K., & Kim, S. H., (2015). Caspase-9 as a therapeutic target for treating cancer. *Expert Opinion on Therapeutic Targets, 19*(1), 113–127.

Kim, J. H., Kang, J. W., Kim, M. S., et al., (2012). The apoptotic effects of the flavonoid N101-2 in human cervical cancer cells. *Toxicology in vitro, 26*(1), 67–73.

Kiraz, Y., Adan, A., Kartal, Y. M., & Baran, Y., (2016). Major apoptotic mechanisms and genes involved in apoptosis. *Tumor Biology, 37*(7), 8471–8486.

Komposch, G., Schenkel, J., Alonso, A., & Tomakidi, P., (2004). The HPV-16 E5 protein inhibits TRAIL- and FasL-mediated apoptosis in human keratinocyte raft cultures. *Intervirology, 47*(1), 48–56.

Kumar, S., & Dorstyn, L., (2009). Analyzing caspase activation and caspase activity in apoptotic cells. *Methods in Molecular Biology, 559*, 3–17.

Kumar, S., Fairmichael, C., Longley, D. B., & Turkington, R. C., (2020). The multiple roles of the IAP super-family in cancer. *Pharmacology and Therapeutics, 214*, 107610.

Lagunas-Martínez, A., Madrid-Marina, V., & Gariglio, P., (2010). Modulation of apoptosis by early human papillomavirus proteins in cervical cancer. *Biochimica et Biophysica Acta, 1805*(1), 6–16.

Li, S., Hong, X., Wei, Z., et al., (2019). Ubiquitination of the HPV oncoprotein E6 is critical for E6/E6AP-mediated p53 degradation. *Frontiers in Microbiology, 10*, 2483.

Li, T. T., Zhao, L. N., Liu, Z. G., Han, Y., & Fan, D. M., (2005). Regulation of apoptosis by the papillomavirus E6 oncogene. *World Journal of Gastroenterology, 11*(7), 931–937.

Liu, L., Wang, M., Li, X., Yin, S., & Wang, B., (2021). An overview of novel agents for cervical cancer treatment by inducing apoptosis: Emerging drugs ongoing clinical trials and preclinical studies. *Frontiers in Medicine, 8*, 682366.

Liu, R. M., Li, Y. B., Liang, X. F., Liu, H. Z., Xiao, J. H., & Zhong, J. J., (2015). Structurally related ganoderic acids induce apoptosis in human cervical cancer HeLa cells: Involvement of oxidative stress and antioxidant protective system. *Chemico-Biological Interactions, 240*, 134–144.

Liu, Y., Liu, Z., Gao, H., Zhou, Y., Androphy, E. J., & Chen, J. J., (2005). Opposing effects of bovine papillomavirus type 1 E6 and E7 genes on Fas-mediated apoptosis. *Oncogene, 24*(24), 3942–3953.

Melillo, R. M., Helin, K., Lowy, D. R., & Schiller, J. T., (1994). Positive and negative regulation of cell proliferation by E2F-1: Influence of protein level and human papillomavirus oncoproteins. *Molecular and Cellular Biology, 14*(12), 8241–8249.

Nagata, S., (1996). Fas-induced apoptosis, and diseases caused by its abnormality. *Genes to Cells, 1*(10), 873–879.

Ogura, H., Tsukumo, Y., Sugimoto, H., Igarashi, M., Nagai, K., & Kataoka, T., (2008). Ectodomain shedding of TNF receptor 1 induced by protein synthesis inhibitors regulates TNF-alpha-mediated activation of NF-kappaB and caspase-8. *Experimental Cell Research, 314*(6), 1406–1414.

Pistritto, G., Trisciuoglio, D., Ceci, C., Garufi, A., & D'Orazi, G., (2016). Apoptosis as anticancer mechanism: Function and dysfunction of its modulators and targeted therapeutic strategies. *Aging, 8*(4), 603–619.

Qi, M., Anderson, A. E., Chen, D. Z., Sun, S., & Auborn, K. J., (2005). Indole-3-carbinol prevents PTEN loss in cervical cancer *in vivo*. *Molecular Medicine, 11*(1–12), 59–63.

Sartorius, U., Schmitz, I., & Krammer, P. H., (2001). Molecular mechanisms of death-receptor-mediated apoptosis. *Chembiochem, 2*(1), 20–29.

Scribner, D. R. Jr., & Benbrook, D. M., (2002). Retinoids enhance cisplatin-based chemoradiation in cervical cancer cells *in vitro*. *Gynecologic Oncology, 85*(1), 223–225.

Solary, E., Plenchette, S., Sordet, O., et al., (2001). Modulation of apoptotic pathways triggered by cytotoxic agents. *Therapie, 56*(5), 511–518.

Straub, C. S., (2011). Targeting IAPs as an approach to anti-cancer therapy. *Current Topics in Medicinal Chemistry, 11*(3), 291–316.

Suvarna, V., Singh, V., & Murahari, V., (2019). Current overview on the clinical update of Bcl-2 anti-apoptotic inhibitors for cancer therapy. *European Journal of Pharmacology, 862*, 172655. https://doi.org/10.1016/j.ejphar.2019.172655.

Thompson, D. A., Zacny, V., Belinsky, G. S., Classon, M., Jones, D. L., Schlegel, R., & Münger, K., (2001). The HPV E7 oncoprotein inhibits tumor necrosis factor alpha-mediated apoptosis in normal human fibroblasts. *Oncogene, 20*(28), 3629–3640.

Thyrell, L., Sangfelt, O., Zhivotovsky, B., Pokrovskaja, K., Wang, Y., Einhorn, S., & Grandér, D., (2005). The HPV-16 E7 oncogene sensitizes malignant cells to IFN-alpha-induced apoptosis. *Journal of Interferon and Cytokine Research, 25*(2), 63–72.

Wang, A., Zhang, Y., & Cao, P., (2019). Inhibition of BAP31 expression inhibits cervical cancer progression by suppressing metastasis and inducing intrinsic and extrinsic apoptosis. *Biochemical and Biophysical Research Communications, 508*(2), 499–506.

Wang, Z. B., Liu, Y. Q., & Cui, Y. F., (2005). Pathways to caspase activation. *Cell Biology International, 29*(7), 489–496.

Wen, X., Li, D., Zhang, Y., Liu, S., Ghali, L., & Iles, R. K., (2012). Arsenic trioxide induces cervical cancer apoptosis, but specifically targets human papillomavirus-infected cell populations. *Anti-Cancer Drugs, 23*(3), 280–287.

Wu, S. F., Zhang, J. W., Qian, W. Y., et al., (2012). Altered expression of survivin, Fas and FasL contributed to cervical cancer development and metastasis. *European Review for Medical and Pharmacological Sciences, 16*(15), 2044–2050.

Wu, S., Wang, L., Ren, X., et al., (2017). Involvement of retinoblastoma-associated protein 48 during photodynamic therapy of cervical cancer cells. *Molecular Medicine Reports, 15*(3), 1393–1400.

Xu, X., Lai, Y., & Hua, Z. C., (2019). Apoptosis and apoptotic body: Disease message and therapeutic target potentials. *Bioscience Reports, 39*(1), BSR20180992.

Zantl, N., Weirich, G., Zall, H., et al., (2007). Frequent loss of expression of the pro-apoptotic protein Bim in renal cell carcinoma: Evidence for contribution to apoptosis resistance. *Oncogene, 26*(49), 7038–7048.

Zhang, B., Spandau, D. F., & Roman, A., (2002). E5 protein of human papillomavirus type 16 protects human foreskin keratinocytes from UV B-irradiation-induced apoptosis. *Journal of Virology, 76*(1), 220–231.

Zhang, Y., Ge, Y., Chen, Y., Li, Q., Chen, J., Dong, Y., & Shi, W., (2012). Cellular and molecular mechanisms of silibinin induces cell-cycle arrest and apoptosis on HeLa cells. *Cell Biochemistry and Function, 30*(3), 243–248.

Zheng, L., Tang, W., Wei, F., et al., (2013). Radiation-inducible protein RbAp48 contributes to radiosensitivity of cervical cancer cells. *Gynecologic Oncology, 130*(3), 601–608.

Zhou, J. H., Chen, H. Z., Ye, F., Lu, W. G., & Xie, X., (2006). Fas-mediated pathway and apoptosis in normal cervix, cervical intraepithelial neoplasia and cervical squamous cancer. *Oncology Reports, 16*(2), 307–311.

Zhou, X., Jiang, W., Liu, Z., Liu, S., & Liang, X., (2017). Virus infection and death receptor-mediated apoptosis. *Viruses, 9*(11), 316.

Zhu, J., Li, Y., Guan, C., & Chen, Z., (2012). Anti-proliferative and pro-apoptotic effects of 3,3'-diindolylmethane in human cervical cancer cells. *Oncology Reports, 28*(3), 1063–1068.

Zucchi, F., da, S. I. D., Ribalta, J. C., et al., (2009). Fas/CD95 promoter polymorphism gene and its relationship with cervical carcinoma. *European Journal of Gynaecological Oncology, 30*(2), 142–144.

CHAPTER 7

NF-κB in Cervical Cancer Management

7.1 AN OVERVIEW OF NF-κB PROTEIN FAMILY AND SIGNALING PATHWAY

NF-κB is a group of nuclear transcription factors that play an important role in inflammation, innate immune response, viral replication, and the process of carcinogenesis. The NF-kB family in mammal comprises of five members, namely RelA (p65), RelB, c-Rel, NF-kB1 (p50/p105), and NF-kB2 (p52/p100) (Rothwarf & Karin, 1999; Karin & Ben-Neriah, 2000). The NF-kB proteins are recognized by an N-terminus conserved Rel Homology Domain (RHD), which helps in the dimerization process, DNA binding, and interaction with specific inhibitors (Li & Vema, 2002; Hayden & Ghosh, 2004). The NF-kB1 and NF-kB2 proteins are produced in it preform as p105 and p100 and thereafter processed to p50 and p52, respectively via proteolytic breakdown. All these five proteins can form different types of homo- and heterodimers by undergoing several posttranslational modifications that are required for their activation and nucleus transportation. After nuclear translocation, active NF-kB molecules bind to specific target DNA and resulted in induction of target genes (Wong et al., 2011; Xing et al., 2013). In absence of specific stimulus, dimeric NF-kB is associated with inhibitory molecules of IkB proteins. These IkB inhibitory molecules are identified by ankyrin repeats that specifically bound to DNA binding domains of different transcription factors and leads to their inactivation. After gets stimulated, NF-kB regulates target gene expressions that performed several cellular and molecular functions

Cervical Cancer: Signaling Pathways, Molecular Mechanisms, Natural Products, and Therapeutic Approaches. Pratibha Pandey, Fahad Khan, Saher Islam, and Devarajan Thangadurai, (Eds.)

such as cell proliferation, inflammatory immune response generation and tumor microenvironment transformations (Rao et al., 2011; Jana et al., 2017; Silva-Gomez et al., 2021).

NF-kB can be stimulated by two different molecular pathways, namely, canonical and alternative pathways. The most common canonical pathway is activated by a variety of stimuli, including toll-like receptors, inflammatory cytokines, and antigen receptors. After gets stimulated by its ligand, this pathway activates the NF-kB dimers, which is composed of p50, p65, c-Rel, and RelB subunits. These NF-kB dimers then transported to the nucleus and bind of specific DNA sequences which resulted in transcription of multiple genes responsible for various biological processes (Chen et al., 2001; Häcker & Karin, 2006). This canonical pathway plays an important role in tumor promotion, anti-apoptotic properties, and has also been associated with the progression of several inflammatory diseases including inflammatory bowel disease, rheumatoid arthritis, and asthma (Ji et al., 2004; Schuliga, 2015).

The second non-canonical or alternative activation pathway is resulted in the activation of NF-kB dimers composed of p100 and RelB subunits (Table 7.1). This pathway is regulated by specific stimuli including receptor activator of NF-kB ligand (RANKL), B cell activating factor (BAFF), lymphotoxin β, CD40 ligand, and tumor necrosis factor (TNF) family members (Neumann & Neumann, 2007; Gaptulbarova et al., 2020). The stimuli activate IKKα catalytic subunit which further phosphorylates p100, undergoes proteolysis and generates p52-containing dimers. These activated NF-kB dimers attach to specific DNA binding locations that are found in the promoter sequences of the target genes and regulate their expression (Baud & Karin, 2009; Liu et al., 2012). Studies suggested that there are some alterations in DNA binding affinities of various NF-kB subunits and the DNA binding regions (kB sites) of target genes. Certain dimers, (like Rel A, p50, and c-Rel homodimers) can attach kB sites that comprise only 50% of the site consensus sequence (Hou et al., 2003; Smith et al., 2019; Vonderach et al., 2019). It has also been reported that this NF-kB dimer can have diverse effects on the transcription of genes on the basis of slight variation in the DNA binding site.

TABLE 7.1 NF-kB Protein Family Members and Their Stimuli

Precursor Molecule	Active Protein	Functional Domains	Precursor Gene Symbol	Stimuli
p105	p50	Subunit RHD	*NFkB1*	Pattern recognition receptors ligands; cytokines, T-cell receptor signals; B-cell receptor signals; oxidative stress, hypoxia; radiation, mitogen-activated protein kinase signals.
p100	p52	Subunit RHD	*NFkB2*	
–	p65 subunit (RelA)	RHD, TAD	*RELA*	
–	c-Rel	RHD, TAD	*REL*	
–	RelB	RHD, TAD	*RELB*	

7.2 ROLE OF NF-κB SIGNALING PATHWAY IN INFLAMMATORY RESPONSES

Numerous research findings showed that canonical NF-kB signaling pathway activation could resulted in elevated expression level of chemokines, inflammatory cytokines and their receptors, thus considered as pro-inflammatory signaling pathway which stimulate the immune system against oxidative stress (Rayet & Gélinas, 1999; Ravi & Bedi, 2004; Yu et al., 2020). On the other hand, inflammatory cytokines can also stimulate NK-kB activity and creates a prospect for positive feedback mechanism (Perkins, 2004; Afonina et al., 2017). In tumor cells with induced NF-kB activity resulted in the deposition of pro-inflammatory cytokines which directly responsible for tumor initiation and development (Chang & Van, 2005; Lee et al., 2011; Xia et al., 2014). NF-kB molecules have the capability to stimulate chemoattractant proteins and various adhesion proteins for the employment of inflammatory cells which helps in combating infectious diseases such as HPV infection (Disis, 2010; Aleixo et al., 2013). A modest increase level of NF-kB activity was also reported in chronic inflammatory disorders. The correlation between hyperactivation of NF-kB with protumorogenic effect is confirmed by the fact that patients having chronic inflammatory disorders have a higher susceptibility of cancer development (Hoesel & Schmid, 2013). In some cases, the p50 protein has also been responsible for promoting immunosuppression by inhibiting M1-polarization and encouraging M2-polarization of macrophages cells (Porta et al., 2009). Few studies reported the inducing role of NF-kB proteins in the expression of anti-inflammatory genes, such as triggering the leucocyte apoptosis during the exhibition of inflammation. Indeed NF-kB prevention can sometimes resulted in a constitutive inflammatory reaction. Altogether, it can be established that on the basis of time and tissue two types of NF-kB associated mediators are formed during the process of inflammation viz., pro- and anti-inflammatory. The balance between these two inflammatory proteins appears to govern the disease progression (Baldwin, 2001; Lawrence, 2009; Kauppinen et al., 2013; Dorrington & Fraser, 2019).

7.3 NF-κB IN TUMOR PROGRESSION

Several preclinical and clinical experimental findings demonstrated that NF-kB signaling pathway mediators are critical players in the cancer initiation and development, which control gene expressions associated with cell proliferation, apoptosis, metastasis, and angiogenesis (Karin, 2006; Khan et al., 2020; Morgan et al., 2020). Activation of both classical and alternative NF-kB pathways is stimulated in various types of carcinomas that can be related with a bad prognosis of disease (Viatour et al., 2005; Gupta et al., 2010). Aberrant mutations in NF-kB genes were firstly reported in B-cell lymphoid cancer but are limited in solid tumors. On the other hand, it has been revealed that mutations in signaling molecules like EGFR, RAS, HER2, PGF generally resulted in constitutive stimulation of NF-kB in solid tumors (Chaturvedi et al., 2011; Espinosa & Marruecos, 2021). Additionally, NF-kB is triggered by continuous production of inflammatory cytokines through macrophages in the tumor microenvironment (Bradford & Baldwin, 2014). NF-kB induction can increase cell proliferation, survival and preventing apoptosis by activating the expression of anti-apoptotic genes (Kucharczak et al., 2003). This forms a basis to combat the physiological stress produced during inflammation, and plays a crucial role as cancer initiation factor (Dutta et al., 2006; Perkins & Gilmore, 2006). NF-kB can also induce upregulated expression of genes associated with cell proliferation, metastasis, angiogenesis, and anti-apoptotic genes (Guttridge et al., 1999; Kim et al., 2006). These findings suggested that NF-kB forms an important connection between chronic inflammation and tumor induction. In solid tumors, the tumor microenvironment releases increased levels of inflammatory cytokines and possess hypoxic atmosphere, both these factors induces activation and movement of NF-kB inside the nucleus (Bharti & Aggarwal, 2002; Perkins, 2004; Chen et al., 2011). Activation of NF-kB proteins can also stimulate the expression of AID (activation-induced cytodine deaminase) and the APOBEC proteins. These AID/APOBEC family proteins are responsible for cancer development and clonal progression of tumor by prompting genomic damage due to their DNA deaminating property (Rebhandl et al., 2015; Bader et al., 2021). The APOBECs can stimulate activating mutations in c-MYC, p53, and other genes, which forms a strong basis for the initiation and development of cervical cancer (Tilborghs et al., 2017). Active STAT3 is a crucial regulator of a variety of genes such as C-MYC, cyclin D1, BCL-xl, surviving, and VEGF that encourage uncontrolled cell growth and inhibit cell death in cervical lesions (Aggarwal et al., 2009). STAT3 works in close association with NF-kB proteins as a network. These two control the expression of genes coding chemokines and cytokines and regulate various kinds of target genes involved in anti-apoptotic pathways and cell cycle regulation.

7.4 THE HPV AND NF-κB

NF-kB is considered as an important precursor in the generation of innate and adaptive immune response. The E6 and E7 proteins in HPV-16 type control the NF-kB expression, but there are contradictory facts whether they activate or suppress NF-kB induction (James et al., 2006; Saidu et al., 2019; Carrillo-Beltrán et al., 2020). The important determinants for activation or suppression are mainly cell type, growth rate, and nature of the signals. The balance between the various types of dimerization of NF-kB family proteins is a crucial aspect. For example, dimerization of p50/p52 and relA/relB do not have a transactivation domain, and as a result dimers of these proteins act as transcriptional repressors (Marienfeld et al., 2003; Alharbi et al., 2021). HPV E6 proteins enhanced the expression levels of functional mediators of the NF-kB pathway and activate the DNA binding activity of NF-kB, which concurrently increase in secretion of pro-inflammatory cytokines (Nees et al., 2001; Gusho & Laimins, 2021). HPV16 LCR (long control region) has a functional DNA binding site for NF-kB that act as a transcriptional repressor of the HPV. The HPV virus requires a mechanism to overcome this suppressive activity for replication. In case of high-risk HPV (HR-HPV), E7 proteins can achieve this by inhibiting the nuclear transfer of NF-kB and binding with the LCR DNA elements of HPV (Struyk et al., 2000; Sizemore et al., 2001; Spitkovsky et al., 2002). Similarly, HR-HPV E6 follows the same mechanism to repress the transcriptional activity of p65 proteins of NF-kB inside the nucleus (Patel et al., 1999; Müller-Schiffmann et al., 2006). A study reported the significant higher NF-kB activation in early phase of HPV; however immortalization resulted in reduced NF-kB activity and its responsive genes expression in the transformation zone cells. Suppression of NF-kB activity via introduction of mutant IkB repressor molecule enhances colony forming ability and immortalization by HPV16. Furthermore, HPV16 E6 and E7 proteins suppress basal and TNF-α-mediated NF-κB activity in transformation zone epithelial cells (Vandermark et al., 2012; Smith et al., 2016). Triggering of NF-kB pathway by continuous expression of p65 molecules inhibits cellular proliferation and immortalization. It therefore appears to be that during the initial stage of HPV infection NF-kB activity is activated in context to the normal host immune response, but later on decreased NF-kB activity related to the promotion of persistent infection of HPV. HPV-16 also negatively regulates the specific NF-kB interrelated pathways that resulted in down regulated expression of major histocompatibility genes, β-defensins, interferons, and cytokines (Georgopoulos et al., 2000; Smahel et al., 2003; Pešut et al., 2021). HPV 16 also abrogates the TLR-9 (Toll-like receptor-9) and represses the host immune response that may contribute to cell immortalization (Diamond et al., 2008; Sannigrahi et al., 2017). NF-κB activation gives rise to important transformations in the tumor microenvironment promoting the process of carcinogenesis (Pikarsky et al., 2004). An interesting case control demonstrated the role of NF-kB in carcinogenesis which reported that HPV-infected postmenopausal women containing insertional mutation were more at risk to develop cervical cancer (Pallavi et al., 2015; Fu et al., 2017).

7.5 ROLE OF NF-κB SIGNALING PATHWAY IN CERVICAL CANCER

Several reports have demonstrated the correlation between persistent chronic inflammation, the prevalence of high-grade squamous intraepithelial neoplasia, and invasive cervical cancer (Schwebke

& Zajackowski, 1997; Georgescu et al., 2018; Lugović-Mihić et al., 2021). The cellular analysis of cervical cancer tissue compared to a healthy cervix tissue, it has been revealed that the augmented movement of macrophages cells in cervical epithelium could aggravate the intensity of HPV induced wounds, which causes inflammatory condition (Hammes et al., 2007; Yildiz et al., 2007). There are different signaling pathways that are responsible for the inflammatory response generation as well as HPV-induced inflammation and release of cytokines and chemokines (Sadri Nahand et al., 2020). One such signaling pathway is NF-κB signaling cascade. Concomitant NF-κB activation with the incorporation of HPV DNA into the host genome, could be an important factor in cervical cancer initiation and progression. In addition to the normal targets of HPV E6 and E7 oncoproteins and successive suppression of p53 and pRB tumor suppressors, these oncoproteins linked with the stimulation of NF-κB, which resulted in uncontrollable cell cycle and cellular alteration (Senba & Mori, 2012). HPV E6 is responsible for the nuclear localization of NF-κB transcription factor in HPV-infected cell. HPV oncoproteins (E6 and E7) are manifested to have a positive correlation with increased expression of NF-κB, which denotes that NF-κB plays an important role in the transformation of chronic inflammation into advanced tumor and metastasis (James et al., 2006; Basukala & Banks, 2021). Besides HPV E6 and E7 oncoproteins, IL-17 also demonstrates a potential to activate the NF-κB signaling pathway, which consequently resulted in enhanced cellular proliferation and invasion. Few studies reported the correlation of elevated level of IL-17 with the induced activity and expression of the HPV E6 oncoprotein (Chang et al., 2010; Sahu et al., 2021). Subsequently, it has been also seen that HPV E7 protein caused a marked increase in the expression of IL-1β and NF-κB. In contrast to this, it is shown that HPV E6 obstructs the expression of IL-1β; however the mechanisms associated with the IL1β-related inflammation following the HPV infection yet remains unveiled (Ainouze et al., 2018). It has been reported that the repression of TNF-α activity and associated antiproliferative efficacy could be responsible for HPV mediated cancer development (Beglin et al., 2009; Jin et al., 2013; Wang et al., 2020). Recently, a research study has demonstrated a remarkable increase in TGF-β, IL-6, IL-10, IL-17, and IL-23 expression, and decrease in IFN-γ (interferon γ) expression in cancer patients (Figure 7.1).

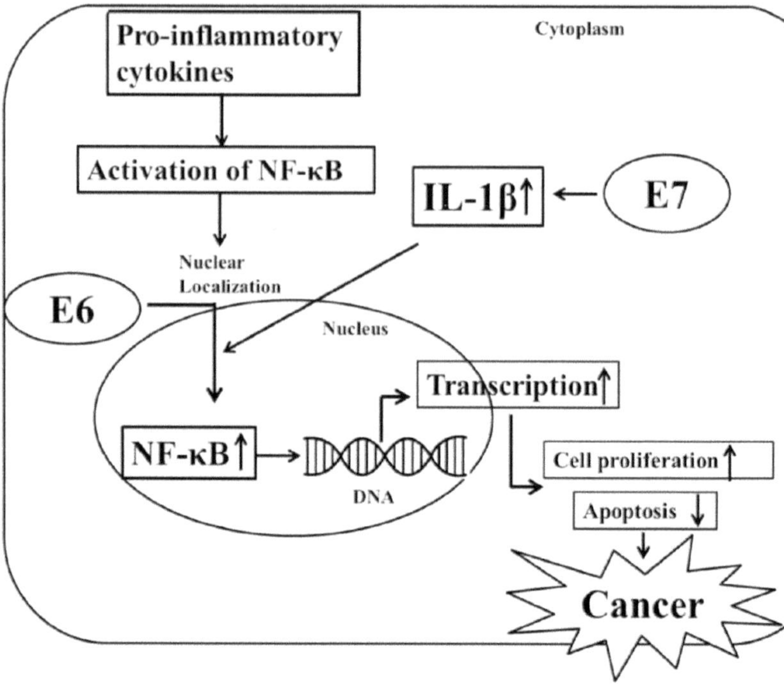

FIGURE 7.1 Mechanism associated with cervical cancer progression and NF-kB signaling cascade.

A direct association was observed between the increase tumor grade of cervical cancer *in situ* and the cytoplasmic NF-kB expression that advocates a tumor-inducing potential of NF-kB during the cervical cancer progression (Branca et al., 2006; Snijders et al., 2006). It has been seen that during normal cervix and low grade cancerous lesions, various forms of NF-kB including p50, RelA (p65) and IkB-α are confined in the cytosol, conversely, in high-grade lesions and squamous cell carcinoma, nuclear translocation of NF-kB is found (Wu et al., 2019; He et al., 2021). This kind of NF-kB upregulation takes place during late-stage carcinogenesis. A study by Nair et al. (2003) revealed that a reduction in the IkB-α level in the cytosol was observed during tumor advancement, indicating degradation of IkB-α in the late stages of cervical cancer progression. There was a positive correlation between gradually rising NF-kB expression inside the nucleus and DNA binding efficacy from normal to advanced stage cervical carcinoma precancerous, though HPV relations were not documented in this research. Another study by Prusty et al. also noticed a continuous increase in NF-kB expression and DNA binding efficacy from primary stage to advanced cervical carcinoma. Additionally, this study exhibited that the p50 appears to form a homodimer (p50/p50) during onset on disease progression instead of normal heterodimer p50/p65 subunit which resulted in inhibition of transcriptional activity because of the absence of a transactivation domain (Burley, 1995; Prusty et al., 2005). There was a successive increase in the nuclear localization and expression of p50 subunit and a subsequent reduction of p65 expression as the tumor progressed. p65 translocation inside the nucleus was observed, but dimerization of p65 was not seen (Prusty et al., 2005). Whereas other research findings did not detect a substantial variation in the activity p52, RelB, and c-Rel activity (Prusty et al., 2005; Hua et al., 2019; Ma et al., 2021). Furthermore, Branca et al. demonstrated that overexpression of nuclear NF-kB is significantly related with the progression of cervical intraepithelial neoplasia (CIN) to carcinoma in 152 CIN lesions and 150 squamous carcinomas patient samples, however a slight increase was observed in cytoplasmic NF-kB activity (Branca et al., 2006). They hypothesized that this can be elucidated through a mechanism in which HPV escapes from the transcriptional regulation of NF-kB. HPV E7 causes deteriorated nuclear transfer of cytosolic NF-kB while E6 attenuate NF-kB (p65 subunit) mediated transcriptional activity. NF-kB expression in the cytoplasmic region remains evident throughout the cervical cancer progression and development. In a few cases, phosphorylation of Ik-B-α takes place during CIN lesions progression that describes the moderate relocation from cytosol to the nucleus in high-grade CIN (Nair et al., 2003). Some studies proposed that the reciprocation between CFTR (cystic fibrosis transmembrane conductance regulator) and NF-kB could be an important factor for the cervical cancer development. Both these mediators are co-expressed during the development of cervical cancer and NF-kB facilitating the CFTR expression (Peng et al., 2012; Wu et al., 2013; Wu et al., 2020). A study performed by Wu Zu et al. revealed that expression of NF-kB and CFTR increased gradually in cervical cancer patients sample compared to normal tissue. Co-expression was an important prognostic marker for cervical carcinoma and elevated level of NF-kB and CFTR expression was substantially linked with poor prognosis (for example, poor histological grade, advanced FIGO stage, lymph node metastasis, deeper invasive growth, and worse survival rate), however these findings required validation in a larger cohort.

In addition to these, NF-KB also impact and closely associated with the functioning of several other transcription factors such as SMAD3, SMAD4, and STAT3 (Maliekal et al., 2003). STAT3 and NK-kB simultaneously control the expression of various target genes, such as anti-apoptotic and cell cycle regulatory genes, and cytokines-chemokines encoding genes (Rossetti et al., 2020). STAT3 mainly controls function and expression of p53 through binding to its promoter; subsequently decrease in de novo expression. It directly affects p53 mediatory genes that inhibit p53-mediated apoptosis in tumor cells. p53 inhibits the STAT3 phosphorylation and thus both these factors negatively influence the expression of each other. In tumor cells, downregulation of p53 leads to the STAT3 mediated cell survival and proliferation without early stage mutation. STAT3 obstruction promotes the p53-mediated cancer cell apoptosis and tumor cell growth inhibition, indicating probabilities for STAT3 as a therapeutic target in cervical cancer (Niu et al., 2005). COX-2 (Cyclooxygenase-2) has been considered as an important factor in cervical cancer development and progression via augmenting lymph node metastasis and apoptotic resistance (Kulkarni et al., 2001; Ishikawa et al., 2006). NF-kB plays a crucial role in the stimulation of COX-2 in tumor cells (Surh et al., 2001). HPV E5 oncoproteins stimulates EGFR (epidermal growth factor receptor) and COX-2 expression through enhancement in COX-2 promoter activity (Crusius et al., 1998). The promoter region of COX-2 has three main binding domains, viz. NF-IL6, NF-kB, and CRE (cyclic adenosine monophosphate-responsive element). E5-regulated EGFR stimulation was accompanied by the phosphorylation of downstream signaling protein targets, including PI3K/Akt and ERK/MAPK, which further induces expression of COX-2 (Branca et al., 2004). E5-EGFR signaling pathway mediated induction of COX-2 expression causes increased level of VEGF (vascular endothelial growth factor), which plays a key role in transforming angiogenic phenotype during cervical cancer advancement. E5 augments the expression of COX-2 by AP-1 and more importantly by the activation of NF-kB. This demonstrated that CRE and NF-kB promoter sites are the important controlling regions for the E5-promoted COX-2 expression (Kim et al., 2006, 2009). HPV E6 and E7 oncoproteins activate COX-2 transcription by increasing the activator protein-1 (AP-1) binding to CRE domain; however, independent of NF-kB signaling pathway (Subbaramaiah & Dannenberg, 2007; Medda et al., 2021). Altogether, it can be concluded that targeting NF-kB signaling pathway with other cross-linking pathway might be a productive approach for the treatment and management of cervical cancer.

KEYWORDS

- **activator protein-1**
- **angiogenic phenotype**
- **cervical cancer**
- **cross-linking pathway**
- **downstream signaling**
- **signaling pathway**

REFERENCES

Afonina, I. S., Zhong, Z., Karin, M., & Beyaert, R., (2017). Limiting inflammation-the negative regulation of NF-κB and the NLRP3 inflammasome. *Nature Immunology, 18*(8), 861–869.

Aggarwal, B. B., Kunnumakkara, A. B., Harikumar, K. B., et al., (2009). Signal transducer and activator of transcription-3, inflammation, and cancer: How intimate is the relationship? *Annals of the New York Academy of Sciences, 1171*, 59–76.

Ainouze, M., Rochefort, P., Parroche, P., et al., (2018). Human papillomavirus type 16 antagonizes IRF6 regulation of IL-1β. *PLoS Pathogens, 14*(8), e1007158.

Aleixo, A. A., Michelin, M. A., & Murta, E. F., (2013). Immunotherapy with dendritic cells as a cancer treatment: Perspectives and therapeutic potential. *Recent Patents on Endocrine, Metabolic and Immune Drug Discovery, 7*(3), 226–232.

Alharbi, K. S., Fuloria, N. K., Fuloria, S., et al., (2021). Nuclear factor-kappa B and its role in inflammatory lung disease. *Chemico-Biological Interactions, 345*, 109568.

Bader, S. B., Ma, T. S., Simpson, C. J., et al., (2021). Replication catastrophe induced by cyclic hypoxia leads to increased APOBEC3B activity. *Nucleic Acids Research, 49*(13), 7492–7506.

Baldwin A. S. Jr., (2001). The transcription factor NF-kappaB and human disease. The *Journal of Clinical Investigation, 107*(1), 3–6.

Basukala, O., & Banks, L., (2021). The not-so-good, the bad and the ugly: HPV E5, E6 and E7 oncoproteins in the orchestration of carcinogenesis. *Viruses, 13*(10), 1892.

Baud, V., & Karin, M., (2009). Is NF-kappaB a good target for cancer therapy? Hopes and pitfalls. *Nature Reviews Drug Discovery, 8*(1), 33–40.

Beglin, M., Melar-New, M., & Laimins, L., (2009). Human papillomaviruses and the interferon response. *Journal of Interferon and Cytokine Research, 29*(9), 629–635.

Bharti, A. C., & Aggarwal, B. B., (2002). Nuclear factor-kappa B and cancer: Its role in prevention and therapy. *Biochemical Pharmacology, 64*(5, 6), 883–888.

Bradford, J. W., & Baldwin, A. S., (2014). IKK/nuclear factor-kappaB and oncogenesis: Roles in tumor-initiating cells and in the tumor microenvironment. *Advances in Cancer Research, 121*, 125–145.

Branca, M., Ciotti, M., Santini, D., et al., (2004). Activation of the ERK/MAP kinase pathway in cervical intraepithelial neoplasia is related to grade of the lesion but not to high-risk human papillomavirus, virus clearance, or prognosis in cervical cancer. *American Journal of Clinical Pathology, 122*(6), 902–911.

Branca, M., Giorgi, C., Ciotti, M., et al., (2006). Upregulation of nuclear factor-kappaB (NF-kappaB) is related to the grade of cervical intraepithelial neoplasia, but is not an independent predictor of high-risk human papillomavirus or disease outcome in cervical cancer. *Diagnostic Cytopathology, 34*(8), 555–563.

Burley, S. K., (1995). Rel revealed: Cocrystal structures of the NF-kappa B p50 homodimer. *Chemistry and Biology, 2*(2), 77–81.

Carrillo-Beltráán, D., Muñoz, J. P., Guerrero-Vásquez, N., et al., (2020). *Human Papillomavirus* 16 E7 promotes EGFR/PI3K/AKT1/NRF2 signaling pathway contributing to PIR/NF-κB activation in oral cancer cells. *Cancers, 12*(7), 1904.

Chang, A. A., & Van, W. C., (2005). Nuclear factor-KappaB as a common target and activator of oncogenes in head and neck squamous cell carcinoma. *Advances in Oto-Rhino-Laryngology, 62*, 92–102.

Chang, Y. H., Yu, C. W., Lai, L. C., et al., (2010). Up-regulation of interleukin-17 expression by human papillomavirus type 16 E6 in nonsmall cell lung cancer. *Cancer, 116*(20), 4800–4809.

Chaturvedi, M. M., Sung, B., Yadav, V. R., Kannappan, R., & Aggarwal, B. B., (2011). NF-κB addiction and its role in cancer: 'one size does not fit all.' *Oncogene, 30*(14), 1615–1630.

Chen, F., Castranova, V., & Shi, X., (2001). New insights into the role of nuclear factor-kappaB in cell growth regulation. *The American Journal of Pathology, 159*(2), 387–397.

Chen, W., Li, Z., Bai, L., & Lin, Y., (2011). NF-kappaB in lung cancer, a carcinogenesis mediator and a prevention and therapy target. *Frontiers in Bioscience, 16*, 1172–1185.

Crusius, K., Auvinen, E., Steuer, B., Gaissert, H., & Alonso, A., (1998). The human papillomavirus type 16 E5-protein modulates ligand-dependent activation of the EGF receptor family in the human epithelial cell line HaCaT. *Experimental Cell Research, 241*(1), 76–83.

Diamond, G., Beckloff, N., & Ryan, L. K., (2008). Host defense peptides in the oral cavity and the lung: Similarities and differences. *Journal of Dental Research, 87*(10), 915–927.

Disis, M. L., (2010). Immune regulation of cancer. *Journal of Clinical Oncology, 28*(29), 4531–4538.

Dorrington, M. G., & Fraser, I., (2019). NF-κB signaling in macrophages: Dynamics, crosstalk, and signal integration. *Frontiers in Immunology, 10*, 705.

Dutta, J., Fan, Y., Gupta, N., Fan, G., & Gélinas, C., (2006). Current insights into the regulation of programmed cell death by NF-kappaB. *Oncogene, 25*(51), 6800–6816.

Espinosa, L., & Marruecos, L., (2021). NF-κB-dependent and –independent (moonlighting) IκBα functions in differentiation and cancer. *Biomedicines, 9*(9), 1278.

Fu, W., Zhuo, Z. J., Chen, Y. C., et al., (2017). NFKB1 -94insertion/deletion ATTG polymorphism and cancer risk: Evidence from 50 case-control studies. *Oncotarget, 8*(6), 9806–9822.

Gaptulbarova, K. A., Tsyganov, M. M., Pevzner, A. M., Ibragimova, M. K., & Litviakov, N. V., (2020). NF-kB as a potential prognostic marker and a candidate for targeted therapy of cancer. *Experimental Oncology, 42*(4), 263–269.

Georgescu, S. R., Mitran, C. I., Mitran, M. I., et al., (2018). New insights in the pathogenesis of HPV infection and the associated carcinogenic processes: The role of chronic inflammation and oxidative stress. *Journal of Immunology Research, 2018*, 5315816.

Georgopoulos, N. T., Proffitt, J. L., & Blair, G. E., (2000). Transcriptional regulation of the major histocompatibility complex (MHC) class I heavy chain, TAP1 and LMP2 genes by the human papillomavirus (HPV) type 6b, 16 and 18 E7 oncoproteins. *Oncogene, 19*(42), 4930–4935.

Gupta, S. C., Sundaram, C., Reuter, S., & Aggarwal, B. B., (2010). Inhibiting NF-κB activation by small molecules as a therapeutic strategy. *Biochimica et Biophysica Acta, 1799*(10–12), 775–787.

Gusho, E., & Laimins, L., (2021). Human papillomaviruses target the DNA damage repair and innate immune response pathways to allow for persistent infection. *Viruses, 13*(7), 1390.

Guttridge, D. C., Albanese, C., Reuther, J. Y., Pestell, R. G., & Baldwin, A. S. Jr., (1999). NF-kappaB controls cell growth and differentiation through transcriptional regulation of cyclin D1. *Molecular and Cellular Biology, 19*(8), 5785–5799.

Häcker, H., & Karin, M., (2006). Regulation and function of IKK and IKK-related kinases. *Science's STKE: Signal Transduction Knowledge Environment, 357*, re13.

Hammes, L. S., Tekmal, R. R., Naud, P., et al., (2007). Macrophages, inflammation and risk of cervical intraepithelial neoplasia (CIN) progression – clinicopathological correlation. *Gynecologic Oncology, 105*(1), 157–165.

Hayden, M. S., & Ghosh, S., (2004). Signaling to NF-kappaB. *Genes and Development, 18*(18), 2195–2224.

He, H., Zheng, C., & Tang, Y., (2021). Overexpression of SMC4 predicts a poor prognosis in cervical cancer and facilitates cancer cell malignancy phenotype by activating NF-κB pathway. *Human Cell, 34*(6), 1888–1898.

Hoesel, B., & Schmid, J. A., (2013). The complexity of NF-κB signaling in inflammation and cancer. *Molecular Cancer, 12*, 86.

Hou, S., Guan, H., & Ricciardi, R. P., (2003). Phosphorylation of serine 337 of NF-kappaB p50 is critical for DNA binding. *The Journal of Biological Chemistry, 278*(46), 45994–45998.

Hua, F., Li, C. H., Gao, Y. C., Li, J., & Meng, F., (2019). Molecular mechanism and role of NF-κB in the early diagnosis of cervical cancer. *Journal of B.U.ON., 24*(2), 720–728.

Ishikawa, H., Ohno, T., Kato, S., et al., (2006). Cyclooxygenase-2 impairs treatment effects of radiotherapy for cervical cancer by inhibition of radiation-induced apoptosis. *International Journal of Radiation Oncology, Biology, Physics, 66*(5), 1347–1355.

James, M. A., Lee, J. H., & Klingelhutz, A. J., (2006). HPV16-E6 associated hTERT promoter acetylation is E6AP dependent, increased in later passage cells and enhanced by loss of p300. *International Journal of Cancer, 119*(8), 1878–1885.

James, M. A., Lee, J. H., & Klingelhutz, A. J., (2006). Human papillomavirus type 16 E6 activates NF-kappaB, induces cIAP-2 expression, and protects against apoptosis in a PDZ binding motif-dependent manner. *Journal of Virology, 80*(11), 5301–5307.

Jana, A., Krett, N. L., Guzman, G., et al., (2017). NFkB is essential for activin-induced colorectal cancer migration via upregulation of PI3K-MDM2 pathway. *Oncotarget, 8*(23), 37377–37393.

Ji, Q., Zhang, L., Jia, H., & Xu, J., (2004). Pentoxifylline inhibits endotoxin-induced NF-kappa B activation and associated production of proinflammatory cytokines. *Annals of Clinical and Laboratory Science, 34*(4), 427–436.

Jin, L., Sturgis, E. M., Zhang, Y., Huang, Z., Song, X., Li, C., Wei, Q., & Li, G., (2013). Association of tumor necrosis factor-alpha promoter variants with risk of HPV-associated oral squamous cell carcinoma. *Molecular Cancer, 12*, 80.

Karin, M., & Ben-Neriah, Y., (2000). Phosphorylation meets ubiquitination: The control of NF-[kappa]B activity. *Annual Review of Immunology, 18*, 621–663.

Karin, M., (2006). Nuclear factor-kappaB in cancer development and progression. *Nature, 441*(7092), 431–436.

Kauppinen, A., Suuronen, T., Ojala, J., Kaarniranta, K., & Salminen, A., (2013). Antagonistic crosstalk between NF-κB and SIRT1 in the regulation of inflammation and metabolic disorders. *Cellular Signaling, 25*(10), 1939–1948.

Khan, H., Ullah, H., Castilho, P., et al., (2020). Targeting NF-κB signaling pathway in cancer by dietary polyphenols. *Critical Reviews in Food Science and Nutrition, 60*(16), 2790–2800.

Kim, H. J., Hawke, N., & Baldwin, A. S., (2006). NF-kappaB and IKK as therapeutic targets in cancer. *Cell Death and Differentiation, 13*(5), 738–747.

Kim, S. H., Oh, J. M., No, J. H., Bang, Y. J., Juhnn, Y. S., & Song, Y. S., (2009). Involvement of NF-kappaB and AP-1 in COX-2 upregulation by human papillomavirus 16 E5 oncoprotein. *Carcinogenesis, 30*(5), 753–757.

Kucharczak, J., Simmons, M. J., Fan, Y., & Gélinas, C., (2003). To be, or not to be: NF-kappaB is the answer--role of Rel/NF-kappaB in the regulation of apoptosis. *Oncogene, 22*(56), 8961–8982.

Kulkarni, S., Rader, J. S., Zhang, F., Liapis, H., Koki, A. T., Masferrer, J. L., Subbaramaiah, K., & Dannenberg, A. J., (2001). Cyclooxygenase-2 is overexpressed in human cervical cancer. *Clinical Cancer Research, 7*(2), 429–434.

Lawrence, T., (2009). The nuclear factor NF-kappaB pathway in inflammation. *Cold Spring Harbor Perspectives in Biology, 1*(6), a001651.

Lee, H., Deng, J., Xin, H., Liu, Y., Pardoll, D., & Yu, H., (2011). A requirement of STAT3 DNA binding precludes Th-1 immunostimulatory gene expression by NF-κB in tumors. *Cancer Research, 71*(11), 3772–3780.

Li, Q., & Verma, I. M., (2002). NF-kappaB regulation in the immune system. *Nature Reviews Immunology, 2*(10), 725–734.

Liu, Y. C., Chiang, I. T., Hsu, F. T., & Hwang, J. J., (2012). Using NF-κB as a molecular target for theranostics in radiation oncology research. *Expert Review of Molecular Diagnostics, 12*(2), 139–146.

Lugović-Mihić, L., Cvitanović, H., Djaković, I., Kuna, M., & Šešerko, A., (2021). The influence of psychological stress on HPV infection manifestations and carcinogenesis. *Cellular Physiology and Biochemistry, 55*(S2), 71–88.

Ma, X., Zhang, Q., Du, J., Tang, J., & Tan, B., (2021). Integrated analysis of ceRNA regulatory network associated with tumor stage in cervical cancer. *Frontiers in Genetics, 12*, 618753.

Maliekal, T. T., Antony, M. L., Nair, A., Paulmurugan, R., & Karunagaran, D., (2003). Loss of expression, and mutations of Smad 2 and Smad 4 in human cervical cancer. *Oncogene, 22*(31), 4889–4897.

Marienfeld, R., May, M. J., Berberich, I., Serfling, E., Ghosh, S., & Neumann, M., (2003). RelB forms transcriptionally inactive complexes with RelA/p65. *The Journal of Biological Chemistry, 278*(22), 19852–19860.

Medda, A., Duca, D., & Chiocca, S., (2021). Human papillomavirus and cellular pathways: Hits and targets. *Pathogens, 10*(3), 262.

Morgan, D., Garg, M., Tergaonkar, V., Tan, S. Y., & Sethi, G., (2020). Pharmacological significance of the non-canonical NF-κB pathway in tumorigenesis. *Biochimica et Biophysica Acta Reviews on Cancer, 1874*(2), 188449.

Müller-Schiffmann, A., Beckmann, J., & Steger, G., (2006). The E6 protein of the cutaneous human papillomavirus type 8 can stimulate the viral early and late promoters by distinct mechanisms. *Journal of Virology, 80*(17), 8718–8728.

Nair, A., Venkatraman, M., Maliekal, T. T., Nair, B., & Karunagaran, D., (2003). NF-kappaB is constitutively activated in high-grade squamous intraepithelial lesions and squamous cell carcinomas of the human uterine cervix. *Oncogene, 22*(1), 50–58.

Nees, M., Geoghegan, J. M., Hyman, T., Frank, S., Miller, L., & Woodworth, C. D., (2001). Papillomavirus type 16 oncogenes downregulate expression of interferon-responsive genes and upregulate proliferation-associated and NF-kappaB-responsive genes in cervical keratinocytes. *Journal of Virology, 75*(9), 4283–4296.

Neumann, M., & Naumann, M., (2007). Beyond IκBs: Alternative regulation of NF-kB activity. *The FASEB Journal, 21*(11), 2642–2654.

Niu, G., Wright, K. L., Ma, Y., Wright, G. M., Huang, M., Irby, R., Briggs, J., et al., (2005). Role of stat3 in regulating p53 expression and function. *Molecular and Cellular Biology, 25*(17), 7432–7440.

Pallavi, S., Anoop, K., Showket, H., Alo, N., & Mausumi, B., (2015). NFKB1/NFKBIa polymorphisms are associated with the progression of cervical carcinoma in HPV-infected postmenopausal women from rural area. *Tumour Biology, 36*(8), 6265–6276.

Patel, D., Huang, S. M., Baglia, L. A., & McCance, D. J., (1999). The E6 protein of human papillomavirus type 16 binds to and inhibits co-activation by CBP and p300. *The EMBO Journal, 18*(18), 5061–5072.

Peng, X., Wu, Z., Yu, L., Li, J., Xu, W., Chan, H. C., Zhang, Y., & Hu, L., (2012). Overexpression of cystic fibrosis transmembrane conductance regulator (CFTR) is associated with human cervical cancer malignancy, progression and prognosis. *Gynecologic Oncology, 125*(2), 470–476.

Perkins, N. D., & Gilmore, T. D., (2006). Good cop, bad cop: The different faces of NF-kappaB. *Cell Death and Differentiation, 13*(5), 759–772.

Perkins, N. D., (2004). NF-kappaB: Tumor promoter or suppressor? *Trends in Cell Biology, 14*(2), 64–69.

Pešut, E., Đukić, A., Lulić, L., Skelin, J., Šimić, I., Milutin, G. N., Tomaić, V., Sabol, I., & Grce, M., (2021). Human papillomaviruses-associated cancers: An update of current knowledge. *Viruses, 13*(11), 2234.

Pikarsky, E., Porat, R. M., Stein, I., et al., (2004). NF-kappaB functions as a tumor promoter in inflammation-associated cancer. *Nature, 431*(7007), 461–466.

Porta, C., Rimoldi, M., Raes, G., et al., (2009). Tolerance and M2 (alternative) macrophage polarization are related processes orchestrated by p50 nuclear factor kappaB. *Proceedings of the National Academy of Sciences of the United States of America, 106*(35), 14978–14983.

Prusty, B. K., Husain, S. A., & Das, B. C., (2005). Constitutive activation of nuclear factor -kB: Preferntial homodimerization of p50 subunits in cervical carcinoma. *Frontiers in Bioscience, 10*, 1510–1519.

Rao, N. A., McCalman, M. T., Moulos, P., et al., (2011). Coactivation of GR and NFKB alters the repertoire of their binding sites and target genes. *Genome Research, 21*(9), 1404–1416.

Ravi, R., & Bedi, A., (2004). NF-kappaB in cancer – a friend turned foe. *Drug Resistance Updates: Reviews and Commentaries in Antimicrobial and Anticancer Chemotherapy, 7*(1), 53–67.

Rayet, B., & Gélinas, C., (1999). Aberrant rel/nfkb genes and activity in human cancer. *Oncogene, 18*(49), 6938–6947.

Rebhandl, S., Huemer, M., Greil, R., & Geisberger, R., (2015). AID/APOBEC deaminases and cancer. *Oncoscience, 2*(4), 320–333.

Rossetti, R., Da Silva-Junior, I. A., Rodríguez, G. R., et al., (2020). Local and systemic STAT3 and p65 NF-KappaB expression as progression markers and functional targets for patients with cervical cancer. *Frontiers in Oncology, 10*, 587132.

Rothwarf, D. M., & Karin, M., (1999). The NF-kappa B activation pathway: A paradigm in information transfer from membrane to nucleus. *Science's STKE: Signal Transduction Knowledge Environment, 1999*(5), RE1.

Sadri, N. J., Moghoofei, M., Salmaninejad, A., et al., (2020). Pathogenic role of exosomes and microRNAs in HPV-mediated inflammation and cervical cancer: A review. *International Journal of Cancer, 146*(2), 305–320.

Sahu, U., Biswas, D., Prajapati, V. K., Singh, A. K., Samant, M., & Khare, P., (2021). Interleukin-17-A multifaceted cytokine in viral infections. *Journal of Cellular Physiology, 236*(12), 8000–8019.

Saidu, N., Filić, V., Thomas, M., Sarabia-Vega, V., Đukić, A., Miljković, F., Banks, L., & Tomaić, V., (2019). PDZ domain-containing protein NHERF-2 is a novel target of human papillomavirus 16 (HPV-16) and HPV-18. *Journal of Virology, 94*(1), e00663–19.

Sannigrahi, M. K., Sharma, R., Singh, V., Panda, N. K., Rattan, V., & Khullar, M., (2017). Role of host miRNA Hsa-miR-139-3p in HPV-16-induced carcinomas. *Clinical Cancer Research, 23*(14), 3884–3895.

Schuliga, M., (2015). NF-kappaB signaling in chronic inflammatory airway disease. *Biomolecules, 5*(3), 1266–1283.

Schwebke, J. R., & Zajackowski, M. E., (1997). Effect of concurrent lower genital tract infections on cervical cancer screening. *Genitourinary Medicine, 73*(5), 383–386.

Senba, M., & Mori, N., (2012). Mechanisms of virus immune evasion lead to development from chronic inflammation to cancer formation associated with human papillomavirus infection. *Oncology Reviews, 6*(2), e17.

Silva-Gomez, J. A., Galicia-Moreno, M., Sandoval-Rodriguez, A., et al., (2021). Hepatocarcinogenesis prevention by pirfenidone is PPARγ mediated and involves modification of nuclear NF-kB p65/p50 Ratio. *International Journal of Molecular Sciences, 22*(21), 11360.

Sizemore, N., Lerner, N., Dombrowski, N., Sakurai, H., & Stark, G. R., (2002). Distinct roles of the Ikappa B kinase alpha and beta subunits in liberating nuclear factor kappa B (NF-kappa B) from Ikappa B and in phosphorylating the p65 subunit of NF-kappa B. *The Journal of Biological Chemistry, 277*(6), 3863–3869.

Smahel, M., Síma, P., Ludvíková, V., Marinov, I., Pokorná, D., & Vonka, V., (2003). Immunization with modified HPV16 E7 genes against mouse oncogenic TC-1 cell sublines with downregulated expression of MHC class I molecules. *Vaccine, 21*(11, 12), 1125–1136.

Smith, E. L., Somma, D., Kerrigan, D., et al., (2019). The regulation of sequence specific NF-κB DNA binding and transcription by IKKβ phosphorylation of NF-κB p50 at serine 80. *Nucleic Acids Research, 47*(21), 11151–11163.

Smith, S. P., Scarpini, C. G., Groves, I. J., Odle, R. I., & Coleman, N., (2016). Identification of host transcriptional networks showing concentration-dependent regulation by HPV16 E6 and E7 proteins in basal cervical squamous epithelial cells. *Scientific Reports, 6*, 29832.

Snijders, P. J., Steenbergen, R. D., Heideman, D. A., & Meijer, C. J., (2006). HPV-mediated cervical carcinogenesis: Concepts and clinical implications. *The Journal of Pathology, 208*(2), 152–164.

Spitkovsky, D., Hehner, S. P., Hofmann, T. G., Möller, A., & Schmitz, M. L., (2002). The human papillomavirus oncoprotein E7 attenuates NF-kappa B activation by targeting the Ikappa B kinase complex. *The Journal of Biological Chemistry, 277*(28), 25576–25582.

Struyk, L., Van, D. M. E., Minnaar, R., Fontaine, V., Meijer, I., & Ter, S. J., (2000). Transcriptional regulation of human papillomavirus type 16 LCR by different C/EBPbeta isoforms. *Molecular Carcinogenesis, 28*(1), 42–50.

Subbaramaiah, K., & Dannenberg, A. J., (2007). Cyclooxygenase-2 transcription is regulated by human papillomavirus 16 E6 and E7 oncoproteins: Evidence of a corepressor/coactivator exchange. *Cancer Research, 67*(8), 3976–3985.

Surh, Y. J., Chun, K. S., Cha, H. H., Han, S. S., Keum, Y. S., Park, K. K., & Lee, S. S., (2001). Molecular mechanisms underlying chemopreventive activities of anti-inflammatory phytochemicals: Down-regulation of COX-2 and iNOS through suppression of NF-kappa B activation. *Mutation Research, 480, 481*, 243–268.

Tilborghs, S., Corthouts, J., Verhoeven, Y., Arias, D., Rolfo, C., Trinh, X. B., & Van, D. P. A., (2017). The role of nuclear factor-kappa B signaling in human cervical cancer. *Critical Reviews in Oncology/Hematology, 120*, 141–150.

Vandermark, E. R., Deluca, K. A., Gardner, C. R., et al., (2012). Human papillomavirus type 16 E6 and E 7 proteins alter NF-kB in cultured cervical epithelial cells and inhibition of NF-kB promotes cell growth and immortalization. *Virology, 425*(1), 53–60.

Viatour, P., Merville, M. P., Bours, V., & Chariot, A., (2005). Phosphorylation of NF-kappaB and IkappaB proteins: Implications in cancer and inflammation. *Trends in Biochemical Sciences, 30*(1), 43–52.

Vonderach, M., Byrne, D. P., Barran, P. E., Eyers, P. A., & Eyers, C. E., (2019). DNA binding and phosphorylation regulate the core structure of the NF-κB p50 transcription factor. *Journal of the American Society for Mass Spectrometry, 30*(1), 128–138.

Wang, Y., Yang, J., Huang, J., & Tian, Z., (2020). Tumor necrosis factor-α polymorphisms and cervical cancer: Evidence from a meta-analysis. *Gynecologic and Obstetric Investigation, 85*(2), 153–158.

Wong, D., Teixeira, A., Oikonomopoulos, S., et al., (2011). Extensive characterization of NF-κB binding uncovers non-canonical motifs and advances the interpretation of genetic functional traits. *Genome Biology, 12*(7), R70.

Wu, Z., Li, J., Zhang, Y., Hu, L., & Peng, X., (2019). Synchronous co-expression of Id-1 and nuclear NF-κB p65 promotes cervical cancer progression and malignancy, and is associated with a poor prognosis and chemosensitivity. *Oncology Reports, 42*(5), 2075–2086.

Wu, Z., Li, J., Zhang, Y., Hu, L., & Peng, X., (2020). CFTR regulates the proliferation, migration and invasion of cervical cancer cells by inhibiting the NF-κB signaling pathway. *Cancer Management and Research, 12*, 4685–4697.

Wu, Z., Peng, X., Li, J., Zhang, Y., & Hu, L., (2013). Constitutive activation of nuclear factor κB contributes to cystic fibrosis transmembrane conductance regulator expression and promotes human cervical cancer progression and poor prognosis. *International Journal of Gynecological Cancer, 23*(5), 906–915.

Xia, Y., Shen, S., & Verma, I. M., (2014). NF-κB, an active player in human cancers. *Cancer Immunology Research, 2*(9), 823–830.

Xing, Y., Yang, Y., Zhou, F., & Wang, J., (2013). Characterization of genome-wide binding of NF-κB in TNFα-stimulated HeLa cells. *Gene, 526*(2), 142–149.

Yildiz, I. Z., Usubütün, A., Firat, P., Ayhan, A., & Küçükali, T., (2007). Efficiency of immunohistochemical p16 expression and HPV typing in cervical squamous intraepithelial lesion grading and review of the p16 literature. *Pathology, Research and Practice, 203*(6), 445–449.

Yu, H., Lin, L., Zhang, Z., Zhang, H., & Hu, H., (2020). Targeting NF-κB pathway for the therapy of diseases: Mechanism and clinical study. *Signal Transduction and Targeted Therapy, 5*(1), 209.

CHAPTER 8

JAK-STAT Pathway in Cervical Cancer Management

8.1 OUTLINE OF JAK/STAT SIGNALING PATHWAY

The JAK/STAT pathway is an important regulator of embryonic development. This pathway plays an important role in the regulation of various key processes like hematopoiesis, stem cell maintenance, and the inflammatory response (Imada & Leonard, 2000). The JAK/STAT pathway transmits signals from various molecules (interleukins, cytokines, and growth factors) that perform its action through a family of transmembrane receptor. The erythropoietin receptor and the granulocyte colony-stimulating factor receptor are classified as type I receptors. The inactive kinases are intrinsically associated with the intracellular domains of these, named as janus kinases (JAKs). Interaction of ligand with receptor induces conformational variations in the receptor that exposes the target site of JAKs for phosphorylation at tyrosine residues and thus activates JAKs (Igaz et al., 2001). In certain cases, signal transduction via STATs can be stimulated by receptors with inherent tyrosine kinase activity for example, platelet-derived growth factor (PDGF) receptor and epidermal growth factor receptor (EGFR) (Silvennoinen et al., 1993); however, this also includes the cytoplasmic tyrosine kinase Src (Olayioye et al., 1999; Niu et al., 2002). After activation, JAKs causes phosphorylation of receptor at tyrosine amino acid residues, generating binding sites for the recruitment of signal transducers and activators of transcriptions (STATs). Further, STATs undergo dimerization and moved to the nucleus after phosphorylation through JAKs or other tyrosine kinases at highly

Cervical Cancer: Signaling Pathways, Molecular Mechanisms, Natural Products, and Therapeutic Approaches. Pratibha Pandey, Fahad Khan, Saher Islam, and Devarajan Thangadurai, (Eds.)

conserved tyrosine residues. These STAT dimers inside nucleus attach to specific promoter sites and alter transcription of genes regulating cellular functions including differentiation, proliferation, and apoptosis (Rawlings et al., 2004) (Figure 8.1).

In humans, JAK family includes mainly four members namely, JAK1, JAK2, JAK3, and TYK2. This family is recognized by the appearance of two adjoining kinase domains (JH1 and JH2), having a resemblance with the two faces of the Roman god Janus and thus named on that (Yamaoka et al., 2004). JH1 domain mainly associated with the phosphorylation while JH2 performs the regulatory function due to inherent kinase activity. Janus kinases are capable to associate and form homodimers and heterodimers (Aringer et al., 1999; Rane & Reddy, 2000).

There are seven members found in STAT family of humans including STAT1, STAT2, STAT3, STAT4, STAT5A, STAT5B, and STAT6. There is no specific relationship is established between these JAK family members and STAT family members in context to their specificity of binding during

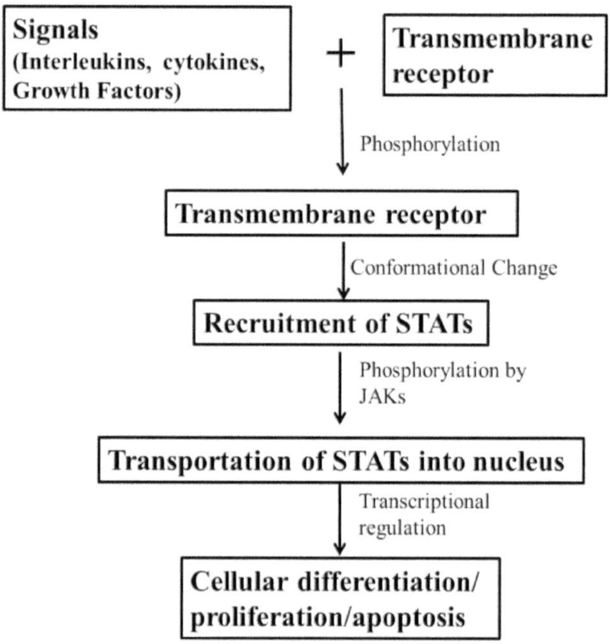

FIGURE 8.1 Summary of JAK/STAT signal transduction pathway.

JAK/STAT signaling. For example, the function of STAT3 and STAT5A/B is to promote the process of carcinogenesis; however, STAT1 function antagonistically (Bowman et al., 2000). STATs contain a functional domain that includes a SH2 domain (Src homology 2) and a C-terminal transactivation domain with specific functions. SH2 domain facilitates in the attachment to phosphorylated tyrosine residues while the C-terminal transactivation domain helps in the transcriptional activation (Bromberg & Darnell, 2000). The regulatory function of the JAK/STAT pathway activation is strictly performed by several negative mediatory molecules acting at different stages (Greenhalgh & Hilton, 2001). Numerous families of phosphatases are responsible for the dephosphorylation from JAKs and STATs. One such inhibitor is PIAS (protein inhibitors of activated STAT) that control STAT cellular location, prevent binding of STAT with DNA, and assist in the post-translational modification process of STATs. Other such protein is SOCS (Suppressor of cytokine signaling) which act as competitive inhibitors of STAT receptor binding domain and also perform the function of ubiquitin ligases that promote proteasomal breakdown of components of target pathway. STATs protein promotes the transcriptional expression of SOCS genes and regulates the fine tuning of pathway by creating a negative feedback loop (Hilton, 1999; Wormald & Hilton, 2004).

Various components of the JAK-STAT signaling cascade also have an impact on the expression of genes that are localized outside the normal signaling pathway by the process of epigenetic modifications related to chromatin. Few studies demonstrated the role of histone modifications by activated JAK2 when it gets entered into the nucleus, but these findings remain controversial (Dawson et al., 2009; Girodon et al., 2011). Dimeric STAT5A in unphosphorylated state can translocate to the nucleus and trigger heterochromatin formation caused by attachment of heterochromatin protein 1 (Hu et al., 2013; Silver-Morse & Li, 2013). In most of the cases, STATs are conventionally found to be responsible for transcription activation, although accumulating evidence from comprehensive gene expression profiling studies revealed that stimulated STATs also decrease the expression level of a large number of genes. In some cells, STATs have also made an impact through transcription-independent manner by modifying mitochondrial function (Wang & Weinman, 2006). Phosphorylation of STAT3 on a specific C-terminus serine residue helps in its localization to the mitochondria, where it promotes the electron transport chain (ETC) activity (Gough et al., 2009). This phosphorylation of STATs is controlled by the Ras/Raf/MEK/ERK signaling pathway, and also needed for Ras-associated transformation (Gough et al., 2013; Garama et al., 2016).

8.2 CONTROLLING FACTORS OF THE JAK-STAT PATHWAY

The main regulatory elements of the JAK/STAT pathway are ligands, receptors, JAKs, STATs, and some inhibitory proteins such as suppressors of cytokine signaling (SOCSs). The ligands or signaling molecules are mainly cytokines or growth factors.

8.2.1 JANUS KINASES

Human Janus kinases are classified into four types namely, JAK1, JAK2, JAK3, and TYK2. These kinases performed the function of catalysis and regulation of JAK-STAT signaling pathway. Each Janus kinase consists of mainly four distinct domains for the execution of specific function (Yeh & Pellegrini, 1999). The four domains of JAKs are N-terminal FERM (protein 4.1, ezrin, radixin, and moesin), SH2 (Src 2 homology) domain, pseudokinase domain, and a protein tyrosine kinase (PTK) domain. The N-terminal FERM domain helps in binding with receptor complexes, while SH2 domain interacts with phosphotyrosine residues. A pseudokinase domain named due to its homology with PTK domain but no catalytic activity and act as regulatory subunit, conversely the protein tyrosine kinase domain with catalytic activity helps in the phosphorylation of downstream targets of signaling pathway (Hou et al., 2002; Thomas et al., 2015; Seif et al., 2017).

8.2.2 RECEPTORS

The receptors of JAK-STAT pathway are mainly cytokine receptors that are categorized into types I and II (Seif et al., 2017). Both types of cytokine receptors specifically bind with different types of JAKs to transduce their signals to the cytoplasmic region as they are devoid of inherent tyrosine kinase activity. The association of the cytokine receptor is important for the phosphorylation of JAK and the subsequent incorporation of STATs and its phosphorylation (Jatiani et al., 2010; Morris et al., 2018).

8.2.3 STATs

The STATs protein family comprising of seven members, and helps in the regulation of diverse cellular and biological processes such as cell proliferation, differentiation, apoptosis, and inflammation (Ivashkiv & Hu, 2004; Bousoik & Montazeri, 2018). These proteins activated by phosphorylation, forms dimer, and act as a transcription factor (Huynh et al., 2019).

8.2.4 CYTOKINE SIGNALING SUPPRESSORS (SOCS)

Another critical regulator of JAK-STAT pathway is SOCS protein which comprises mainly eight protein members including SOCS1, SOCS2, SOCS3, SOCS4, SOCS5, SOCS6, SOCS7 and the protein-inducible SH2 domain cytokines (Malemud, 2017; Yoshimura et al., 2018). Each SOCS consists of mainly four distinct domains for the execution of specific function. The SOCS protein comprises of central SH2 domain, an amino-terminal domain, and a carboxy-terminal module (SOCS box), however SOCS1 and SOCS3 also have a KIR (kinase inhibitory region). The SH2 domain interacts with the phosphorylated tyrosine residue of stimulated JAKs and suppresses STAT activation. The inhibitory domain of the SOCS protein functions as a pseudosubstrate and prevents the activity of JAK. The carboxy-terminal domain binds with different enzymes of the ubiquitination machinery and helps in the proteasomal breakdown of JAKs (Inagaki-Ohara et al., 2013; La et al., 2022).

8.2.5 OTHER REGULATORY ELEMENTS

Besides JAKs, STATs, ligands, receptors, and SOCS, the protein inhibitor of activated STAT (PIAS) and protein tyrosine phosphatases (PTPs) also plays an important role in the regulation of the JAK/STAT pathway (Wu et al., 2019). The PIAS protein family includes mainly five members namely, PIAS1, PIASx, PIASx, PIAS3, and PIASy (Niu et al., 2018). These PIAS proteins can control the transcription process in four different ways:

- Inhibiting the DNA-binding activity of a transcription factor
- Recruitment of co-regulators such as histone deacetylases
- Promoting the SUMOylation process of a transcription factor, and
- Confiscating the transcription factors

PTPs are also classified into different classes, such as CD45, SHP1, SHP2 PTP1B, T cell PTP, PTPBL, and PTPRT. These PTPs are involved in the dephosphorylation of tyrosine residues of JAKs and thus inhibits the activation of the JAK/STAT signaling pathway. It has been noticed that SHP2 can control JAK/STAT signaling in a positive manner. Some studies reported that SHP2 could dephosphorylate JAK2 and prevents the binding of JAK2-SOCS1, thus repressing the JAK2 breakdown (Shuai & Liu, 2005; Xu & Qu, 2008; Zhang et al., 2015; Zehender et al., 2018). Recent studies observed the dual role of SHP2 in the various signaling pathways involved in the carcinogenesis process. For example, SHP2 regulates the JAK/STAT3 signaling in a negative manner, however, some studies have revealed the stimulating role of SHP2 through the Grb2 and Gab proteins (Figure 8.2). Association of SHP2 with different types of cancers has been largely investigated and therefore can be considered as a potential target strategy for cancer therapy (Liu et al., 2020; Liu et al., 2021).

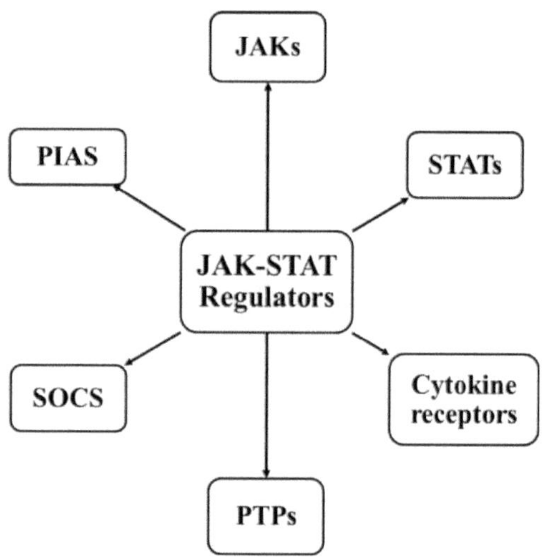

FIGURE 8.2 Critical regulators of JAK-STAT signaling pathway.

8.3 ABERRANT ACTIVATION OF JAK/STAT SIGNALING PATHWAY IN CANCER

The abnormal activation of the JAK-STAT signaling as a result of genetic polymorphisms and/or mutations caused a consistent stimulation of JAKs without cytokine signaling. This process may then lead to tumorigenesis or carcinogenesis induction (Banerjee et al., 2017; Lokau et al., 2019). Still, in several types of cancers where the responsible factor for carcinogenesis is JAK/STAT pathway activation, the exact mechanism behind the abnormal activation of the pathway is not identified. Accumulating evidence exploring the mechanistic approach suggested that cancerous cells utilize a different kind of strategies to stimulate the signaling (Hu et al., 2021). In case of head and neck carcinoma, increased secretion of IL-6 by tumor cells resulted in STAT3 phosphorylation (Sriuranpong et al., 2003; Johnson et al., 2018) while overexpression of the G-CSF receptor is detected in high-grade ovarian epithelial carcinoma and G-CSF receptor further promotes activation of JAK/STAT pathway in ovarian cancer (Kumar et al., 2014; Wu et al., 2020).

In hematological carcinomas, activating mutations in JAKs have been found to be responsible for pathway activation in an aberrant manner (Vainchenker & Constantinescu, 2013). In recent studies, large-scale sequencing data recognized the genetic variations impacting the activity of JAKs in some solid tumors. JAK1-related missense mutations have been documented in 9% of patient sample of Hepatitis B-related hepatocellular carcinoma. *In vitro* studies demonstrated that these mutations could enhance JAK1 and STAT3 phosphorylation, and assist in cytokine-independent cell growth and proliferation (Kan et al., 2013; Zucman-Rossi et al., 2015). A comprehensive molecular characterization study has shown frequent augmentation of the chromosomal locus comprising JAK2 in gastric adenocarcinoma that correspond to increases in JAK2 expression levels and thus activation of JAK-STAT pathway (The Cancer Genome Atlas Research Network, 2014).

STATs-related activating mutations were also reported in several cancers (Loh et al., 2019). Mutations targeting the SH2 domain of STAT3 were observed in 40% of the patient sample having large granular lymphocytic leukemia. These types of mutations incorporate hydrophobic residues supposed to STAT dimers stabilization and resulted in elevated STAT-mediated transcription (Koskela et al., 2012). In prostate cancer, STAT5A/B locus amplification has been identified which is related with overexpression and nuclear translocation of STAT5 in cancer samples. These amplifications are further responsible for increase cell growth and survival in culture and support tumor growth in a xenograft animal model (Haddad et al., 2013; Erb et al., 2020). Promoter hypermethylation in tumor samples of non-small cell lung cancer (NSCLC) has been found to be associated with inhibition of SOCS3 expression followed by reduced gene transcription. This study was validated by using a NSCLC cell line in which restoration of SOCS3 activity decreases phosphorylation of STAT3 (He et al., 2003). In glioblastoma, the PIAS3 protein expression has been reported to be attenuated, may be due to enhanced protein breakdown. Decrease PIAS3 levels are related with elevated pSTAT3 and concomitantly augmented protein expression generated from STAT target genes in glioblastoma patient samples (Brantley et al., 2008; Bian et al., 2021).

8.4 ROLE OF JAK/STAT PATHWAY IN CERVICAL CANCER

The involvement of the activated JAK/STAT signaling pathway in the carcinogenesis process has become more evident in different types of cancers such as liver, breast, lung, prostate, cervical, ovarian, and pancreatic cancer. The hyperactivation of JAK/STAT proteins and down-regulation of various SOCS are closely involved in cellular proliferation, survival, and metastasis in different kinds of cancer cells (Sabaawy et al., 2021). The JAK/STAT signaling is also correlated with the occurrence of tumor tolerance, due to a persistent association between JAK/STAT over-activation and increase transcription of genes engaged in the Tregs cells regulation (Chang & Lai, 2019). Studies revealed that more than 90% of samples of cervical cancer possess HR HPV DNA, and their oncoproteins E5, E6, and E7 can modify multiple signal transduction pathways required for the initiation and progression of disease. Although, it has recently been observed that HPV infection may also influence the expression of various machineries of the JAK/STAT signaling and its repressor molecules (Walboomers et al., 1999; Chen, 2015; Campos-Parra et al., 2016; Ezeonwumelu et al., 2021).

8.4.1 IMPLICATION OF STAT1 PROTEINS IN CERVICAL CANCER

The expression of STAT1 in cervical lesions and cervical cancer has been reported in several research. A study performed by Rajkumar et al. observed STAT1 overexpression in initial cervical intraepithelial neoplasia (CIN) stages, and a significantly elevated level in invasive carcinomas (Rajkumar et al., 2011). In accordance with this study, Ding et al. also detected significantly increased levels of STAT1 in samples of cervical cancer in comparison with normal tissue samples (Ding et al., 2015). Elevated expression level of STAT1 is associated with all three stages of

CIN as well as with malignant cervical cancer; however, STAT1 expression has no significant impact on overall survival rate (Yi et al., 2020; Raspaglio et al., 2021; Yuan et al., 2021).

Additionally, there are studies related to the impact of HPV on STAT1 protein. Infection of keratinocytes with HR-HPV E6 or E7 oncoproteins demonstrated downregulated expression of STAT1α/β (Chang & Laimins, 2000; Hong et al., 2011). HPV16 E6 has the potential of decreasing the quantity of STAT1 and attachment with ISREs (IFN-stimulated response elements). Simultaneously, both these oncoproteins (E6 and E7) decrease the movement of STAT1 to the nucleus (Nees et al., 2001). Lei et al. (2015) reported that the cisplatin-treated HeLa cells show increased expression of STAT1 and, siRNA-mediated (small interfering RNA) silencing of STAT1 stimulates cellular proliferation and reducing the adverse effect of cisplatin on tumor cells, thus suggested the potential of STAT1 in cell death initiation in tumor cells. Similarly, Buttarelli et al. (2019) revealed that locally advanced cervical cancer patients were responsive to chemoradiation therapy with increased STAT1 levels in comparison to resistant patients, which recommends the correlation of STAT1 expression with improved sensitivity towards radiotherapy (Shi & Bonner, 2021). Altogether, these facts suggested that STAT1 could possess a dual role in HPV-mediated carcinogenesis, displaying a protective role in the initial stage of HPV infection, while as a proto-oncogene during the invasive stages of cervical cancer development.

8.4.2 IMPLICATION OF STAT2 PROTEINS IN CERVICAL CANCER

A study done by Liang et al. observed that the tissue samples of CIN shows overexpression of STAT2 in comparison to the cervicitis samples, however no such substantial increased expression level was found with the severity of cervical lesions. Thus, they proposed that the elevated expression of STAT2 initiates in premalignant dysplasia and continues in cervical cancer. This study also observed no significant variation in the five-year survival rate of cervical cancer patients with down regulated and upregulated expression of STAT2 (Liang et al., 2012; Yue et al., 2015; Ho et al., 2016). In contrast to this, HPV identified to repress STAT2 in an indirect manner. The HPV E6 oncoprotein can bind with Tyk2 and stop its interaction with IFNAR1, thus inhibiting the STAT1 and STAT2 phosphorylation (Li et al., 1999). The HPV 16 E7 oncoprotein interacts with IFR9 and prevents its attachment to STAT1/STAT2 heterodimers, thus obstructing the generation of the ISGF3 complex and its nuclear translocation.

8.4.3 IMPLICATION OF STAT3 PROTEINS IN CERVICAL CANCER

STAT3 aberrant activation has been demonstrated in various types of carcinomas, including bladder, cervical, bone, colon, esophagus, breast, brain, head and neck, lung, ovary, pancreas, kidney, liver, uterus, stomach, and prostate cancer (Zou et al., 2020). Important factors of STAT3 hyper-activation are the occurrence of increased levels of cytokines and growth factors, lack of negative regulatory molecules, and the stimulation of protein tyrosine kinases with inherent catalytic activity (Verhoeven et al., 2020). STAT3 protein considered as an important player in cancer development due to its regulatory role in the transcription of the genes related to cell cycle (cyclin D, cyclin E, RAC1), cell death (BCL2, BCLXL, FAS, HSP70), cellular metabolism (OCT1, HIF1A), immunosuppression (IL-10, IL-23, IL-6), chemoresistance (COX-2, MYC, ABCC2, ABCC6), cell migration and invasion (MMP1-3, TWIST1), angiogenesis (VEGFA and bFGF), and other mechanisms (Demaria et al., 2010; Carpenter & Lo, 2014).

In cervical cancer, STAT3 has attained specific attention from research findings displaying that its incidence and activity are strongly related with the malignant transformation of cervical lesions (Page et al., 2000). HR HPV-infected cells display a greater expression level of active STAT3 in comparison to HPV-negative cells (Shukla et al., 2013). HPV-associated cervical cancer cells are able to produce an increase number of IL-6 that resulted in enhanced STAT3 activation (Morgan & Macdonald, 2019). It is a well-established fact that the HPV genome expression mainly depends upon host transcription factors as well as some other transcription factors such as AP-1, NF-κB, and STAT3. These transcription factors might play an important role in HPV infection regulation due to the occurrence of some specific sites (cis-related elements) in the upstream regulatory regions (URRs) which involved in carcinogenesis (Roca et al., 2018; Shukla et al., 2019). A study by Arany et al. elucidated that binding of STAT3 to HPV16 upstream of the URR promotes the expression of E7 oncoprotein (Arany et al., 2002). However, various studies showed the correlation of STAT3 expression with the expression of E6. The suppression of STAT3 with the STAT3 inhibitors like cryptotanshinone

STAT3-specific siRNA AG490 curcumin resulted in reduced expression of E6 and E7 oncoproteins (Morgan et al., 2018; Ashrafizadeh et al., 2020). The downregulated expression of STAT3 in cervical cancer cells have diverse stringent effects, which includes an increase expression of cell cycle regulatory proteins (p21, pRB, p53) and concomitant increase in apoptosis induction via decreased expression of pro-apoptotic proteins and the activation of effector caspases (Shukla et al., 2013; Morgan et al., 2018). In conclusion, the repression of STAT3 in cervical cancer cells resulted in a significant reduction in the E6 and E7 oncoproteins thus STAT3 inhibition could serve as a potential therapeutic target in the treatment of and management of cervical cancer.

8.4.4 IMPLICATION OF STAT4 PROTEINS IN CERVICAL CANCER

The association of STAT4 protein has been has been poorly understood in cervical cancer pathogenesis (Wurster et al., 2000; Nishi et al., 2017; Zhao et al., 2017; Anderson et al., 2020). However, some studies reported the prevalence of STAT4 in cervical cancer development. One such study done by Luo et al. assessed the STAT4 expression in histological lesions, and reported elevated STAT4 expression in adenocarcinoma and squamous cell carcinoma (SCC) patient samples in comparison to non-cancerous tissue samples. This study also demonstrated that approximately 95.83% of the metastasis cancerous samples isolated from the lymph nodes were expressing upregulated level of STAT4 and established a correlation between the STAT4 with carcinogenesis and the severity of disease (Luo et al., 2016). These experimental findings suggested a positive relation between STAT4 with cancer progression, and metastasis/invasion in cervical cancer cells, as well as the impact of HPV E7 oncoproteins on STAT4 expression. Though, there are very few reports, thus further research is required to understand the mechanistic role of STAT4 expression in cervical cancer initiation and development.

8.4.5 IMPLICATION OF STAT5 PROTEINS IN CERVICAL CANCER

STAT5 protein overexpression is reported in most of the stages of cervical cancer progression and development (Schwaller et al., 2000; Li et al., 2004; Xiong et al., 2009; Chen et al., 2012; Feng & Cao, 2014). However, studies suggested an unusual expression pattern of STAT5a and STAT5b isoforms was observed in cervical tumor. A study done by Sobti et al. observed a positive relationship between elevated expressions of STAT5b with disease severity, whereas STAT5a expression was significantly lowers in cervical cancer tissue samples (Sobti et al., 2010). Morgan and Macdonald demonstrated that phosphorylation of STAT5 rises with the disease progression from CIN1 to CIN3 in HPV16+ and HPV18+ cervical cancer cell lines. Additionally, this study revealed that repression of STAT5b promotes a significant decrease in cell proliferation and survival due to downregulation of cyclin D1 and upregulation of p21. Moreover, they reported an upsurge in early and late apoptosis induction because of activation of caspase, PARP cleavage, and downregulated expression of the anti-apoptotic protein (Bcl-xL). siRNA-mediated STAT5b inhibition leads to the decrease in the HPV E6 and E7 oncoproteins expression. These studies suggested a significant role of STAT5b in the cervical tumorigenesis and viral oncoproteins regulation (Hong & Laimins, 2013; Morgan & Macdonald, 2019).

8.4.6 IMPLICATION OF STAT6 PROTEINS IN CERVICAL CANCER

Reports established the associations of STAT6 protein with cervical cancer progression are very limited (Das et al., 2009; Goenka & Kaplan, 2011; Cao et al., 2016; Xu et al., 2019). Li et al. revealed that exposure of cervical tumor cells with IFN-γ/TNF-α in conjugation with nanoparticles enhanced the STAT6 expression and activation. They also found the inverse association between STAT6 activation and tumor size in tumor models. Moreover, the STAT6 silencing in cervical cancer HeLa cells decreases the expression of p53 and Bax, and inhibition of apoptotic pathway. This experimental evidence could suggest a significant role of STAT6 in apoptosis induction in cancerous cells through IFN-γ and TNF-α (Li et al., 2014). Some research studies revealed that HPV oncoproteins modulates the expression of STAT6 in various ways. HPV E6 and E7 oncoproteins have significant ability to induce activation and expression of STAT6 (Figure 8.3). A study showed that HPV16 genome transfection increase STAT6 and STAT1 activation (Scott et al., 2020). Altogether, there is very limited research in this context, and further research must be conducted to confirm the potential of STAT6 in tumor progression and development.

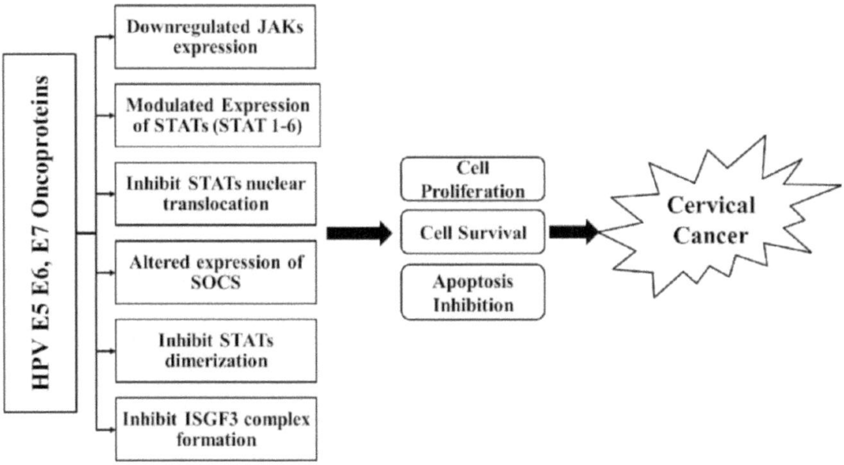

FIGURE 8.3 HPV oncoproteins mediated aberrant activation of JAK-STAT pathway and their association in the cervical cancer development.

8.5 ASSOCIATION OF SOCS AND CERVICAL CANCER PROGRESSION

A negative relationship has been established between SOCS proteins and JAK-STAT signal transduction pathway. It has been found that inhibition of SOCS associated with enhanced tumor development and poor survival in several types of cancer, including breast, prostate liver, lung, ovarian cancer, and others (Yoshikawa et al., 2001; Neuwirt et al., 2009; Lv et al., 2018; Yang et al., 2020, 2021). HPV and their oncoproteins can alter the expression of different types of SOCS proteins in cervical tumor; in HPV16/18 positive cervical cell lines, a downregulated expression of SOCS1, SOCS3, and SOCS5 was observed (Kim et al., 2015). Reduced expression of SOCS1 has also been found in precancerous lesions as well as in the various stages of cervical cancer progression, which exhibited a correlation between disease severity and SOCS1 downregulation (Sobti et al., 2011). Various studies revealed that the SOCS1 inhibition is mediated by HPV via promoter hypermethylation. SOCS1 can bind with the HPV E7 oncoprotein and encourages its breakdown, which subsequently resulted in upregulation of Rb protein and reduced tumor proliferation and survival (Kamio et al., 2004).

KEYWORDS

- **hypermethylation**
- **precancerous lesions**
- **Rb protein**
- **SOCS proteins**
- **SOCS1 downregulation**
- **tumor proliferation**
- **upregulation**

REFERENCES

Anderson, K., Ryan, N., Volpedo, G., Varikuti, S., Satoskar, A. R., & Oghumu, S., (2020). Immune suppression mediated by STAT4 deficiency promotes lymphatic metastasis in HNSCC. *Frontiers in Immunology, 10*, 3095.

Arany, I., Grattendick, K. G., & Tyring, S. K., (2002). Interleukin-10 induces transcription of the early promoter of human papillomavirus type 16 (HPV16) through the 5'-segment of the upstream regulatory region (URR). *Antiviral Research, 55*(2), 331–339.

Aringer, M., Cheng, A., Nelson, J. W., Chen, M., Sudarshan, C., Zhou, Y. J., & O'Shea, J. J., (1999). Janus kinases and their role in growth and disease. *Life Sciences, 64*(24), 2173–2186.

Ashrafizadeh, M., Rafiei, H., Mohammadinejad, R., Afshar, E. G., Farkhondeh, T., & Samarghandian, S., (2020). Potential therapeutic effects of curcumin mediated by JAK/STAT signaling pathway: A review. *Phytotherapy Research, 34*(8), 1745–1760.

Banerjee, S., Biehl, A., Gadina, M., Hasni, S., & Schwartz, D. M., (2017). JAK–STAT signaling as a target for inflammatory and autoimmune diseases: Current and future prospects. *Drugs, 77*(5), 521–546.

Bian, Z., Ji, W., Xu, B., Huo, Z., Huang, H., Huang, J., Jiao, J., Shao, J., & Zhang, X., (2021). Noncoding RNAs involved in the STAT3 pathway in glioma. *Cancer Cell International, 21*(1), 445.

Bousoik, E., & Montazeri, A. H., (2018). "Do we know jack" about JAK? A closer look at JAK/STAT signaling pathway. *Frontiers in Oncology, 8*, 287.

Bowman, T., Garcia, R., Turkson, J., & Jove, R., (2000). STATs in oncogenesis. *Oncogene, 19*(21), 2474–2488.

Brantley, E. C., Nabors, L. B., Gillespie, G. Y., et al., (2008). Loss of protein inhibitors of activated STAT-3 expression in glioblastoma multiforme tumors: Implications for STAT-3 activation and gene expression. *Clinical Cancer Research, 14*(15), 4694–4704.

Bromberg, J., & Darnell, J. E., (2000). The role of STATs in transcriptional control and their impact on cellular function. *Oncogene, 19*(21), 2468–2473.

Buttarelli, M., Babini, G., Raspaglio, G., et al., (2019). A combined ANXA2-NDRG1-STAT1 gene signature predicts response to chemoradiotherapy in cervical cancer. *Journal of Experimental and Clinical Cancer Research, 38*(1), 279.

Campos-Parra, A. D., Padua-Bracho, A., Pedroza-Torres, A., et al., (2016). Comprehensive transcriptome analysis identifies pathways with therapeutic potential in locally advanced cervical cancer. *Gynecologic Oncology, 143*(2), 406–413.

Cancer Genome Atlas Research Network, (2014). Comprehensive molecular characterization of gastric adenocarcinoma. *Nature, 513*(7517), 202–209.

Cao, H., Zhang, J., Liu, H., et al., (2016). IL-13/STAT6 signaling plays a critical role in the epithelial-mesenchymal transition of colorectal cancer cells. *Oncotarget, 7*(38), 61183–61198.

Carpenter, R. L., & Lo, H. W., (2014). STAT3 target genes relevant to human cancers. *Cancers, 6*(2), 897–925.

Chang, W. H., & Lai, A. G., (2019). An immunoevasive strategy through clinically-relevant pan-cancer genomic and transcriptomic alterations of JAK-STAT signaling components. *Molecular Medicine, 25*(1), 46.

Chang, Y. E., & Laimins, L. A., (2000). Microarray analysis identifies interferon-inducible genes and Stat-1 as major transcriptional targets of human papillomavirus type 31. *Journal of Virology, 74*(9), 4174–4182.

Chen, H. H., Chou, C. Y., Wu, Y. H., et al., (2012). Constitutive STAT5 activation correlates with better survival in cervical cancer patients treated with radiation therapy. *International Journal of Radiation Oncology, Biology, Physics, 82*(2), 658–666.

Chen, J., (2015). Signaling pathways in HPV-associated cancers and therapeutic implications. *Reviews in Medical Virology, 25*(1), 24–53.

Das, S., Roth, C. P., Wasson, L. M., & Vishwanatha, J. K., (2007). Signal transducer and activator of transcription-6 (STAT6) is a constitutively expressed survival factor in human prostate cancer. *The Prostate, 67*(14), 1550–1564.

Dawson, M. A., Bannister, A. J., Göttgens, B., Foster, S. D., Bartke, T., Green, A. R., & Kouzarides, T., (2009). JAK2 phosphorylates histone H3Y41 and excludes HP1α from chromatin. *Nature, 461*(7265), 819–822.

Demaria, M., Giorgi, C., Lebiedzinska, M., et al., (2010). A STAT3-mediated metabolic switch is involved in tumour transformation and STAT3 addiction. *Aging, 2*(11), 823–842.

Ding, Y., Yang, M., She, S., Min, H., Xv, X., Ran, X., Wu, Y., Wang, W., Wang, L., Yi, L., & Yang, Y., (2015). iTRAQ-based quantitative proteomic analysis of cervical cancer. *International Journal of Oncology, 46*(4), 1748–1758.

Erb, H., Bodenbender, J., Handle, F., et al., (2020). Assessment of STAT5 as a potential therapy target in enzalutamide-resistant prostate cancer. *PLoS One, 15*(8), e0237248.

Ezeonwumelu, I. J., Garcia-Vidal, E., & Ballana, E., (2021). JAK-STAT pathway: A novel target to tackle viral infections. *Viruses, 13*(12), 2379.

Feng, C., & Cao, S., (2014). Activation of STAT5 contributes to proliferation in U87 human glioblastoma multiforme cells. *Molecular Medicine Reports, 10*(1), 203–210.

Garama, D. J., White, C. L., Balic, J. J., & Gough, D. J., (2016). Mitochondrial STAT3: Powering up a potent factor. *Cytokine, 87*, 20–25.

Girodon, F., Mara, P., Steinkamp, C. C., Sylvie, H., & Bridget, S. W., (2011). Confocal imaging studies cast doubt on nuclear localization of JAK2 V617F. *Blood, 118*(9), 2633, 2634.

Goenka, S., & Kaplan, M. H., (2011). Transcriptional regulation by STAT6. *Immunologic Research, 50*(1), 87–96.

Gough, D. J., Corlett, A., Schlessinger, K., Wegrzyn, J., Larner, A. C., & Levy, D. E., (2009). Mitochondrial STAT3 supports Ras-dependent oncogenic transformation. *Science, 324*(5935), 1713–1716.

Gough, D. J., Koetz, L., & Levy, D. E., (2013). The MEK-ERK pathway is necessary for serine phosphorylation of mitochondrial STAT3 and Ras-mediated transformation. *PLoS One, 8*(11), e83395.

Greenhalgh, C. J., & Hilton, D. J., (2001). Negative regulation of cytokine signaling. *Journal of Leukocyte Biology, 70*(3), 348–356.

Haddad, B. R., Gu, L., Mirtti, T., et al., (2013). STAT5A/B gene locus undergoes amplification during human prostate cancer progression. *The American Journal of Pathology, 182*(6), 2264–2275.

He, B., You, L., Uematsu, K., et al., (2003). SOCS-3 is frequently silenced by hypermethylation and suppresses cell growth in human lung cancer. *Proceedings of the National Academy of Sciences of the United States of America, 100*(24), 14133–14138.

Hilton, D. J., (1999). Negative regulators of cytokine signal transduction. *Cellular and Molecular Life Sciences, 55*(12), 1568–1577.

Ho, J., Pelzel, C., Begitt, A., Mee, M., Elsheikha, H. M., Scott, D. J., & Vinkemeier, U., (2016). STAT2 is a pervasive cytokine regulator due to its inhibition of STAT1 in multiple signaling pathways. *PLoS Biology, 14*(10), e2000117.

Hong, S., & Laimins, L. A., (2013). The JAK-STAT transcriptional regulator, STAT-5, activates the ATM DNA damage pathway to induce HPV 31 genome amplification upon epithelial differentiation. *PLoS Pathogens, 9*(4), e1003295.

Hong, S., Mehta, K. P., & Laimins, L. A., (2011). Suppression of STAT-1 expression by human papillomaviruses is necessary for differentiation-dependent genome amplification and plasmid maintenance. *Journal of Virology, 85*(18), 9486–9494.

Hou, S. X., Zheng, Z., Chen, X., & Perrimon, N., (2002). The Jak/STAT pathway in model organisms: Emerging roles in cell movement. *Developmental Cell, 3*(6), 765–778.

Hu, X., Dutta, P., Tsurumi, A., Li, J., Wang, J., & Li, W. X., (2013). Unphosphorylated STAT5A stabilizes heterochromatin and suppresses tumor growth. *Proceedings of the National Academy of Sciences of the United States of America, 110*(25), 10213–10218.

Hu, X., Fu, M., Zhao, X., & Wang, W., (2021). The JAK/STAT signaling pathway: From bench to clinic. *Signal Transduction and Targeted Therapy, 6*(1), 1–33.

Huynh, J., Chand, A., Gough, D., & Ernst, M., (2019). Therapeutically exploiting STAT3 activity in cancer – using tissue repair as a road map. *Nature Reviews Cancer, 19*(2), 82–96.

Igaz, P., Toth, S., & Falus, A., (2001). Biological and clinical significance of the JAK-STAT pathway; lessons from knockout mice. *Inflammation Research, 50*(9), 435–441.

Imada, K., & Leonard, W. J., (2000). The jak-STAT pathway. *Molecular Immunology, 37*(1, 2), 1–11.

Inagaki-Ohara, K., Kondo, T., Ito, M., & Yoshimura, A., (2013). SOCS, inflammation, and cancer. *JAK-STAT, 2*(3), e24053.

Ivashkiv, L. B., & Hu, X., (2004). Signaling by STATs. *Arthritis Research and Therapy, 6*(4), 159–168.

Jatiani, S. S., Baker, S. J., Silverman, L. R., & Reddy, E. P., (2010). Jak/STAT pathways in cytokine signaling and myeloproliferative disorders: Approaches for targeted therapies. *Genes and Cancer, 1*(10), 979–993.

Johnson, D. E., O'Keefe, R. A., & Grandis, J. R., (2018). Targeting the IL-6/JAK/STAT3 signaling axis in cancer. *Nature Reviews Clinical Oncology, 15*(4), 234–248.

Kamio, M., Yoshida, T., Ogata, H., et al., (2004). SOCS1 [corrected] inhibits HPV-E7-mediated transformation by inducing degradation of E7 protein. *Oncogene, 23*(17), 3107–3115.

Kan, Z., Zheng, H., Liu, X., et al., (2013). Whole-genome sequencing identifies recurrent mutations in hepatocellular carcinoma. *Genome Research, 23*(9), 1422–1433.

Kim, M. H., Kim, M. S., Kim, W., et al., (2015). Suppressor of cytokine signaling (SOCS) genes are silenced by DNA hypermethylation and histone deacetylation and regulate response to radiotherapy in cervical cancer cells. *PLoS One, 10*(4), e0123133.

Koskela, H. L., Eldfors, S., Ellonen, P., et al., (2012). Somatic STAT3 mutations in large granular lymphocytic leukemia. *The New England Journal of Medicine, 366*(20), 1905–1913.

Kumar, J., Fraser, F. W., Riley, C., Ahmed, N., McCulloch, D. R., & Ward, A. C., (2014). Granulocyte colony-stimulating factor receptor signaling via Janus kinase 2/signal transducer and activator of transcription 3 in ovarian cancer. *British Journal of Cancer, 110*(1), 133–145.

La, M. S., De Benedictis, I., & Marasco, D., (2022). Proteomimetics of natural regulators of JAK-STAT pathway: Novel therapeutic perspectives. *Frontiers in Molecular Biosciences, 8*, 792546.

Lei, R. L., Xiao, S. S., & Xue, M., (2015). Nan fang yi ke da Xue Xue bao. *Journal of Southern Medical University, 35*(1), 88–92.

Li, H., Ahonen, T. J., Alanen, K., et al., (2004). Activation of signal transducer and activator of transcription 5 in human prostate cancer is associated with high histological grade. *Cancer Research, 64*(14), 4774–4782.

Li, S., Labrecque, S., Gauzzi, M. C., et al., (1999). The human papilloma virus (HPV)-18 E6 oncoprotein physically associates with Tyk2 and impairs Jak-STAT activation by interferon-alpha. *Oncogene, 18*(42), 5727–5737.

Li, Z., Guan, Y. Q., & Liu, J. M., (2014). The role of STAT-6 as a key transcription regulator in HeLa cell death induced by IFN-γ/TNF-α co-immobilized on nanoparticles. *Biomaterials, 35*(18), 5016–5027.

Liang, Z., Gao, L. H., Cao, L. J., et al., (2012). Detection of STAT2 in early stage of cervical premalignancy and in cervical cancer. *Asian Pacific Journal of Tropical Medicine, 5*(9), 738–742.

Liu, M., Gao, S., Elhassan, R. M., Hou, X., & Fang, H., (2021). Strategies to overcome drug resistance using SHP2 inhibitors. *Acta Pharmaceutica Sinica B, 11*(12), 3908–3924.

Liu, Q., Qu, J., Zhao, M., Xu, Q., & Sun, Y., (2020). Targeting SHP2 as a promising strategy for cancer immunotherapy. *Pharmacological Research, 152*, 104595.

Loh, C. Y., Arya, A., Naema, A. F., Wong, W. F., Sethi, G., & Looi, C. Y., (2019). Signal transducer and activator of transcription (STATs) proteins in cancer and inflammation: Functions and therapeutic implication. *Frontiers in Oncology, 9*, 48.

Lokau, J., Schoeder, V., Haybaeck, J., & Garbers, C., (2019). Jak-Stat signaling induced by interleukin-6 family cytokines in hepatocellular carcinoma. *Cancers, 11*(11), 1704.

Luo, J., Huang, Q., Lin, X., et al., (2016). STAT4 expression is correlated with clinicopathological characteristics of cervical lesions. *Int. J. Clin. Exp. Pathol., 9*, 3751–3758.

Lv, Y., Song, G., & Li, P., (2018). Correlation of SOCS-1 gene with onset and prognosis of breast cancer. *Oncology Letters, 16*(1), 383–387.

Malemud, C. J., (2017). Negative regulators of JAK/STAT signaling in rheumatoid arthritis and osteoarthritis. *International Journal of Molecular Sciences, 18*(3), 484.

Morgan, E. L., & Macdonald, A., (2019). Autocrine STAT3 activation in HPV positive cervical cancer through a virus-driven Rac1-NFκB-IL-6 signaling axis. *PLoS Pathogens, 15*(6), e1007835.

Morgan, E. L., & Macdonald, A., (2019). JAK2 inhibition impairs proliferation and sensitizes cervical cancer cells to cisplatin-induced cell death. *Cancers, 11*(12), 1934.

Morgan, E. L., Wasson, C. W., Hanson, L., et al., (2018). STAT3 activation by E6 is essential for the differentiation-dependent HPV18 life cycle. *PLoS Pathogens, 14*(4), e1006975.

Morris, R., Kershaw, N. J., & Babon, J. J., (2018). The molecular details of cytokine signaling via the JAK/STAT pathway. *Protein Science, 27*(12), 1984–2009.

Nees, M., Geoghegan, J. M., Hyman, T., Frank, S., Miller, L., & Woodworth, C. D., (2001). Papillomavirus type 16 oncogenes downregulate expression of interferon-responsive genes and upregulate proliferation-associated and NF-kappaB-responsive genes in cervical keratinocytes. *Journal of Virology, 75*(9), 4283–4296.

Neuwirt, H., Puhr, M., Santer, F. R., et al., (2009). Suppressor of cytokine signaling (SOCS)-1 is expressed in human prostate cancer and exerts growth-inhibitory function through down-regulation of cyclins and cyclin-dependent kinases. *The American Journal of Pathology, 174*(5), 1921–1930.

Nishi, M., Batsaikhan, B. E., Yoshikawa, K., et al., (2017). High STAT4 expression indicates better disease-free survival in patients with gastric cancer. *Anticancer Research, 37*(12), 6723–6729.

Niu, G. J., Xu, J. D., Yuan, W. J., et al., (2018). Protein inhibitor of activated STAT (PIAS) negatively regulates the JAK/STAT pathway by inhibiting STAT phosphorylation and translocation. *Frontiers in Immunology, 9*, 2392.

Niu, G., Bowman, T., Huang, M., et al., (2002). Roles of activated Src and Stat3 signaling in melanoma tumor cell growth. *Oncogene, 21*(46), 7001–7010.

Olayioye, M. A., Beuvink, I., Horsch, K., Daly, J. M., & Hynes, N. E., (1999). ErbB receptor-induced activation of stat transcription factors is mediated by Src tyrosine kinases. *Journal of Biological Chemistry, 274*(24), 17209–17218.

Page, C., Huang, M., Jin, X., Cho, K., Lilja, J., Reynolds, R. K., & Lin, J., (2000). Elevated phosphorylation of AKT and Stat3 in prostate, breast, and cervical cancer cells. *International Journal of Oncology, 17*(1), 23–28.

Rajkumar, T., Sabitha, K., Vijayalakshmi, N., Shirley, S., Bose, M. V., Gopal, G., & Selvaluxmy, G., (2011). Identification and validation of genes involved in cervical tumorigenesis. *BMC Cancer, 11*, 80.

Rane, S. G., & Reddy, E. P., (2000). Janus kinases: Components of multiple signaling pathways. *Oncogene, 19*(49), 5662–5679.

Raspaglio, G., Buttarelli, M., Filippetti, F., Battaglia, A., Buzzonetti, A., Scambia, G., & Gallo, D., (2021). Stat1 confers sensitivity to radiation in cervical cancer cells by controlling Parp1 levels: A new perspective for Parp1 inhibition. *Cell Death and Disease, 12*(10), 933.

Rawlings, J. S., Rosler, K. M., & Harrison, D. A., (2004). The JAK/STAT signaling pathway. *Journal of Cell Science, 117*(8), 1281–1283.

Roca, S. A. A., Van, R. N., Baumert, T. F., & Lupberger, J., (2018). Viral manipulation of STAT3: Evade, exploit, and injure. *PLoS Pathogens, 14*(3), e1006839.

Sabaawy, H. E., Ryan, B. M., Khiabanian, H., & Pine, S. R., (2021). JAK/STAT of all trades: Linking inflammation with cancer development, tumor progression and therapy resistance. *Carcinogenesis, 42*(12), 1411–1419.

Schwaller, J., Parganas, E., Wang, D., et al., (2000). Stat5 is essential for the myelo- and lymphoproliferative disease induced by TEL/JAK2. *Molecular Cell, 6*(3), 693–704.

Scott, M. L., Woodby, B. L., Ulicny, J., Raikhy, G., Orr, A. W., Songock, W. K., & Bodily, J. M., (2020). *Human Papillomavirus* 16 E5 inhibits interferon signaling and supports episomal viral maintenance. *Journal of Virology, 94*(2), e01582–19.

Seif, F., Khoshmirsafa, M., Aazami, H., Mohsenzadegan, M., Sedighi, G., & Bahar, M., (2017). The role of JAK-STAT signaling pathway and its regulators in the fate of T helper cells. *Cell Communication and Signaling, 15*(1), 1–13.

Shi, L. Z., & Bonner, J. A., (2021). Bridging radiotherapy to immunotherapy: The IFN–JAK–STAT axis. *International Journal of Molecular Sciences, 22*(22), 12295.

Shuai, K., & Liu, B., (2005). Regulation of gene-activation pathways by PIAS proteins in the immune system. *Nature Reviews Immunology, 5*(8), 593–605.

Shukla, S., Jadli, M., Thakur, K., et al., (2019). Level of phospho-STAT3 (Tyr705) correlates with copy number and physical state of human papillomavirus 16 genome in cervical precancer and cancer lesions. *PLoS One, 14*(9), e0222089.

Shukla, S., Mahata, S., Shishodia, G., et al., (2013). Functional regulatory role of STAT3 in HPV16-mediated cervical carcinogenesis. *PLoS One, 8*(7), e67849.

Silvennoinen, O., Witthuhn, B. A., Quelle, F. W., Cleveland, J. L., Yi, T., & Ihle, J. N., (1993). Structure of the murine Jak2 protein-tyrosine kinase and its role in interleukin 3 signal transduction. *Proceedings of the National Academy of Sciences of the United States of America, 90*(18), 8429–8433.

Silver-Morse, L., & Li, W. X., (2013). JAK-STAT in heterochromatin and genome stability. *JAK-STAT, 2*(3), e26090.

Sobti, R. C., Singh, N., Hussain, S., Suri, V., Bharadwaj, M., & Das, B. C., (2010). Deregulation of STAT-5 isoforms in the development of HPV-mediated cervical carcinogenesis. *Journal of Receptor and Signal Transduction Research, 30*(3), 178–188.

Sobti, R. C., Singh, N., Hussain, S., Suri, V., Nijhawan, R., Bharti, A. C., Bharadwaj, M., & Das, B. C., (2011). Aberrant promoter methylation and loss of suppressor of cytokine signaling-1 gene expression in the development of uterine cervical carcinogenesis. *Cellular Oncology, 34*(6), 533–543.

Sriuranpong, V., Park, J. I., Amornphimoltham, P., Patel, V., Nelkin, B. D., & Gutkind, J. S., (2003). Epidermal growth factor receptor-independent constitutive activation of STAT3 in head and neck squamous cell carcinoma is mediated by the autocrine/paracrine stimulation of the interleukin 6/gp130 cytokine system. *Cancer Research, 63*(11), 2948–2956.

Thomas, S. J., Snowden, J. A., Zeidler, M. P., & Danson, S. J., (2015). The role of JAK/STAT signaling in the pathogenesis, prognosis and treatment of solid tumors. *British Journal of Cancer, 113*(3), 365–371.

Vainchenker, W., & Constantinescu, S. N., (2013). JAK/STAT signaling in hematological malignancies. *Oncogene, 32*(21), 2601–2613.

Verhoeven, Y., Tilborghs, S., Jacobs, J., et al., (2020). The potential and controversy of targeting STAT family members in cancer. *Seminars in Cancer Biology, 60*, 41–56.

Walboomers, J. M., Jacobs, M. V., Manos, M. M., et al., (1999). *Human papillomavirus* is a necessary cause of invasive cervical cancer worldwide. *The Journal of Pathology, 189*(1), 12–19.

Wang, T., & Weinman, S. A., (2006). Causes and consequences of mitochondrial reactive oxygen species generation in hepatitis C. *Journal of Gastroenterology and Hepatology, 21*, S34–S37.

Wormald, S., & Hilton, D. J., (2004). Inhibitors of cytokine signal transduction. *Journal of Biological Chemistry, 279*(2), 821–824.

Wu, C. J., Sundararajan, V., Sheu, B. C., Huang, R. Y. J., & Wei, L. H., (2020). Activation of STAT3 and STAT5 signaling in epithelial ovarian cancer progression: Mechanism and therapeutic opportunity. *Cancers, 12*(1), 24.

Wu, M., Song, D., Li, H., Yang, Y., Ma, X., Deng, S., Ren, C., & Shu, X., (2019). Negative regulators of STAT3 signaling pathway in cancers. *Cancer Management and Research, 11*, 4957–4969.

Wurster, A. L., Tanaka, T., & Grusby, M. J., (2000). The biology of Stat4 and Stat6. *Oncogene, 19*(21), 2577–2584.

Xiong, H., Su, W. Y., Liang, Q. C., et al., (2009). Inhibition of STAT5 induces G1 cell cycle arrest and reduces tumor cell invasion in human colorectal cancer cells. *Laboratory Investigation, 89*(6), 717–725.

Xu, B., Lu, X., Zhao, Y., et al., (2019). MicroRNA-135a induces prostate cancer cell apoptosis via inhibition of STAT6. *Oncology Letters, 17*(2), 1889–1895.

Xu, D., & Qu, C. K., (2008). Protein tyrosine phosphatases in the JAK/STAT pathway. *Frontiers in Bioscience, 13*, 4925–4932.

Yamaoka, K., Saharinen, P., Pesu, M., Holt, V. E., Silvennoinen, O., & O'Shea, J. J., (2004). The Janus kinases (jaks). *Genome Biology, 5*(12), 1–6.

Yang, M., Chen, H., Zhou, L., Huang, X., Su, F., & Wang, P., (2020). Identification of SOCS family members with prognostic values in human ovarian cancer. *American Journal of Translational Research, 12*(5), 1824–1838.

Yang, S., Wang, B., Liu, C., et al., (2021). THAP9-AS1 promotes tumorigenesis and reduces ROS generation through the JAK2/STAT3 signaling pathway by increasing SOCS3 promoter methylation in osteosarcoma. *Oxidative Medicine and Cellular Longevity, 2021*, 5620475.

Yeh, T. C., & Pellegrini, S., (1999). The Janus kinase family of protein tyrosine kinases and their role in signaling. *Cellular and Molecular Life Sciences, 55*(12), 1523–1534.

Yi, Y., Fang, Y., Wu, K., Liu, Y., & Zhang, W., (2020). Comprehensive gene and pathway analysis of cervical cancer progression. *Oncology Letters, 19*(4), 3316–3332.

Yoshikawa, H., Matsubara, K., Qian, G. S., Jackson, P., Groopman, J. D., Manning, J. E., Harris, C. C., & Herman, J. G., (2001). SOCS-1, a negative regulator of the JAK/

STAT pathway, is silenced by methylation in human hepatocellular carcinoma and shows growth-suppression activity. *Nature Genetics, 28*(1), 29–35.

Yoshimura, A., Ito, M., Chikuma, S., Akanuma, T., & Nakatsukasa, H., (2018). Negative regulation of cytokine signaling in immunity. *Cold Spring Harbor Perspectives in Biology, 10*(7), a028571.

Yuan, Y., Cai, X., Shen, F., & Ma, F., (2021). HPV post-infection microenvironment and cervical cancer. *Cancer Letters, 497*, 243–254.

Yue, C., Xu, J., Tan, E., et al., (2015). Host STAT2/type I interferon axis controls tumor growth. *International Journal of Cancer, 136*(1), 117–126.

Zehender, A., Huang, J., Györfi, A. H., et al., (2018). The tyrosine phosphatase SHP2 controls TGFβ-induced STAT3 signaling to regulate fibroblast activation and fibrosis. *Nature Communications, 9*(1), 3259.

Zhang, J., Zhang, F., & Niu, R., (2015). Functions of Shp2 in cancer. *Journal of Cellular and Molecular Medicine, 19*(9), 2075–2083.

Zhao, L., Ji, G., Le, X., et al., (2017). An integrated analysis identifies STAT4 as a key regulator of ovarian cancer metastasis. *Oncogene, 36*(24), 3384–3396.

Zou, S., Tong, Q., Liu, B., Huang, W., Tian, Y., & Fu, X., (2020). Targeting STAT3 in cancer immunotherapy. *Molecular Cancer, 19*(1), 145.

Zucman-Rossi, J., Villanueva, A., Nault, J. C., & Llovet, J. M., (2015). Genetic landscape and biomarkers of hepatocellular carcinoma. *Gastroenterology, 149*(5), 1226–1239.

CHAPTER 9

Role of Micro-RNA in Cervical Cancer Progression and Its Therapeutic Implications

9.1 AN OVERVIEW OF Micro-RNAs

MicroRNAs (miRNAs) are single-stranded noncoding RNAs of 19–22 nucleotides that have evolved over time. miRNAs are made up of immature primary transcripts (primary miRNAs) that can be several kilobases long and are encoded within the genome from intronic, exonic, or intergenic sequences (Weiss & Ito, 2017). The RNAse enzyme Drosha cleaves primary miRNAs before transcription into 60–100 nucleotide hairpin precursor RNAs, which is how miRNA is made (precursor miRNA). The nuclear export factor exportin-5 transports the precursor miRNA to the cytoplasm, where it is excised by the RNA polymerase enzyme Dicer to form 70-nucleotide-long precursor miRNAs. Subsequently, a putative helicase unwinds the precursor miRNAs into mature miRNAs of 18–24 nucleotides (Pillai, 2005). Single-stranded mature miRNAs interact with argonaute proteins to produce a multisubunit gene regulation complex, the RNA-induced silencing complex (RISC). This RISC allows miRNA-associated gene regulation via base pairing among miRNA and sequence(s) inside the 39 untranslated regions (UTR) of the target messenger RNA (mRNA) (Stavast & Erkeland, 2019). The interaction of miRNA to mRNA slows down translation and/or promotes mRNA degradation (Figure 9.1). However, emerging evidence indicates that miRNAs can promote mRNA translation in cells that are undergoing cell cycle arrest (Vasudevan et al.,

Cervical Cancer: Signaling Pathways, Molecular Mechanisms, Natural Products, and Therapeutic Approaches. Pratibha Pandey, Fahad Khan, Saher Islam, and Devarajan Thangadurai, (Eds.)

2008). The half-life of miRNA varies based on organs, biological samples, and types of cells and can range from hours to days (van Rooij et al., 2007). In comparison to mRNA, miRNAs are extremely stable in formalin-fixed paraffin-embedded tissue blocks or biobank-stored animal and human biological samples, enabling them to be used for biomarker research even after years of preservation (Samirand & Pessler, 2016; Keshavarz et al., 2018).

miRNAs serve as a crucial mediator in almost every biological function (Diener et al., 2022). The concept that hosts miRNAs may play a crucial role in host responses to invading pathogens has been confirmed by the differential gene expression of host miRNAs upon infection (Ojha et al., 2016). The regulatory role of miRNAs has been found to be significantly more complex than previously thought due to their cooperativity (i.e., many miRNA species can target the same mRNA) and diversity of targets (i.e., one miRNA can target hundreds of mRNA species). The three main mechanisms of miRNA-related gene regulation are translation suppression, direct mRNA destruction, and miRNA-mediated mRNA degradation (Engels & Hutvagner, 2006; Nilsen, 2007). According to new findings, the

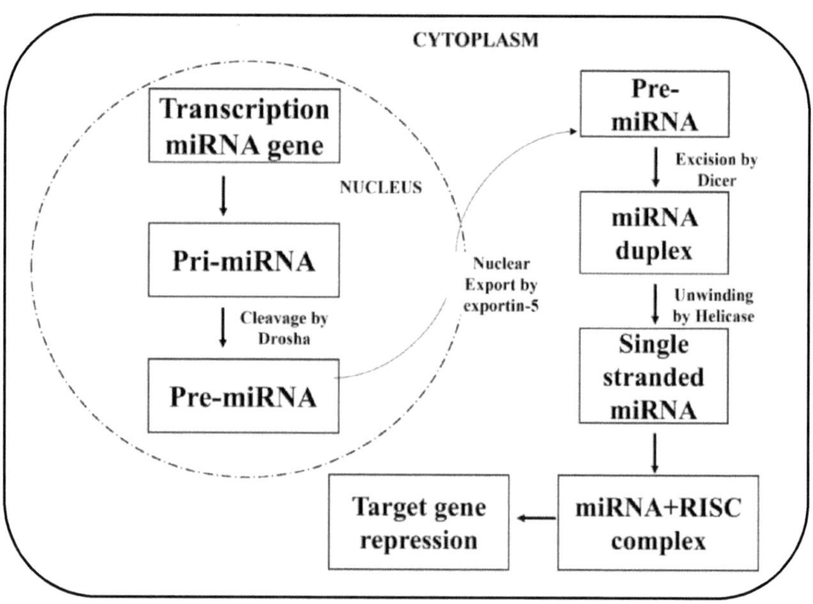

FIGURE 9.1 A schematic diagram of process of miRNA biogenesis.

repression mechanism is predominantly triggered by a decrease in mRNA target stability. Markedly, miRNAs have been involved in a variety of functions, such as cell cycle and differentiation, metabolic pathway regulation, inflammation, and cardiovascular, neurologic, and metabolic diseases, apoptosis, tumor progression, and metastasis (Christensen & Schratt, 2009; Lynam-Lennon et al., 2009; Baranwal & Alahari, 2010; Bueno & Malumbres, 2011; Price et al., 2014; Nouraee & Mowla, 2015).

9.2 DISCOVERY OF miRNA

In the early 1990s, Lee et al. (1993) noticed that RNA expressed from the lin-4 locus did not generate a protein, but rather silenced the gene encoding Lin-14 (a crucial protein in larval development) during a study focused on the sequence of embryonic development of different larval stages of the *Caenorhabditis elegans* worm. The existence of complementary sequences in the 39 UTR region of lin-14 mRNA indicated that lin-4 may regulate lin-14 mRNA translation in *C. elegans*, leading in the formation of temporal patterns during development (Lee et al., 2002, 2003). Furthermore, the finding that miRNAs are implicated in sensing nutrient stress in plants or mediating responses to environmental stress as one of the strategies used to reconfigure gene expression so that cells can adapt to environmental changes has opened up new prospects in terms of determining their roles in human diseases (Chiou, 2007; Yang et al., 2007; Zhu et al., 2011; Islam et al., 2022). miRNA-mediated translational repression has been found to be associated in practically every cellular activity. The regulatory patterns of various other miRNAs have now been revealed in species ranging from viruses to humans (Berezikov et al., 2006; Hammond, 2015). The newest version of the miRBase database (v22) comprises 38,589 entries from 271 organisms that represent hairpin precursor microRNAs. This is more than a third increase in sequences over the previous release. There are 48,860 distinct mature microRNA sequences produced by these hairpin precursors. Thousands of microRNAs can be found in vertebrate genomes: the human genome, for example, has 1917 identified hairpin precursors and 2,654 mature sequences. Hundreds of microRNAs can be found in both invertebrates and plants with well-annotated genomes (Griffiths-Jones et al., 2006; Van Peer et al., 2014; Kozomara et al., 2019). This finding raised questions about gene cluster cistronic expression regulating patterns (Persson et al.,

2011; Tahiri et al., 2014). Deregulation of one member of the cluster is thought to be followed by comparable deregulations of other miRNAs from the same cluster. As a result, determining whether one miRNA in a cluster can be regulated independently of others is critical, particularly in connection to miRNAs involved in the pathogenesis of human disorders (Vishnoi & Rani, 2017). miRNAs are thought to target roughly one-third of human mRNAs, and a single miRNA can target up to 200 transcripts at once due to variable target binding patterns (Brennecke et al., 2005; Brodersen & Voinnet, 2009). As a result, a detailed analysis of miRNA regulation may yield useful ways for controlling multiple genes at the same time.

9.3 MICRO-RNA AND CANCER

Cancer is a complex genetic disorder involving structural and expression anomalies associated with coding and noncoding transcripts. The first evidence of a link between miRNAs and cancer was discovered in 2002 when recurrent deletions in a miRNA-coding sequence were detected in 50% of patients with B-cell chronic lymphocytic leukemia (Calin et al., 2004). Since then, scientists have shown that miRNA dysregulation is highly important and plays a role in cancer progression and development (Pereira et al., 2013). Furthermore, various tumor suppressor or oncogenic miRNAs have been discovered (Wang et al., 2010; Gambari et al., 2016). It is now apparent that the genomic complexity of cancer cells is substantially higher than reported. After this substantial research, the identification of over 1,000 miRNAs has been made possible by the characterization and cloning of short, noncoding RNAs with a length of less than 22 nucleotides long. Through precise base-pairing with target transcript or protein molecules, transcriptional and post-transcriptional control of their expression, miRNAs regulate cellular activities, such as cell proliferation, differentiation, apoptosis, and genomic stability (Landau & Slack, 2011). According to the GENCODE data (v.29), around 2,600 mature miRNAs are encoded by 1,872 identified miRNA precursor genes in humans; however, roles of many of these miRNAs are still unknown (Hsu et al., 2006). A single miRNA can interact with hundreds of distinct transcripts (Slezak-Prochazka et al., 2010). Furthermore, a single mRNA can bind to many miRNAs at the same time or in a situation-dependent manner (Xie et al., 2013). miRNAs play a direct role in tumorigenesis process in various tissues since they either act as tumor suppressors (miR-15a and miR-16-1) or oncogenes (miR-17–92 cluster and miR-155) (Shenouda & Alahari, 2009; Xiang & Wu, 2010). Furthermore, miRNAs have been considered as biomarkers for cancer susceptibility (Mo et al., 2012). According to molecular studies, the activity of miRNAs is affected by genomic abnormalities such as chromosomal rearrangements, deletions, mutations, or genomic amplifications (Urbanek-Trzeciak et al., 2020). Besides their impact on cancer cell biological activities, miRNAs can regulate the function of some of the other cells in the tumor. Extracellular miRNAs can influence intercellular communications by collaborating with stromal cells and extracellular matrix constituents to produce an appropriate microenvironment for tumor cells to proliferate and evade from immune surveillance (Munir et al., 2020). For example, miR-200c reduces PTEN and FOG2 expression, increasing the PI3K/Akt signaling pathway and resulting in the accumulation of myeloid-derived suppressor cells and immune response suppression in the tumor microenvironment (Mei et al., 2015). Furthermore, macrophages have been demonstrated to release miRNA-containing exosomes that help breast cancer cells to invade more effectively. Among these miRNAs, miR-223 was found to be predominant, which is specific for interleukin-4-induced macrophages (Yang et al., 2011). Additionally, exosomal transfer of miR-144 and miR-126 also plays a key role in the formation of a novel metabolic system that promotes tumor progression (Das & Halushka, 2015).

9.4 miRNAs IN DUAL ROLE AS Onco-miRs AND TUMOR-SUPPRESSOR

Different viewpoints on miRNA involvement in human malignancies have been suggested by genome expression analysis. miRNAs have been implicated in a variety of biological processes, such as cell proliferation, differentiation, and programmed cell death (Conti et al., 2020). miRNAs have been reported to act as tumor suppressor genes by targeting oncogenic miRNAs (oncomiRs) by a variety of mechanisms, including the inactivation of tumor suppressor proteins. For example, miR-125b acts as a tumor suppressor in many solid tumors, since its expression reduces the levels of LIPA, PCTP, HK2 GSS, ACCS1, SCD1, IKZF4, and TP53 (Tili et al., 2012). However, miR-125b is an act as oncomiR in most human leukemias, such as AML, AMKL, CML, and ALL (Bousquet et al.,

2008; Gefen et al., 2010; Klusmann et al., 2010; Enomoto et al., 2011). Interestingly, miR-125b primarily acts as an oncogene by repressing hematopoietic differentiation factors (PRDM1, CBFB, IRF4, IL10RA, IL2RB) or by directly targeting metastasis gene promoters (LIN28B, ARID3B, MMP13), metastasis inhibitors (STARD13, TP53INP1), and pro-apoptotic regulators (BAK1, TP53, BBC3, BMF, MAPK) (Chaudhuri et al., 2012; Shaham et al., 2012). Another example is miR-155, which plays an oncogenic role in a variety of hematological and solid cancers and is thus categorized as an oncomiR (Babar et al., 2012). miR-155 at high levels specifically targets SHIP1 and the IL-6 pathway, a negative regulator of B-cell development that promotes the aggregation of apoptosis-resistant pre-BI cells (Costinean et al., 2009). Despite its powerful oncogenic effects, Levati et al. reported that miR-155 inhibits cancer proliferation and promotes apoptosis in various melanoma cell lines where it functions as a tumor suppressor by silencing the SKI gene (Levati et al., 2011). Likewise, Suardi et al. and Li et al. demonstrated that miR-155 works as a tumor suppressor in ovarian and gastric tumor-initiating cells, by directly targeting CLDN1 and SMAD2, respectively (Li et al., 2012; Suardi et al., 2020). Alteration in genomic miRNA within target locations could be a key cause of cancer risk genetic variations. Polymorphisms and mutations have been found to cause the functional loss or modification of existing miRNA target locations as well as the emergence of new miRNA binding sites (Agirre et al., 2012; Preskill & Weidhaas, 2013). Figures 9.2 and 9.3 summarizes major oncosuppressor and oncogenic miRNAs and their targets associated with metastasis inhibition.

9.5 CERVICAL CANCER AND miRNA

There are various factors which are required for the progression of cervical carcinoma, such as the association of viral and environmental factors and the host's immune ability (Pal & Kundu, 2020). Furthermore, knowledge about epigenetic regulatory mechanisms has progressively expanded over the last two decades, with a focus on the deregulation of oncogene and tumor suppressor gene as the primary cause of the malignant phenotype (Razavi et al., 2021). In this way, miRNAs are considered as an essential regulator of biological processes such as apoptosis, cell cycle progression, metastases, migration, and drug resistance (Kumar et al., 2007; Grzywa

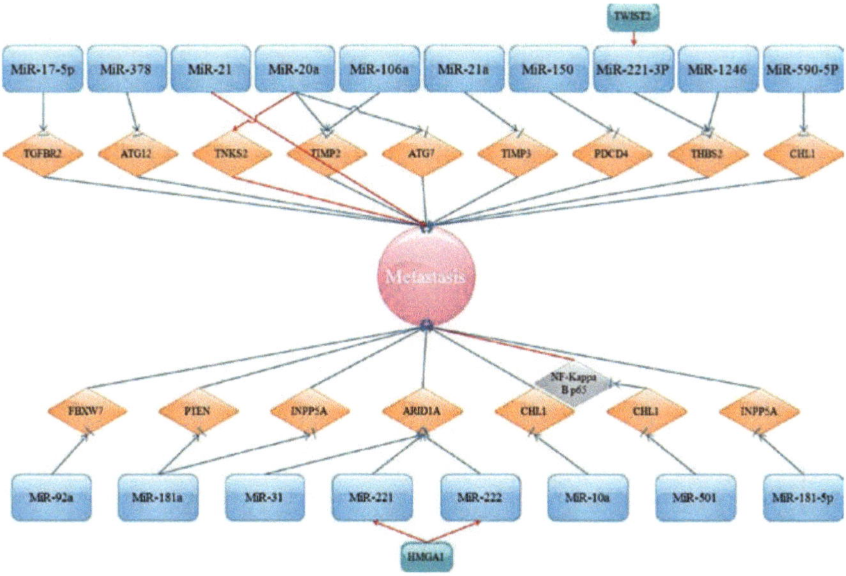

FIGURE 9.2 Oncogenic miRNAs and their targets in promoting metastasis.

Source: Adapted from Wang & Chen (2019); https://creativecommons.org/licenses/by/4.0/

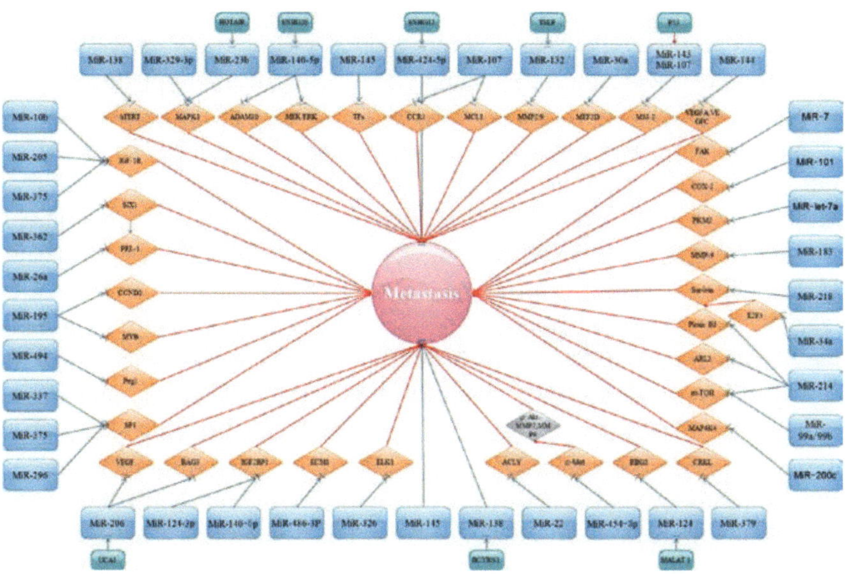

FIGURE 9.3 Oncosuppressor miRNAs and their targets in inhibiting metastasis.

Source: Adapted from Wang & Chen (2019); https://creativecommons.org/licenses/by/4.0/

et al., 2020). In order to better understand their importance, many investigations have been performed to establish the precise regulatory role of different miRNAs during cervical carcinogenesis. On the basis of their function, miRNA can be categorized into oncogenic miRNAs (oncomiRs) and tumor suppressor miRNAs (tsmiRs) (Svoronos et al., 2016). To employ miRNAs as potential therapeutic targets in personalized medicine for the treatment of cervical cancer, firstly, we have to understand the oncogenic or tumor suppressive function of miRNAs, as well as their regulatory mechanism in disease development and progression. OncomiR inhibition and downregulation may be significant in the treatment of this tumor, while tsmiR overexpression may have antitumor therapeutic effects (Kota & Balasubramanian, 2010; Zheng et al., 2010; Parasramka et al., 2012). In cervical cancer, several oncomiRs and tumor suppressor miRNAs have been detected (Tables 9.1 and 9.2). miR-21 is a negative regulator of the tumor suppressor gene programmed cell death 4 (PDCD4) and is overexpressed in many types of cancer. Because PDCD4 expression is linked to apoptosis and also suppresses tumor growth by blocking translation, miR-21 interaction to the PDCD4 3′-UTR promotes cell growth (Calin et al., 2004). CCL20, a critical regulator of tumor progression and nodular metastasis, is also targeted and regulated by miR-21 (He & Hannon, 2004). miR-10a promotes tumor growth, and metastasis by limiting CHL1 expression, whereas overexpression of miR-19a and miR-19b was reported in cervical cancer HeLa and C33A cells and are implicated in the process of cytopoiesis (Ferracin & Negrini, 2015). miR-19a and miR-19b promote cell proliferation and metastasis, however miR-19a and miR-19b null cells are non-malignant. Both miR-19a and miR-19b target Cullin 5 (CUL5), although expression of CUL5 without the 3′-UTR reduces tumor growth and migration mediated by miR-19a and miR-19b (Iorio & Croce, 2012). The expression level of oncogene tyrosine kinase nonreceptor-2 (TNKS2) is stimulated by miR-20. The suppression of TNKS2 inhibits cervical cancer cell metastasis and invasion. But at the other hand, miR-20 positively controls TNKS2, leading to increased metastasis and invasion (He et al., 2016). miR-133b controls CDC42, MST2 (mammalian sterile 20-like kinase), and RHOA (ras homolog gene family member A), which promotes MAPK1/AKT1 signaling cascade and facilitates tumor progression. Injecting cervical cancer cells with upregulation of miR-133b resulted in lung tumorigenesis and invasion (Almeida et al., 2009). The latency period of cervical neoplasms decreases as expression of miR-133b rises, making miR-133b a biomarker for early cervical carcinoma. Several investigations also reported the role of tumor suppressor miRNAs (Zhang et al., 2007). miR-138, for example, is implicated in the regulation of telomerase enzyme that is closely linked to cell immortality and cancer progression via the elongation of telomeres in chromosomal ends. Human telomerase reverse transcriptase (hTERT) production is required for telomerase activity, and miR-138 decreases mRNA expression of hTERT, thus suppress telomerase activity. The expression of miR-138 in cervical cancer cells is much less than in normal tissues, which leads to telomerase activation and tumorigenesis (Chakrabarti et al., 2013). Overexpression of miR-7 decreases cell development and increases apoptosis in HeLa and C33-A cervical cancer cells, but inhibition of miR-7 expression has the inverse result. miR-7 also targets and regulates XIAP (X-linked inhibitor of apoptosis protein) (Liu et al., 2013), thus considered as a tumor suppressor miRNA. miR-17-5p suppresses cell development and leads to death by targeting the tumor protein p53-induced nuclear protein-1 (TP53INP1). TP53INP1 is involved in stress reactions in cells, and ectopically produced TP53INP1 interferes with miR-17-5p-stimulated cell growth reduction. In cervical cancer tissues, a similar correlation between TP53INP1 and miR-17-5p has been identified. As a result, miR-17-5p could function as a tumor suppressor miRNA (Wei et al., 2012). Cui et al. having found that upregulation of miR-125b suppressed cellular proliferation, promoted apoptosis, and significantly reduced tumorigenesis by repressing the PIK3CD (phosphoinositide-3-kinase catalytic subunit delta) via targeting the PI3K/Akt/mTOR pathway (Cui et al., 2012).

9.6 miRNA AS A DIAGNOSTIC AND PROGNOSIS BIOMARKER

Secreted miRNA contained in exosomes and granular vesicles have been detected circulating in blood since 2007. These miRNAs have since been established to transfect via signal transduction and cell communication via placental and breast milk transfer. miRNA can be isolated from a broad range of samples, such as blood, plasma, urine, serum, fresh tissues and cell lines, using specific reagents, and their expression can subsequently be evaluated employing quantitative RT-PCR and microarray study. Thus, based on plasma and serum testing, miRNA with particular expression alterations with malignancy might be employed as diagnostic and prognostic biomarkers (Banno et al., 2014; Grimaldi et al., 2018). Various patterns of miRNA expression, even just a single miRNA, have been employed as cancer biomarkers for early diagnosis, classification, prognosis, and prediction (Gao et al., 2017). A growing number of studies have revealed the use of miRNA as potential cancer biomarkers and antitumor therapeutics (de Planell-Saguer & Rodicio, 2011). Tang et al. (2013) quantified miRNA levels in cervical cancer by using TaqMan RT-PCR and investigated the level of miRNA-182 in cervical cancer and normal cervix. miRNA-182 and -183 were constantly up-regulated in cervical cancer, while miRNA-142-5p, -142-3p, -145, -150, -211, -223, -195, -199b, and -328 were constantly downregulated. Lin et al. used miRNA microarray, RT-PCR, and *in situ* hybridization to investigate the miRNA patterns of cervical cancer in Uygur women for use in early diagnosis. They observed that miRNA-101 expression was substantially lower in cervical cancer tissues than in normal tissues (Lin et al., 2014). Li et al. (2014) reported that cervical cancer tissues have 195 up-regulated miRNAs and 96 down-regulated miRNAs, specifically up-regulated miRNAs being miRNA-10a, 21, -15b, -20b, -141, -200a, and -224, and down-regulated miRNAs being miRNA-126, -143, -145, and -203. Hu et al. investigated two miRNAs (miRNA-200a and -9) that could be utilized to predict survival rates and had significant cervical cancer regulatory effects (Hu et al., 2010). Han et al. identified miRNA-21 and assessed its efficacy as a cervical cancer prognostic biomarker. They found that miRNA-21 expression was linked to clinicopathological factors like the extent of invasion and lymph node metastases (Han et al., 2015). Yang et al. (2014) observed that miRNA-126 expression in cervical cancer tissues was relatively low than in adjacent non-tumorous tissues, and this inadequate level was closely linked with lymphatic invasion, metastasis, and tumor grade. Similarly, miRNA-142-3p and -138 were identified (Liu et al., 2016; Li et al., 2017). On the other hand, miRNA-31 is considerably overexpressed in cell lines and tissues of cervical cancer, and its high expression has been linked to a greater FIGO stage, nodal metastases, vascular engagement, and profound stromal invasion (Wang et al., 2014). Li et al. effectively created a multivariate Cox's model using both clinical data and miRNA patterns of cervical carcinoma patients and identified 7 miRNA that were involved in the development, progression, and prognosis of the disease (Li et al., 2017). As previously indicated, identifiable anomalies in several miRNA expression patterns have been validated, thus allowing them to be used as potent diagnostic or prognostic biomarkers in cervical cancer (Shen et al., 2020).

TABLE 9.1 List of Tumor Suppressor/Downregulated miRNA and Their Associated Mechanism in the Development and Progression of Cervical Cancer

miRNA	Cell Line/Model	Molecular Target	Mechanism	References
miRNA-7	Human cervical cancer tissue, HeLa, C33A	XIAP, EGFR	Reduced cell growth, invasion, and induced apoptosis.	Liu et al. (2013)
miRNA-9	Human cervical cancer tissue, HeLa, C33A, SiHa	FOXO-1, FOXO-3	Reduced cell growth, invasion, and apoptosis induction.	Jin & Wang (2016); Aishanjiang et al. (2018); Zhang et al. (2018)
miRNA-26a	ME-180, CaSki, HeLa, SiHa, human cervical cancer tissue, Xenograft mice of HeLa cervical cancer cells	PRL-1	Cell and tumor growth inhibition.	Dong et al. (2014)
miRNA-30e	Hela, SiHa, and Caski	GALN T7	Cell growth inhibition, suppressed invasion.	Wu et al. (2017)
miRNA-101	HeLa, human cervical cancer tissue	Cox-2, Fos	Cell growth inhibition, decreased invasion, G1/S phase arrest.	Lin et al. (2015)
miRNA-124	HeLa, SiHa, CaSKi, and C33A	AEG-1, Amot L1	Cell growth inhibition, suppressed migration and invasion.	Zhang et al. (2016)
miRNA-124-3p	HeLa	IGF2B P	Cell growth and metastasis inhibition.	Wang et al. (2022)
miRNA-125a-5 p	Human cervical cancer tissues, HeLa, SiHa, CaSki, C33-A, DoTc24510, HT-3, and C-4I	ABL2	Cell growth and migration inhibition.	Qin et al. (2015)
miRNA-130a	HeLa, C33A	PTEN, TNF-α, NF-kB	Suppressed tumor growth.	Feng et al. (2016)
miRNA-132	Human cervical cancer tissues, HeLa, C33A cells	SMAD 2, CCND 1, CDK2, CDK4, cyclin E	Cell growth and migration inhibition, apoptosis induction, G1/S phase cell cycle arrest.	Liu et al. (2017)

TABLE 9.1 *(Continued)*

miRNA	Cell Line/Model	Molecular Target	Mechanism	References
miRNA-136	Human cervical cancer tissues	E2F1, TFCP2	Inhibited proliferation, migration, and invasion, cell cycle arrest.	Zhang et al. (2018)
miRNA-433	HeLa, C33A, SiHa, and CaSki	Metadherin (MTDH)	Reduced cell growth, invasion, and apoptosis induction, targeting AKT and β-catenin pathways.	Liang et al. (2017)
miRNA-454-3p	HeLa	C-met	Cell growth and metastasis inhibition.	Guo et al. (2018)
miRNA-484	HeLa	ZEB1, SMAD 2	Induced cell growth and apoptosis, suppressed invasion and migration.	Hu et al. (2017)
miRNA-485	HeLa, SiHa, CaSKi, and C33A, human cervical cancer tissue	MACC 1	Cell growth and invasion inhibition, Met/AKT signaling pathway inhibition.	Wang et al. (2018)
miRNA-486-3p	Human cervical cancer tissue	ECM1	Cell growth and metastasis inhibition.	Ye et al. (2016)
miRNA-491-5p	HeLa, SiHa, CaSKi, and C33A, human cervical cancer tissue, female athymic nude (nu/nu) mice.	JMJD2A	Retarded cell growth and induced apoptosis.	Li et al. (2019)
miRNA-634	Human cervical cancer tissues, HeLa, and SiHa.	mTOR	Inhibited proliferation, migration, and invasion.	Cong et al. (2016)
miRNA-847	Human cervical cancer tissues, HeLa, SiHa, CaSki, C33A.	ETS1	Inhibited cell proliferation and invasiveness and induces apoptosis.	Liao et al. (2018)
miRNA-1284	Human cervical cancer tissues, MS751, HeLa, SiHa, and C33 A	HMGB 1	Inhibited proliferation, migration, and invasion, and induces apoptosis.	Chen & Li (2018)
miRNA-2861	Human cervical cancer tissues, HeLa, SiHa	EGFR, AKT2, CCND1	Inhibited proliferation, migration, and invasion, induced apoptosis.	Xu et al. (2016)

TABLE 9.1 *(Continued)*

miRNA	Cell Line/Model	Molecular Target	Mechanism	References
miRNA-let-7a	Human cervical cancer tissues, HeLa, SiHa	PKM2, HAS2	Inhibited proliferation, migration, and invasion.	Guo et al. (2017)
miRNA-138	Human cervical cancer tissues, HeLa, SiHa	TCF3, hTERT, c-Met, RMN D5A	Inhibited proliferation, migration, and invasion.	Song et al. (2015)
miRNA-139-3p	Human cervical cancer tissues, HeLa	NOB1	Inhibited proliferation, migration, and invasion, induced apoptosis.	Huang et al. (2016)
miRNA-142	Human cervical cancer tissues, HeLa, SiHa.	HMGB 1	Inhibited cell proliferation and invasiveness and induces apoptosis.	Jiang et al. (2017)
miRNA-142-3p	SiHa xenograft female nude Balb-c mice, HeLa, SiHa.	FZD7	Inhibited cell proliferation and invasiveness and induces apoptosis.	Deng et al. (2015)
miRNA-143	Human cervical cancer tissues, HeLa, SiHa.	GOLM1, Bcl-2, HIF-1α	Inhibited proliferation, migration, and invasion, G0/G-1 phase cell cycle arrest.	Zhou et al. (2018)
miRNA-146b-5p	CaSki cells	CXCR4	Inhibited cell growth, suppressed invasion and migration, G0/G1 cell cycle arrest.	Shen et al. (2015)
miRNA-183	Human cervical cancer tissues, HeLa, SiHa.	MMP-9	Inhibited proliferation, migration, and invasion.	Fan et al. (2016)
miRNA-187	Human cervical cancer tissues, HeLa, SiHa, CaSki, C33A.	E6, FGF9	Inhibited proliferation, migration, and invasion.	Liang et al. (2017)
miRNA-196b	Human cervical cancer tissues, ME-180, SiHa, and HT-3.	HOXB7, VEGF	Inhibited proliferation, migration, and invasion, reduced tumor growth, tumor angiogenesis.	How et al. (2013)

TABLE 9.1 *(Continued)*

miRNA	Cell Line/Model	Molecular Target	Mechanism	References
miRNA-202	Human cervical cancer tissues, HeLa, SiHa, CaSki	Cyclin D1	Inhibited proliferation, migration, and invasion.	Yi et al. (2016)
miRNA-203	Human cervical cancer tissues, HeLa, CaSki.	VEGF-A, surviving, BANF1	Inhibited proliferation, migration, and invasion.	Zhu et al. (2013)
miRNA-204	Human cervical cancer tissues, HeLa, SiHa, CaSki, C33A.	TCF12	Inhibited proliferation, migration, and invasion.	Shu et al. (2018)
miRNA-206	Human cervical cancer tissues, HeLa, SiHa.	G6PD, Notch3	Inhibited proliferation, migration, and invasion.	Song et al. (2009)
miRNA-211	Human cervical cancer tissues, HeLa, SiHa, CaSki, C33A.	ZEB1	Inhibited proliferation, migration, and invasion.	Chen et al. (2018)
miRNA-214	Human cervical cancer tissues, HeLa, C33A.	EZH2, ARL2, GALNT7, Bcl-212	Inhibited proliferation, migration, and invasion.	Peng et al. (2017); Yang et al. (2018)
miRNA-320	Human cervical cancer tissues, HeLa, SiHa, CaSki, C33A.	FOXM 1, Mcl-1	Decreased cell viability, migration, and invasion.	Yang et al. (2016); Shi & Zhang (2017a)
miRNA-329-3p	Human cervical cancer tissues, HeLa, SiHa, CaSki, C33A.	MAPK 1	Inhibited proliferation, migration, and invasion.	Li et al. (2017)
miRNA-342-3p	Human cervical cancer tissues, HeLa, CaSki.	FOXM 1	Inhibited cell growth, suppressed invasion and migration.	Li et al. (2014)
miRNA-362	Human cervical cancer tissue, SiHa, HeLa, C33a, and CaSki.	SIX1	Inhibited cell growth, suppressed invasion and migration.	Shi & Zhang (2017b)
miRNA-362-3p	Human cervical cancer tissues.	MCM5	Inhibited cell growth, suppressed invasion and migration.	Wang et al. (2018)

TABLE 9.1 *(Continued)*

miRNA	Cell Line/Model	Molecular Target	Mechanism	References
miRNA-377	Human cervical cancer tissue, SiHa, HeLa, C33a, and CaSki.	ZEB2	Inhibited cell proliferation and invasion.	Ye et al. (2019)
miRNA-411	Human cervical cancer tissue, SiHa, HeLa, C33a, and CaSki.	STAT3	Inhibited cell proliferation and invasion.	Shan et al. (2019)
miRNA-429	CaSki, SiHa, male BALB/c nu/nu nude mice.	IKKβ, ZEB1, CRKL	Inhibited cell growth, suppressed invasion and migration.	Wang et al. (2016)
miRNA-506	CaSki, HeLa	Gli3	Cell growth inhibition, G1/S phase cell cycle arrest, hedgehog pathway.	Wen et al. (2015)
miRNA-195	Human cervical cancer tissue, SiHa, HeLa, C33a, and CaSki.	HDGF, Cyclin D1a, pRb, PCNA	Inhibited proliferation, migration, and invasion, G1 phase cell cycle arrest.	Song et al. (2017)
miRNA-375	Human cervical cancer tissue, SiHa, and CaSki.	SP1	Inhibited proliferation, migration, and invasion, arrested G1/S phase transition.	Wang et al. (2011)
miRNA-126	Human cervical cancer tissue, SiHa, Hela, ME180, C33a, and CaSki.	ZEB1, MMP2, MMP9	Inhibited proliferation, migration, and invasion, inactivated JAK2/STAT3 signaling pathway.	Zhang et al. (2017)
miR-503	Human cervical cancer tissue, SiHa, Hela.	AKT2	Inhibited proliferation, migration, and invasion.	Yin et al. (2015)
miR-638	Human cervical cancer tissues, HeLa, SiHa, CaSki, C33-A.	Beta-catenin, cyclin D1, c-myc	Inhibited proliferation, migration, and invasion.	Wei et al. (2017)
miRNA-664	Human cervical cancer tissues, SiHa, Hela, Caski, C-33A and Hela-229.	E-cadherin	Reduced cell migration and increased drug chemosensitivity.	Zhang et al. (2016)
miR-144	Human cervical cancer tissues, Hela, C33A.	VEGFA, and VEGFC	Inhibited proliferation, migration, and invasion.	Tao et al. (2018)

TABLE 9.1 *(Continued)*

miRNA	Cell Line/Model	Molecular Target	Mechanism	References
miRNA-145	Human cervical cancer tissues, HeLa, SiHa, CaSki, C33-A.	HLTF	Inhibited tumor growth, cell proliferation, migration, and invasion.	Yan et al. (2016); Sathyanarayanan et al. (2017); Lv & Zhang (2020)
miRNA-200c	Human cervical cancer tissues, C33A, HeLa, HeLa229, HCC94, HT-3 and ME-180.	MAP4 K4	Inhibited proliferation, migration, and invasion.	Mei et al. (2018)
miRNA-337	Human cervical cancer tissues, HeLa, SiHa, CaSki, C33A.	Specificity protein 1	Inhibited proliferation, migration, and invasion.	Dong et al. (2017)
miRNA-338-3p	Human cervical cancer tissues, HeLa, CaSki.	MACC1, HIF-1α	Inhibited proliferation, migration, and invasion, induced apoptosis.	Hua et al. (2017); Qian et al. (2020); Wang et al. (2021)
miRNA-494	Human cervical cancer tissues, HeLa.	SOCS6, HCCR1	Inhibited proliferation, migration, and invasion.	Yang et al. (2015)

TABLE 9.2 List of Onco/Upregulated miRNA and Their Associated Mechanism in the Development and Progression of Cervical Cancer

miRNA	Cell Line/Model	Molecular Target	Mechanism	References
miRNA-21	HeLa	PDCD4, PTEN	Induced cell proliferation and apoptosis inhibition.	Zhang et al. (2018)
miR-9-5p	Human cervical cancer tissues, HeLa, SiHa, CaSki.	TWIST1	Promoted tumor growth.	Babion et al. (2019); Wei et al. (2019); Xie et al. (2019); Ma et al. (2021)
miRNA-20a	Human cervical cancer tissues, HeLa, SiHa, CaSki, HCC94 and C33A cells, nude female mice (SiHa).	TNKS2, PDCD6, ATG7, TIMP2, THBS2	Promoted cell growth, migration, and invasion.	Kang et al. (2012); Zhao et al. (2015); Liu (2018); Zhou et al. (2019)
miRNA-31	HeLa, CaSki, C33A	ARID1A	Promoted cell growth, migration, and invasion.	Wang et al. (2014); Zheng et al. (2015)
miRNA-92	Human cervical cancer tissues, SiHa, C33A.	PTEN	Promoted cell growth, migration, and invasion.	Yu et al. (2013)
miRNA-92a	Human cervical cancer tissues, HeLa, SiHa, CaSki, C33A.	FBXW7	Promoted cell growth, migration, and invasion and G1/S transition.	Zhou et al. (2015); Su et al. (2017)
miRNA-96	Human cervical cancer tissues, HeLa cells.	PTPN9, CAV1	Promoted cellular proliferation and tumorigenicity.	Chen et al. (2019); Yang et al. (2020)
miRNA-146a	Human cervical cancer tissues, SiHa, and C33A.	CTNNB1, STAT3, RELA, CCND1 and SNAI1	Promoted cell growth, migration, and invasion.	Wang et al. (2011); Sathyanarayanan et al. (2016)
miRNA-155	Human cervical cancer tissues.	LKB1	Induced cell proliferation.	Lao et al. (2014) Fang et al. (2016); Wang et al. (2016)
miRNA-196a	Human cervical cancer tissues, MS751, C33A, HeLa, HeLa229, SiHa, HCC94, CaSKi, HT-3 and ME-180.	FOXO1, p27kip1, Netrin 4	Induced cell proliferation, and G1/S transition.	Zhang et al. (2013); Hou et al. (2014); Chen et al. (2016)

TABLE 9.2 *(Continued)*

miRNA	Cell Line/Model	Molecular Target	Mechanism	References
miRNA-199b-5p	Human cervical cancer tissues, Hela, CaSki, SiHa, ME180, MS-751 and C33 A.	KLK10	Induced cell proliferation, migration, invasion and apoptosis inhibition.	Xu et al. (2018)
miRNA-205	Human cervical cancer tissues, CaSki, HeLa, SW756, ME-180, SiHa, C4I and C33A.	CYR61, CTGF	Promoted cell growth, migration, and invasion.	Xie et al. (2012); Ma et al. (2014)
miRNA-361-5p	Human cervical cancer tissues, C33A, HeLa, SiHa, CaSki, and C4-1 cells.	circ-MYBL2	Promoted cell growth, migration, and invasion.	Wu et al. (2013); Liu et al. (2018)
miRNA-373	Human cervical cancer tissues, HeLa, SiHa, CaSki, C33A.	YOD1	Induced cell proliferation.	Wang et al. (2015)
miRNA-501	Human cervical cancer tissues, HeLa.	CYLD	Induced cell proliferation, migration, invasion and apoptosis inhibition.	Sanches et al. (2018)
miRNA-590	Human cervical cancer tissues, HeLa, and C33A.	CHL1	Induced cell proliferation, migration, invasion and apoptosis inhibition.	Chu et al. (2014)
miR-944	Human cervical cancer tissues, CaSki, HeLa, SW756, ME-180, SiHa, C4I and C33A.	HECW2 (HECT domain ligase W2) and S100PBP (S100P binding protein).	Promoted cell growth, migration, and invasion.	Xie et al. (2015); Chen et al. (2021); Zhang & Zhang (2022)

9.7 THE CORRELATION BETWEEN HPV AND miRNA IN CERVICAL CANCER

HPV-16, -18, -31, -52, and -58 subtypes were previously divided into high-risk and low-risk variants based on the correlation between cervical cancer and precursor lesions (Chen et al., 2019). Dürst et al. revealed the association between HPV and cervical cancer for the first time in 1983 (Dürst et al., 1983). The presence of DNA from high-risk HPV types was found to be responsible for between 79% and 100% of invasive cervical cancer cases worldwide, with HPV-16 and -18 accounting for over 70% of all instances. HPV contains eight open reading frames in its genome which encodes for 8 proteins. These are separated into those with early-stage activity (E1, E2, E4-7) and those with late-stage activity (L1 and L2). Oncoproteins E6 and E7 are recognized to disrupt cell-cycle control, altering signaling pathways involved in cell repair and apoptotic cell death. E6 has been investigated for its inhibitory action on cell-cycling proliferation and repair (Tomaić 2016; Almeida et al., 2019). A chronic HPV infection causes aberrant expression of a wide number of miRNAs in cervical cancer (Lajer et al., 2017). Most of these miRNAs are downstream targets of the transcription factors c-Myc, p53, and E2F, and their expression is generally influenced by carcinogenic HPV E6 and E7. Wang et al. discovered 12 up-regulated miRNA and 9 down-regulated miRNA in HPV-infected cervical cells, with up-regulated miRNA being miRNA-15b, -16, -17-5p, -20a, -20b, -21, -93, -106, -155, -182, -185, and -224, and down-regulated miRNA being miRNA-29a, -34a, -126, -miRNA-34a, -23b, -125a, and -218, which are closely connected to E6 and p53 proteins, may increase the cervical carcinogenesis (Martinez et al., 2008; Wang et al., 2008; Li et al., 2010). In high-risk HPV cervical cancer tissues, the expression level of miRNA-34a and -218 is decreased (Wang et al., 2009). Furthermore, E7 oncoprotein may suppress miRNA-203 expression by inhibiting the MAPK/PKC pathway, as it does for miRNA-15a and -16 (Melar-New & Laiminins, 2010). High-risk oncoproteins E6 and E7 engage with different cellular components in various ways, which might result in up- or down-regulation of cellular miRNA expression. Both E6 and E7 are responsible for miRNA-21 expression in cervical carcinoma (Zheng & Wang, 2011). In HPV-16 and -18-positive cancer cell lines, aberrant miRNA expression might also directly suppress E6 and E7 activity. For example, upregulation of miRNA-375 could suppress E6 and E7 expression, thus restoring the p53 and pRB signaling cascade (Jayamohan et al.,

2019). Some miRNAs have been found to silent E6 and E7 expression as well as suppressed other overexpressed oncogenic proteins in cervical cancer. As a result, future research into therapeutic approaches that affect miRNA expression to modulate HPV-16 and -18 expression and stimulate tumor suppressor protein expression could be a potential alternative for treating HPV-induced cervical cancer (Chiantore et al., 2016).

9.8 miRNAs LINKED WITH DRUG RESISTANCE IN CERVICAL CANCER

Several findings reveal that various dysregulated miRNAs are key regulators in the commencement of drug and radio resistance in cervical cancer. In cervical cancer, many miRNAs are up- or downregulated, and their expression levels can affect susceptibility to chemotherapy and radiotherapy (Masadah et al., 2021). Phuah et al. reported the expression profiles of 25 miRNAs, including miR-138, miR-210, and miR-744, which were found to affect susceptibility to 1′S-1′-acetoxychavicol (ACA) and cisplatin (Phuah et al., 2013, 2017). As a result, miRNAs could play a key role in the chemotherapeutic response. Lei et al. showed that miR-155 suppresses growth, metastasis, and EMT transition, as well as increasing cisplatin sensitivity (Li et al., 2012). By suppressing Bcl2l2 expression, miR-214 induces apoptosis cell death and reduces tumor growth, and increases sensitivity to cisplatin (Shen et al., 2013) while miR-218 induces apoptosis, suppresses tumor growth, and increases sensitivity to cisplatin in cervical cancer cells via targeting AKT/mTOR signaling cascade (Sato et al., 2009). Furthermore, miRNA may augment the resistance to chemotherapeutic cervical cancer treatment. miR-375 has been found to have a role in the acquisition of paclitaxel resistance in cervical cancer cells (Karimi & Mollaei, 2021). Another example is miR-181a, which has been demonstrated to enhance cellular resistance to irradiation by decreasing radiation-induced apoptosis and reducing G2/M stage block by downregulating proapoptotic protein kinase (PRKCD). If miRNA expression is particularly susceptible to cisplatin or paclitaxel resistant miRNA is overexpressed, cisplatin may be the best option. This treatment technique could be effective in cervical cancer personalized treatment or targeted therapy. Numerous recent findings revealed that aberrant expression of miRNAs has been linked to the development of cervical cancer (Di Leva et al., 2012; Feng et al., 2018; Sharma & Vashist, 2019), where they alter cancer cell growth, migration, immune evasion, and drug resistance. miR-145 was identified as a component of a p53-miR-145 axis regulating the IGF signaling pathway implicated in mitomycin resistance in cervical cancer (Shi et al., 2012; Zhou et al., 2017). Several research have recently contributed to understanding the role of miRNAs in cisplatin resistance in cervical cancer. Fekete and colleagues explored the possibility of miRNAs serving as markers of platinum-based chemotherapy for squamous cell carcinoma (Fekete et al., 2020). *In vitro* findings suggested that miR-7-5p upregulated in HeLa and SiHa cervical cancer cells with acquired cisplatin resistance. The results of Feng and colleagues are another example of the dual involvement of miRNAs in cisplatin resistance, in which a SOX9/miR-130a/CTR1 axis was discovered to participate in drug resistance (Feng et al., 2018). Chen and colleagues found that miR-499a-5p transfection enhanced migration, metastasis, and cisplatin resistance in both cervical cancer cells and mice models (Chen et al., 2020). Increasing evidence demonstrated that miR-218 is considerably downregulated in human cancer tissues relative to adjacent non-cancerous tissues (Liu et al., 2016; Yang et al., 2017), including cervical cancer, where it acts as a tumor suppressor miRNA (Liu et al., 2020). miR-144 is another example of miRNA that is differentially expressed in cisplatin-resistant cells (Shi et al., 2019).

9.9 miRNA AS A THERAPEUTIC TOOL IN CERVICAL CANCER

Regulating the expression level of miRNAs can be used to treat cancer. This could include administering complementary nucleic acid sequences or lowering the overall levels of expression of miRNAs (oncomiRs) over-expressed in tumor to block their function. Besides this, supplementing the miRNA itself, the function of miRNAs (tumor suppressor miRs) with lower levels in cancer can be restored (Pardini et al., 2018; Miao et al., 2020). Both procedures rely on synthetic nucleic acid-based medications that need to be delivered. Simultaneous administration of synthetic nucleic acids is also a major concern in the use of siRNAs as therapeutic agents, and delivery challenges are one of the reasons why *in vitro* results are frequently not reproduced *in vivo*. To maintain stability *in vivo* and to transport nucleic acid-based medications into cells efficiently and safely, a delivery method is necessary. Atelocollagen, a protein that forms the terminal section (telopeptide) of collagen type I, is being investigated as a possible drug delivery mechanism (Ochiya et al., 1999). This protein is isolated from calf dermis, processed, and then treated with protease to minimize antigenicity. Under physiological settings, atelocollagen is positively charged and forms a compound with negatively charged nucleic-acid-based agents. This compound can be delivered into tissues and cells in a stable manner. Because no adverse gross or biological findings were discovered after high dosage intravenous administration to rabbits and monkeys, this delivery technique may be suitable for clinical development. In a mouse model, an inhibitory impact of miR-143 on metastasis was observed after intravenous injection of a combination with atelocollagen (Liu et al., 2012). MiR-34 levels have been replenished using this strategy. Although distribution to the brain is problematic, a delivery strategy based on RGD peptide that can cross the blood-brain barrier may be possible. As a result, a variety of nucleic-acid-based pharmaceutical delivery techniques are being developed for both general and clinical applications (Córdova-Rivas et al., 2019). One therapy method for cancer patients with low miRNA expression is to restore function by supplementing the miRNA itself. Because the RISC complex does not recognize single-stranded mature miRNA, extracellular injection is ineffective. As a result, synthesized nucleic acid molecules that can be transformed into mature miRNA via the intrinsic cellular pathway must be delivered. Although this method resembles gene therapy, it should be safer because synthetic nucleic acid molecules are used instead of viral vectors. The process for producing siRNAs as medicines is useful as a reference since therapy based on miRNA administration utilizes *in vivo* RNAi functionalities. Supplementary agents are divided into two structural types: hairpin single-stranded pre-miRNA, which is the structure before Dicer; and double-stranded RNA, which is formed by cleaving the loop of a single stranded hairpin pre-miRNA and has a shape similar to siRNA. Hairpins must be delivered as long-strand RNAs with at least 50 bases. The creation of a 110-mer miRNA precursor with miR-196a activity indicated that 2-cyanoethoxymethyl (CEM) technology can be used to produce long RNAs (Shilba et al., 2007). Double-stranded RNA is identical to the RNA used in siRNA medicines and may be created employing current technologies. In contrast to siRNAs, miRNAs can have effects even if they are not fully complementary to the target mRNA; hence, one miRNA can repress several targets. In the pharmaceutical industry, this is a disadvantage because specificity is lowered. The many targets of developed miRNAs, on the other hand, are not random gene groups with a shared function. Thus, introducing one miRNA inhibits several genes in the same signaling pathway, and one miRNA may have an effect similar to introducing numerous siRNAs for these genes at the same time (Linsley et al., 2007). In this context, a therapeutic strategy using double-stranded RNA to complement miR34 is being developed. Osaki et al. evaluated the influence of miR-143 supplementation on the suppression of lung metastasis from osteosarcoma. After transplanting human osteosarcoma cells into mice, miR-143 was detected in miRNA microarray assay of human osteosarcoma cells either with or without frequent lung metastasis (Osaki et al., 2008). In an *in vitro* study, miR-143 decreased infiltration of human osteosarcoma cells but had no effect on cell proliferation. It was the miRNA with the lowest expression level in cells with recurrent metastasis. In an osteosarcoma spontaneous lung metastasis model, intravenous injection of miR-143 decreased lung metastasis but had no impact on primary lesion size. MMP-13 expression in osteosarcoma cells of the initial lesion was reduced in cells with high expression level of miR-143, and the expression of miR-143 in the human primary osteosarcoma lesion was decreased in cells with metastasis as compared to cells without metastasis. As a result, MMP13 overexpression caused by miR-143 downregulation increased lung metastasis, implying that supplementing osteosarcoma cells with miR-143 decreased their invasive and metastatic ability. Therefore, a s a tumor suppressor miRNA, miR-143 supplementation may aid in the treatment of cervical cancer (Osaki et al., 2011; Zhao et al., 2019). With increased miR-143 expression, Liu et al. found that cell proliferation was suppressed, and apoptosis was enhanced in HeLa cervical cancer cells. Even when pre-miR-143-treated HeLa cells were transplanted into female nude mice, carcinogenesis was suppressed by miR-143 expression. In comparison to normal tissue, Bcl2 expression enhanced in tissues with reduced miR-143 expression. In HeLa cells, upregulated miR-143 expression suppressed Bcl2, while miR-143 knockdown increased Bcl2 expression level (Liu et al., 2012). As a result, miR-143 is linked to Bcl2, and therapeutic strategies targeting this pathway could be an effective treatment method (Chen et al., 2014).

9.10 CONCLUSION

In conclusion, a great deal of evidence suggests that miRNA has a variety of functions in diagnosis, treatment, radio-sensitivity, chemo-sensitivity, and chemo-resistance, mostly through their targeting of related genes and interactions with diverse signal transduction (Figure 9.4). In this chapter, miRNAs were collected based on their expression level, functional classification, potential target, and molecular mechanisms. This report indicates that miRNA has an impact on a variety of biological processes in cervical carcinoma and can be used to improve prognosis, diagnosis, and therapeutic strategies. To understand more about therapeutically essential miRNA for cervical cancer treatment, more research needs to be done. With the rapid development of miRNA as a therapeutic tool for cervical cancer, several technologies will be employed such as next-generation sequencing technology. More miRNA will be unearthed, allowing a more comprehensive understanding of miRNA expression profiles in cervical carcinoma to be portrayed. A representation like this will allow us to understand the molecular events that govern the phenotypes of cervical cancer. The next task is to figure out the regulatory association between miRNA, target genes, and proteins. Thus, miRNAs seem to have a strong possibility to be employed as prognostic, diagnostic, and therapeutic biomarkers in the management of cervical cancer.

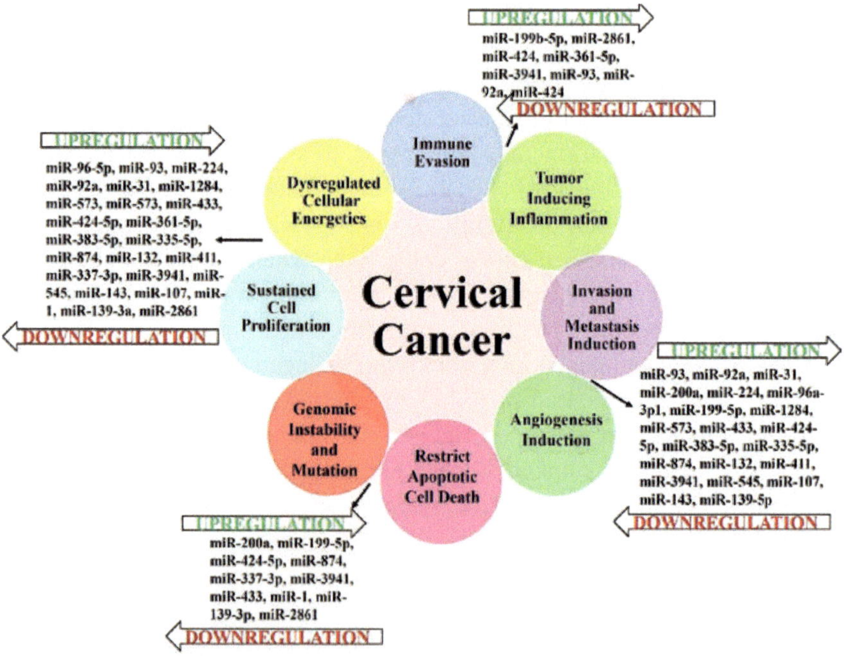

FIGURE 9.4 Different miRNAs and their association with various regulatory mechanisms in the process of cervical cancer carcinogenesis.

KEYWORDS

- **cervical cancer treatment**
- **cervical carcinoma**
- **diagnosis**
- **microRNAs**
- **miRNA expression profiles**
- **therapeutic biomarkers**

REFERENCES

Agirre, X., Martínez-Climent, J. Á., Odero, M. D., & Prósper, F., (2012). Epigenetic regulation of miRNA genes in acute leukemia. *Leukemia, 26*(3), 395–403.

Aishanjiang, A., Rouzi, N., Jiao, Z., et al., (2018). MicroRNA-9 enhances invasion and migration of cervical carcinomas by directly targeting FOXO1. *Eur. Rev. Med. Pharmacol. Sci., 22*(8), 2253–2260.

Almeida, A. M., Queiroz, J. A., Sousa, F., & Sousa, Â., (2019). Cervical cancer and HPV infection: Ongoing therapeutic research to counteract the action of E6 and E7 oncoproteins. *Drug Discovery Today, 24*(10), 2044–2057.

Almeida, M. I., Reis, R. M., & Calin, G. A., (2011). MicroRNA history: Discovery, recent applications, and next frontiers. *Mutation Research, 717*(1, 2), 1–8.

Babar, I. A., Cheng, C. J., Booth, C. J., Liang, X., Weidhaas, J. B., Saltzman, W. M., & Slack, F. J., (2012). Nanoparticle-based therapy in an *in vivo* microRNA-155 (miR-155)-dependent mouse model of lymphoma. *Proceedings of the National Academy of Sciences of the United States of America, 109*(26), E1695–E1704.

Babion, I., Jaspers, A., Van, S. A. P., Van, D. H. I., Wilting, S. M., & Steenbergen, R., (2019). miR-9–5p exerts a dual role in cervical cancer and targets transcription factor TWIST1. *Cells, 9*(1), 65.

Banno, K., Iida, M., Yanokura, M., Kisu, I., Iwata, T., Tominaga, E., Tanaka, K., & Aoki, D., (2014). MicroRNA in cervical cancer: OncomiRs and tumor suppressor miRs in diagnosis and treatment. *The Scientific World Journal*, 178075.

Baranwal, S., & Alahari, S. K., (2010). miRNA control of tumor cell invasion and metastasis. *International Journal of Cancer, 126*(6), 1283–1290.

Berezikov, E., Cuppen, E., & Plasterk, R. H., (2006). Approaches to microRNA discovery. *Nature Genetics, 38*(6), S2–S7.

Bousquet, M., Quelen, C., Rosati, R., et al., (2008). Myeloid cell differentiation arrest by miR-125b-1 in myelodysplastic syndrome and acute myeloid leukemia with the translocation. *The Journal of Experimental Medicine, 205*(11), 2499–2506.

Brennecke, J., Stark, A., Russell, R. B., Cohen, S. M., & Carrington, J. C., (2005). Principles of microRNA–target recognition. *PLoS Biology, 3*(3), e85.

Brodersen, P., & Voinnet, O., (2009). Revisiting the principles of microRNA target recognition and mode of action. *Nature Reviews Molecular Cell Biology, 10*(2), 141–148.

Bueno, M. J., & Malumbres, M., (2011). MicroRNAs and the cell cycle. *Biochimica et Biophysica Acta (BBA) – Molecular Basis of Disease, 1812*(5), 592–601.

Calin, G. A., Liu, C. G., Sevignani, C., et al., (2004). MicroRNA profiling reveals distinct signatures in B cell chronic lymphocytic leukemias. *Proceedings of the National Academy of Sciences of the United States of America, 101*(32), 11755–11760.

Calin, G. A., Sevignani, C., Dumitru, C. D., et al., (2004). Human microRNA genes are frequently located at fragile sites and genomic regions involved in cancers. *Proceedings of the National Academy of Sciences of the United States of America, 101*(9), 2999–3004.

Chakrabarti, M., Banik, N. L., & Ray, S. K., (2013). miR-138 overexpression is more powerful than hTERT knockdown to potentiate apigenin for apoptosis in neuroblastoma *in vitro* and *in vivo*. *Experimental Cell Research, 319*(10), 1575–1585.

Chaudhuri, A. A., So, A. Y., Mehta, A., et al., (2012). Oncomir miR-125b regulates hematopoiesis by targeting the gene Lin28A. *Proceedings of the National Academy of Sciences of the United States of America, 109*(11), 4233–4238.

Chen, G., Huang, P., Xie, J., & Li, R., (2018). microRNA-211 suppresses the growth and metastasis of cervical cancer by directly targeting ZEB1. *Molecular Medicine Reports, 17*(1), 1275–1282.

Chen, J., & Li, G., (2018). MiR-1284 enhances the sensitivity of cervical cancer cells to cisplatin via downregulating HMGB1. *Biomedicine and Pharmacotherapy, 107*, 997–1003.

Chen, J., Deng, Y., Ao, L., et al., (2019). The high-risk HPV oncogene E7 upregulates miR-182 expression through the TGF-β/Smad pathway in cervical cancer. *Cancer Letters, 460*, 75–85.

Chen, Y., Gu, Y., Gu, Y., & Wu, J., (2021). Long noncoding RNA LINC00899/miR-944/ESR1 axis regulates cervical cancer cell proliferation, migration, and invasion. *Journal of Interferon and Cytokine Research, 41*(6), 220–233.

Chen, Y., Liu, C., Xie, B., Chen, S., Zhuang, Y., & Zhang, S., (2020). miR-96 exerts an oncogenic role in the progression of cervical cancer by targeting CAV-1. *Molecular Medicine Reports, 22*(1), 543–550.

Chen, Y., Ma, C., Zhang, W., Chen, Z., & Ma, L., (2014). Down regulation of miR-143 is related with tumor size, lymph node metastasis and HPV16 infection in cervical squamous cancer. *Diagnostic Pathology, 9*(1), 1–11.

Chen, Y., Song, Y., Mi, Y., et al., (2020). microRNA-499a promotes the progression and chemoresistance of cervical cancer cells by targeting SOX6. *Apoptosis: An International Journal on Programmed Cell Death, 25*(3, 4), 205–216.

Chen, Z. Y., Chen, X., & Wang, Z. X., (2016). The role of microRNA-196a in tumorigenesis, tumor progression, and prognosis. *Tumor Biology, 37*(12), 15457–15466.

Chiantore, M. V., Mangino, G., Iuliano, M., et al., (2016). Human papillomavirus E6 and E7 oncoproteins affect the expression of cancer-related microRNAs: Additional evidence in HPV-induced tumorigenesis. *Journal of Cancer Research and Clinical Oncology, 142*(8), 1751–1763.

Chiou, T. J., (2007). The role of microRNAs in sensing nutrient stress. *Plant, Cell and Environment, 30*(3), 323–332.

Christensen, M., & Schratt, G. M., (2009). microRNA involvement in developmental and functional aspects of the nervous system and in neurological diseases. *Neuroscience Letters, 466*(2), 55–62.

Chu, Y., Ouyang, Y., Wang, F., Zheng, A., Bai, L., Han, L., Chen, Y., & Wang, H., (2014). MicroRNA-590 promotes cervical cancer cell growth and invasion by targeting CHL1. *Journal of Cellular Biochemistry, 115*(5), 847–853.

Cong, J., Liu, R., Wang, X., Jiang, H., & Zhang, Y., (2016). MiR-634 decreases cell proliferation and induces apoptosis by targeting mTOR signaling pathway in cervical cancer cells. *Artificial Cells, Nanomedicine, and Biotechnology, 44*(7), 1694–1701.

Conti, I., Varano, G., Simioni, C., Laface, I., Milani, D., Rimondi, E., & Neri, L. M., (2020). miRNAs as influencers of cell-cell communication in tumor microenvironment. *Cells, 9*(1), 220.

Córdova-Rivas, S., Fraire-Soto, I., Mercado-Casas, T. A., et al., (2019). 5p and 3p strands of miR-34 family members have differential effects in cell proliferation, migration, and invasion in cervical cancer cells. *International Journal of Molecular Sciences, 20*(3), 545.

Costinean, S., Sandhu, S. K., Pedersen, I. M., et al., (2009). Src homology 2 domain-containing inositol-5-phosphatase and CCAAT enhancer-binding protein beta are targeted by miR-155 in B cells of emicro-MiR-155 transgenic mice. *Blood, 114*(7), 1374–1382.

Cui, F., Li, X., Zhu, X., et al., (2012). MiR-125b inhibits tumor growth and promotes apoptosis of cervical cancer cells by targeting phosphoinositide 3-kinase catalytic subunit delta. *Cellular Physiology and Biochemistry, 30*(5), 1310–1318.

Das, S., & Halushka, M. K., (2015). Extracellular vesicle microRNA transfer in cardiovascular disease. *Cardiovascular Pathology, 24*(4), 199–206.

De Planell-Saguer, M., & Rodicio, M. C., (2011). Analytical aspects of microRNA in diagnostics: A review. *Analytica Chimica Acta, 699*(2), 134–152.

Deng, B., Zhang, Y., Zhang, S., Wen, F., Miao, Y., & Guo, K., (2015). MicroRNA-142–3p inhibits cell proliferation and invasion of cervical cancer cells by targeting FZD7. *Tumor Biology, 36*(10), 8065–8073.

Di Leva, G., Briskin, D., & Croce, C. M., (2012). MicroRNA in cancer: New hopes for antineoplastic chemotherapy. *Upsala Journal of Medical Sciences, 117*(2), 202–216.

Diener, C., Keller, A., & Meese, E., (2022). Emerging concepts of miRNA therapeutics: From cells to clinic. *Trends in Genetics, 38*(6), 613–626.

Dong, J., Sui, L., Wang, Q., Chen, M., & Sun, H., (2014). MicroRNA-26a inhibits cell proliferation and invasion of cervical cancer cells by targeting protein tyrosine phosphatase type IVA 1. *Molecular Medicine Reports, 10*(3), 1426–1432.

Dong, W., Li, B., Wang, J., Song, Y., Zhang, Z., & Fu, C., (2017). MicroRNA-337 inhibits cell proliferation and invasion of cervical cancer through directly targeting specificity protein 1. *Tumor Biology, 39*(6), 1010428317711323.

Dürst, M., Gissmann, L., Ikenberg, H., & Zur, H. H., (1983). A papillomavirus DNA from a cervical carcinoma and its prevalence in cancer biopsy samples from different geographic regions. *Proceedings of the National Academy of Sciences of the United States of America, 80*(12), 3812–3815.

Engels, B. M., & Hutvagner, G., (2006). Principles and effects of microRNA-mediated post-transcriptional gene regulation. *Oncogene, 25*(46), 6163–6169.

Enomoto, Y., Kitaura, J., Hatakeyama, K., et al., (2011). Eμ/miR-125b transgenic mice develop lethal B-cell malignancies. *Leukemia, 25*(12), 1849–1856.

Fan, D., Wang, Y., Qi, P., et al., (2016). MicroRNA-183 functions as the tumor suppressor via inhibiting cellular invasion and metastasis by targeting MMP-9 in cervical cancer. *Gynecologic Oncology, 141*(1), 166–174.

Fang, H., Shuang, D., Yi, Z., Sheng, H., & Liu, Y., (2016). Up-regulated microRNA-155 expression is associated with poor prognosis in cervical cancer patients. *Biomedicine and Pharmacotherapy, 83*, 64–69.

Fekete, J. T., Welker, Á., & Győrffy, B., (2020). miRNA expression signatures of therapy response in squamous cell carcinomas. *Cancers, 13*(1), 63.

Feng, C., Ma, F., Hu, C., et al., (2018). SOX9/miR-130a/CTR1 axis modulates DDP-resistance of cervical cancer cell. *Cell Cycle, 17*(4), 448–458.

Feng, X., Zhang, C., Yang, Y., Hou, D., & Zhu, A., (2018). Role of miR-181a in the process of apoptosis of multiple malignant tumors: A literature review. *Adv. Clin. Exp. Med., 27*(2), 263–270.

Feng, Y., Zhou, S., Li, G., Hu, C., Zou, W., Zhang, H., & Sun, L., (2016). Nuclear factor-κB-dependent microRNA-130a upregulation promotes cervical cancer cell growth by targeting phosphatase and tensin homolog. *Archives of Biochemistry and Biophysics, 598*, 57–65.

Ferracin, M., & Negrini, M., (2015). Micromarkers 2.0: An update on the role of microRNAs in cancer diagnosis and prognosis. *Expert Review of Molecular Diagnostics, 15*(10), 1369–1381.

Gambari, R., Brognara, E., Spandidos, D. A., & Fabbri, E., (2016). Targeting oncomiRNAs and mimicking tumor suppressor miRNAs: New trends in the development of miRNA therapeutic strategies in oncology. *International Journal of Oncology, 49*(1), 5–32.

Gao, Y., Lin, L., Li, T., Yang, J., & Wei, Y., (2017). The role of miRNA-223 in cancer: Function, diagnosis and therapy. *Gene, 616*, 1–7.

Gefen, N., Binder, V., Zaliova, M., et al., (2010). Hsa-mir-125b-2 is highly expressed in childhood ETV6/RUNX1 (TEL/AML1) leukemias and confers survival advantage to growth inhibitory signals independent of p53. *Leukemia, 24*(1), 89–96.

Griffiths-Jones, S., Grocock, R. J., Van, D. S., Bateman, A., & Enright, A. J., (2006). miRBase: MicroRNA sequences, targets and gene nomenclature. *Nucleic Acids Research, 34*, 140–144.

Grimaldi, A., Zarone, M. R., Irace, C., Zappavigna, S., Lombardi, A., Kawasaki, H., Caraglia, M., & Misso, G., (2018). Noncoding RNAs as a new dawn in tumor diagnosis. *Seminars in Cell and Developmental Biology, 78*, 37–50.

Grzywa, T. M., Klicka, K., & Włodarski, P. K., (2020). Regulators at every step-how microRNAs drive tumor cell invasiveness and metastasis. *Cancers, 12*(12), 3709.

Guo, M., Zhao, X., Yuan, X., Jiang, J., & Li, P., (2017). MiR-let-7a inhibits cell proliferation, migration, and invasion by down-regulating PKM2 in cervical cancer. *Oncotarget, 8*(17), 28226–28236.

Guo, Y., Tao, M., & Jiang, M., (2018). MicroRNA-454-3p inhibits cervical cancer cell invasion and migration by targeting c-Met. *Experimental and Therapeutic Medicine, 15*(3), 2301–2306.

Hammond, S. M., (2015). An overview of microRNAs. *Advanced Drug Delivery Reviews, 87*, 3–14.

Han, Y., Xu, G. X., Lu, H., et al., (2015). Dysregulation of miRNA-21 and their potential as biomarkers for the diagnosis of cervical cancer. *International Journal of Clinical and Experimental Pathology, 8*(6), 7131–7139.

He, L., & Hannon, G. J., (2004). MicroRNAs: Small RNAs with a big role in gene regulation. *Nature Reviews, 5*(7), 522–531.

Hou, T., Ou, J., Zhao, X., Huang, X., Huang, Y., & Zhang, Y., (2014). MicroRNA-196a promotes cervical cancer proliferation through the regulation of FOXO1 and p27Kip1. *British Journal of Cancer, 110*(5), 1260–1268.

How, C., Hui, A. B., Alajez, N. M., et al., (2013). MicroRNA-196b regulates the homeobox B7-vascular endothelial growth factor axis in cervical cancer. *PLoS One, 8*(7), e67846.

Hsu, P. W., Huang, H. D., Hsu, S. D., et al., (2006). miRNAMap: Genomic maps of microRNA genes and their target genes in mammalian genomes. *Nucleic Acids Research, 34*(1), D135-D139.

Hu, X., Schwarz, J. K., Lewis, J. S., Huettner, P. C., Rader, J. S., Deasy, J. O., Grigsby, P. W., & Wang, X., (2010). A microRNA expression signature for cervical cancer prognosis. *Cancer Research, 70*(4), 1441–1448.

Hu, Y., Xie, H., Liu, Y., Liu, W., Liu, M., & Tang, H., (2017). miR-484 suppresses proliferation and epithelial-mesenchymal transition by targeting ZEB1 and SMAD2 in cervical cancer cells. *Cancer Cell International, 17*, 36.

Hua, F. F., Liu, S. S., Zhu, L. H., Wang, Y. H., Liang, X., Ma, N., & Shi, H. R., (2017). MiRNA-338-3p regulates cervical cancer cells proliferation by targeting MACC1 through MAPK signaling pathway. *European Review for Medical and Pharmacological Sciences, 21*(23), 5342–5352.

Huang, P., Xi, J., & Liu, S., (2016). MiR-139-3p induces cell apoptosis and inhibits metastasis of cervical cancer by targeting NOB1. *Biomedicine and Pharmacotherapy, 83*, 850–856.

Iorio, M. V., & Croce, C. M., (2012). Causes and consequences of microRNA dysregulation. *Cancer Journal, 18*(3), 215–222.

Islam, W., Tauqeer, A., Waheed, A., & Zeng, F., (2022). MicroRNA mediated plant responses to nutrient stress. *International Journal of Molecular Sciences, 23*(5), 2562.

Jayamohan, S., Kannan, M., Moorthy, R. K., Rajasekaran, N., Jung, H. S., Shin, Y. K., & Arockiam, A. J. V., (2019). Dysregulation of miR-375/AEG-1 axis by human papillomavirus 16/18-E6/E7 promotes cellular proliferation, migration, and invasion in cervical cancer. *Frontiers in Oncology, 9*, 847.

Jiang, D., Wang, H., Li, Z., Li, Z., Chen, X., & Cai, H., (2017). MiR-142 inhibits the development of cervical cancer by targeting HMGB1. *Oncotarget, 8*(3), 4001–4007.

Jin, H., & Wang, C., (2016). MicroRNA-9 functions as an oncogene and targets PDCD4 gene in cervical cancer. *International Journal of Clinical and Experimental Pathology, 9*(2), 2726–2734.

Kang, H. W., Wang, F., Wei, Q., Zhao, Y. F., Liu, M., Li, X., & Tang, H., (2012). miR-20a promotes migration and invasion by regulating TNKS2 in human cervical cancer cells. *FEBS Letters, 586*(6), 897–904.

Karimi, F., & Mollaei, H., (2021). Potential of miRNAs in cervical cancer chemoresistance. *Gene Reports, 23*, 101109.

Keshavarz, M., Dianat-Moghadam, H., Sofiani, V. H., et al., (2018). miRNA-based strategy for modulation of influenza A virus infection. *Epigenomics, 10*(6), 829–844.

Klusmann, J. H., Li, Z., Böhmer, K., et al., (2010). miR-125b-2 is a potential oncomiR on human chromosome 21 in megakaryoblastic leukemia. *Genes and Development, 24*(5), 478–490.

Kota, S. K., & Balasubramanian, S., (2010). Cancer therapy via modulation of micro-RNA levels: A promising future. *Drug Discovery Today, 15*(17, 18), 733–740.

Kozomara, A., Birgaoanu, M., & Griffiths-Jones, S., (2019). miRBase: From microRNA sequences to function. *Nucleic Acids Research, 47*(D1), D155–D162.

Kumar, M. S., Lu, J., Mercer, K. L., Golub, T. R., & Jacks, T., (2007). Impaired microRNA processing enhances cellular transformation and tumorigenesis. *Nature Genetics, 39*(5), 673–677.

Lajer, C. B., Garnæs, E., Friis-Hansen, L., et al., (2017). The role of miRNAs in human papilloma virus (HPV)-associated cancers: Bridging between HPV-related head and neck cancer and cervical cancer. *British Journal of Cancer, 117*(5), e2.

Landau, D. A., & Slack, F. J., (2011). MicroRNAs in mutagenesis, genomic instability, and DNA repair. *Seminars in Oncology, 38*(6), 743–751.

Lao, G., Liu, P., Wu, Q., Zhang, W., Liu, Y., Yang, L., & Ma, C., (2014). Mir-155 promotes cervical cancer cell proliferation through suppression of its target gene LKB1. *Tumor Biology, 35*(12), 11933–11938.

Lee, Y., Ahn, C., Han, J., et al., (2003). The nuclear RNase III drosha initiates microRNA processing. *Nature, 425*(6956), 415–419.

Lee, Y., Jeon, K., Lee, J. T., Kim, S., & Kim, V. N., (2002). MicroRNA maturation: Stepwise processing and subcellular localization. *The EMBO Journal, 21*(17), 4663–4670.

Levati, L., Pagani, E., Romani, S., et al., (2011). MicroRNA-155 targets the SKI gene in human melanoma cell lines. *Pigment Cell and Melanoma Research, 24*(3), 538–550.

Li, B., Hu, Y., Ye, F., Li, Y., Lv, W., & Xie, X., (2010). Reduced miR-34a expression in normal cervical tissues and cervical lesions with high-risk human papillomavirus infection. *International Journal of Gynecological Cancer, 20*(4), 597–604.

Li, C. L., Nie, H., Wang, M., et al., (2012). microRNA-155 is downregulated in gastric cancer cells and involved in cell metastasis. *Oncology Reports, 27*(6), 1960–1966.

Li, H., Sheng, Y., Zhang, Y., Gao, N., Deng, X., & Sheng, X., (2017). MicroRNA-138 is a potential biomarker and tumor suppressor in human cervical carcinoma by reversely correlated with TCF3 gene. *Gynecologic Oncology, 145*(3), 569–576.

Li, J., Hu, L., Tian, C., Lu, F., Wu, J., & Liu, L., (2015). microRNA-150 promotes cervical cancer cell growth and survival by targeting FOXO4. *BMC Molecular Biology, 16*(1), 1–9.

Li, J., Ping, Z., & Ning, H., (2012). MiR-218 impairs tumor growth and increases chemosensitivity to cisplatin in cervical cancer. *International Journal of Molecular Sciences, 13*(12), 16053–16064.

Li, M. Y., & Hu, X. X., (2015). Meta-analysis of microRNA expression profiling studies in human cervical cancer. *Medical Oncology, 32*(6), 510.

Li, M., Li, B. Y., Xia, H., & Jiang, L. L., (2017). Expression of microRNA-142-3p in cervical cancer and its correlation with prognosis. *European Review for Medical and Pharmacological Sciences, 21*(10), 2346–2350.

Li, W., Liang, J., Zhang, Z., Lou, H., Zhao, L., Xu, Y., & Ou, R., (2017). MicroRNA-329-3p targets MAPK1 to suppress cell proliferation, migration and invasion in cervical cancer. *Oncology Reports, 37*(5), 2743–2750.

Li, X. R., Chu, H. J., Lv, T., Wang, L., Kong, S. F., & Dai, S. Z., (2014). miR-342-3p suppresses proliferation, migration and invasion by targeting FOXM1 in human cervical cancer. *FEBS Letters, 588*(17), 3298–3307.

Li, Y., Wang, Y., Xie, Z., & Hu, H., (2019). JMJD2A facilitates growth and inhibits apoptosis of cervical cancer cells by downregulating tumor suppressor miR-491-5p. *Molecular Medicine Reports, 19*(4), 2489–2496.

Liang, C., Ding, J., Yang, Y., Deng, L., & Li, X., (2017). MicroRNA-433 inhibits cervical cancer progression by directly targeting metadherin to regulate the AKT and β-catenin signaling pathways. *Oncology Reports, 38*(6), 3639–3649.

Liang, H., Luo, R., Chen, X., Zhao, Y., & Tan, A., (2017). miR-187 inhibits the growth of cervical cancer cells by targeting FGF9. *Oncology Reports, 38*(4), 1977–1984.

Liao, H., Pan, Y., Pan, Y., et al., (2018). MicroRNA-874 is downregulated in cervical cancer and inhibits cancer progression by directly targeting ETS1. *Oncology Reports, 40*, 2389–2398.

Lin, C., Huang, F., Shen, G., & Yiming, A., (2015). MicroRNA-101 regulates the viability and invasion of cervical cancer cells. *International Journal of Clinical and Experimental Pathology, 8*(9), 10148–10155.

Lin, C., Huang, F., Zhang, Y. J., Tuokan, T., & Kuerban, G., (2014). Roles of MiR-101 and its target gene Cox-2 in early diagnosis of cervical cancer in Uygur women. *Asian Pacific Journal of Cancer Prevention, 15*(1), 45–48.

Linsley, P. S., Schelter, J., Burchard, J., et al., (2007). Transcripts targeted by the microRNA-16 family cooperatively regulate cell cycle progression. *Molecular and Cellular Biology, 27*(6), 2240–2252.

Liu, B., Ding, J. F., Luo, J., Lu, L., Yang, F., & Tan, X. D., (2016). Seven protective miRNA signatures for prognosis of cervical cancer. *Oncotarget, 7*(35), 56690–56698.

Liu, B., Tian, Y., Li, F., et al., (2016). Tumor-suppressing roles of miR-214 and miR-218 in breast cancer. *Oncology Reports, 35*(6), 3178–3184.

Liu, G. F., Zhang, S. H., Li, X. F., Cao, L. Y., Fu, Z. Z., & Yu, S. N., (2017). Overexpression of microRNA-132 enhances the radio sensitivity of cervical cancer cells by down-regulating Bmi-1. *Oncotarget, 8*(46), 80757–80769.

Liu, L., Yu, X., Guo, X., et al., (2012). miR-143 is downregulated in cervical cancer and promotes apoptosis and inhibits tumor formation by targeting Bcl-2. *Molecular Medicine Reports, 5*(3), 753–760.

Liu, S., Song, L., Yao, H., Zhang, L., Xu, D., Li, Q., & Li, Y., (2018). Preserved miR-361-3p expression is an independent prognostic indicator of favorable survival in cervical cancer. *Disease Markers, 8949*606.

Liu, S., Zhang, P., Chen, Z., Liu, M., Li, X., & Tang, H., (2013). MicroRNA-7 downregulates XIAP expression to suppress cell growth and promote apoptosis in cervical cancer cells. *FEBS Letters, 587*(14), 2247–2253.

Liu, X., (2018). Up-regulation of miR-20a by HPV16 E6 exerts growth-promoting effects by targeting PDCD6 in cervical carcinoma cells. *Biomedicine and Pharmacotherapy, 102*, 996–1002.

Liu, Z., Mao, L., Wang, L., Zhang, H., & Hu, X., (2020). miR-218 functions as a tumor suppressor gene in cervical cancer. *Molecular Medicine Reports, 21*(1), 209–219.

Lv, R., & Zhang, Q. W., (2020). The long noncoding RNA FTH1P3 promotes the proliferation and metastasis of cervical cancer through microRNA-145. *Oncology Reports, 43*(1), 31–40.

Lynam-Lennon, N., Maher, S. G., & Reynolds, J. V., (2009). The roles of microRNA in cancer and apoptosis. *Biological Reviews, 84*(1), 55–71.

Ma, N., Li, X., Wei, H., Zhang, H., & Zhang, S., (2021). Circular RNA circNFATC3 acts as a miR-9-5p sponge to promote cervical cancer development by upregulating SDC2. *Cellular Oncology, 44*(1), 93–107.

Ma, Q., Wan, G., Wang, S., Yang, W., Zhang, J., & Yao, X., (2014). Serum microRNA-205 as a novel biomarker for cervical cancer patients. *Cancer Cell International, 14*(1), 1–7.

Martinez, I., Gardiner, A. S., Board, K. F., Monzon, F. A., Edwards, R. P., & Khan, S. A., (2008). Human papillomavirus type 16 reduces the expression of microRNA-218 in cervical carcinoma cells. *Oncogene, 27*(18), 2575–2582.

Masadah, R., Rauf, S., Pratama, M. Y., Tiribelli, C., & Pascut, D., (2021). The role of microRNAs in the cisplatin- and radio-resistance of cervical cancer. *Cancers, 13*(5), 1168.

Mei, S., Xin, J., Liu, Y., et al., (2015). MicroRNA-200c promotes the suppressive potential of myeloid-derived suppressor cells by modulating PTEN and FOG2 expression. *PLoS One, 10*(8), e0135867.

Melar-New, M., & Laimins, L. A., (2010). Human papillomaviruses modulate expression of microRNA 203 upon epithelial differentiation to control levels of p63 proteins. *Journal of Virology, 84*(10), 5212–5221.

Miao, J., Regenstein, J. M., Xu, D., et al., (2020). The roles of microRNA in human cervical cancer. *Archives of Biochemistry and Biophysics, 690*, 108480.

Mo, M. H., Chen, L., Fu, Y., Wang, W., & Fu, S. W., (2012). Cell-free circulating miRNA biomarkers in cancer. *Journal of Cancer, 3*, 432.

Munir, J., Yoon, J. K., & Ryu, S., (2020). Therapeutic miRNA-enriched extracellular vesicles: Current approaches and future prospects. *Cells, 9*(10), 2271.

Nilsen, T. W., (2007). Mechanisms of microRNA-mediated gene regulation in animal cells. *Trends in Genetics, 23*(5), 243–249.

Nouraee, N., & Mowla, S. J., (2015). miRNA therapeutics in cardiovascular diseases: Promises and problems. *Frontiers in Genetics, 6*, 232.

Ochiya, T., Takahama, Y., Nagahara, S., et al., (1999). New delivery system for plasmid DNA *in vivo* using atelocollagen as a carrier material: The minipellet. *Nature Medicine, 5*(6), 707–710.

Ojha, C. R., Rodriguez, M., Dever, S. M., Mukhopadhyay, R., & El-Hage, N., (2016). Mammalian microRNA: An important modulator of host-pathogen interactions in human viral infections. *Journal of Biomedical Science, 23*(1), 1–11.

Osaki, M., Takeshita, F., & Ochiya, T., (2008). MicroRNAs as biomarkers and therapeutic drugs in human cancer. *Biomarkers, 13*(7), 658–670.

Osaki, M., Takeshita, F., Sugimoto, Y., et al., (2011). MicroRNA-143 regulates human osteosarcoma metastasis by regulating matrix metalloprotease-13 expression. *Molecular Therapy, 19*(6), 1123–1130.

Pal, A., & Kundu, R., (2020). Human papillomavirus E6 and E7: The cervical cancer hallmarks and targets for therapy. *Frontiers in Microbiology, 10*, 3116.

Parasramka, M. A., Ho, E., Williams, D. E., & Dashwood, R. H., (2012). MicroRNAs, diet, and cancer: New mechanistic insights on the epigenetic actions of phytochemicals. *Molecular Carcinogenesis, 51*(3), 213–230.

Pardini, B., De Maria, D., Francavilla, A., Di Gaetano, C., Ronco, G., & Naccarati, A., (2018). MicroRNAs as markers of progression in cervical cancer: A systematic review. *BMC Cancer, 18*(1), 1–17.

Peng, R., Men, J., Ma, R., Wang, Q., Wang, Y., Sun, Y., & Ren, J., (2017). miR-214 down-regulates ARL2 and suppresses growth and invasion of cervical cancer cells. *Biochemical and Biophysical Research Communications, 484*(3), 623–630.

Pereira, D. M., Rodrigues, P. M., Borralho, P. M., & Rodrigues, C. M., (2013). Delivering the promise of miRNA cancer therapeutics. *Drug Discovery Today, 18*(5, 6), 282–289.

Persson, H., Kvist, A., Rego, N., et al., (2011). Identification of new microRNAs in paired normal and tumor breast tissue suggests a dual role for the ERBB2/Her2 gene. *Cancer Research, 71*(1), 78–86.

Phuah, N. H., Azmi, M. N., Awang, K., & Nagoor, N. H., (2017). Down-regulation of microRNA-210 confers sensitivity towards 1'S-1'-acetoxychavicol acetate (ACA) in cervical cancer cells by targeting SMAD4. *Molecules and Cells, 40*(4), 291–298.

Phuah, N. H., In, L. L., Azmi, M. N., Ibrahim, H., Awang, K., & Nagoor, N. H., (2013). Alterations of microRNA expression patterns in human cervical carcinoma cells (Ca Ski) toward 1'S-1'-acetoxychavicol acetate and cisplatin. *Reproductive Sciences, 20*(5), 567–578.

Pillai, R. S., (2005). MicroRNA function: Multiple mechanisms for a tiny RNA? *RNA, 11*(12), 1753–1761. https://doi.org/10.1261/rna.2248605.

Preskill, C., & Weidhaas, J. B., (2013). SNPs in microRNA binding sites as prognostic and predictive cancer biomarkers. *Critical Reviews in Oncogenesis, 18*(4), 327–340.

Price, N. L., Ramirez, C. M., & Fernández-Hernando, C., (2014). Relevance of microRNA in metabolic diseases. *Critical Reviews in Clinical Laboratory Sciences, 51*(6), 305–320.

Qian, W., Huang, T., & Feng, W., (2020). Circular RNA HIPK3 promotes EMT of cervical cancer through sponging miR-338-3p to up-regulate HIF-1α. *Cancer Management and Research, 12*, 177–187.

Qin, X., Wan, Y., Wang, S., & Xue, M., (2015). MicroRNA-125a-5p modulates human cervical carcinoma proliferation and migration by targeting ABL2. *Drug Design, Development and Therapy, 10*, 71–79.

Razavi, Z. S., Tajiknia, V., Majidi, S., et al., (2021). Gynecologic cancers and noncoding RNAs: Epigenetic regulators with emerging roles. *Critical Reviews in Oncology/Hematology, 157*, 103192.

Samir, M., & Pessler, F., (2016). Small noncoding RNAs associated with viral infectious diseases of veterinary importance: Potential clinical applications. *Frontiers in Veterinary Science, 3*, 22.

Sanches, J., Xu, Y., Yabasin, I. B., et al., (2018). miR-501 is upregulated in cervical cancer and promotes cell proliferation, migration and invasion by targeting CYLD. *Chemico-Biological Interactions, 285*, 85–95.

Sathyanarayanan, A., Chandrasekaran, K. S., & Karunagaran, D., (2016). microRNA-146a inhibits proliferation, migration and invasion of human cervical and colorectal cancer cells. *Biochemical and Biophysical Research Communications, 480*(4), 528–533.

Sathyanarayanan, A., Chandrasekaran, K. S., & Karunagaran, D., (2017). microRNA-145 modulates epithelial-mesenchymal transition and suppresses proliferation, migration and invasion by targeting SIP1 in human cervical cancer cells. *Cellular Oncology, 40*(2), 119–131.

Sato, F., Tsuchiya, S., Terasawa, K., & Tsujimoto, G., (2009). Intra-platform repeatability and inter-platform comparability of microRNA microarray technology. *PLoS One, 4*(5), e5540.

Shaham, L., Binder, V., Gefen, N., Borkhardt, A., & Izraeli, S., (2012). MiR-125 in normal and malignant hematopoiesis. *Leukemia, 26*(9), 2011–2018.

Shan, D., Shang, Y., & Hu, T., (2019). MicroRNA-411 inhibits cervical cancer progression by directly targeting STAT3. *Oncology Research, 27*(3), 349–358.

Sharma, S., & Vashist, M., (2019). MicroRNA in cervical carcinogenesis: Window of therapeutic potential. *Current Women's Health Reviews, 15*(3), 171–178.

Shen, C., Yang, H., Liu, H., Wang, X., Zhang, Y., & Xu, R., (2015). Inhibitory effect and mechanisms of microRNA-146b-5p on the proliferation and metastatic potential of Caski human cervical cancer cells. *Molecular Medicine Reports, 11*(5), 3955–3961.

Shen, S., Zhang, S., Liu, P., Wang, J., & Du, H., (2020). Potential role of microRNAs in the treatment and diagnosis of cervical cancer. *Cancer Genetics, 248*–249.

Shen, Y., Wang, P., Li, Y., et al., (2013). miR-375 is upregulated in acquired paclitaxel resistance in cervical cancer. *British Journal of Cancer, 109*(1), 92–99.

Shenouda, S. K., & Alahari, S. K., (2009). MicroRNA function in cancer: Oncogene or a tumor suppressor? *Cancer and Metastasis Reviews, 28*(3), 369–378.

Shi, C., & Zhang, Z., (2017a). MicroRNA-320 suppresses cervical cancer cell viability, migration and invasion via directly targeting FOXM1. *Oncology Letters, 14*(3), 3809–3816.

Shi, C., & Zhang, Z., (2017b). MicroRNA-362 is downregulated in cervical cancer and inhibits cell proliferation, migration and invasion by directly targeting SIX1. *Oncology Reports, 37*(1), 501–509.

Shi, F., Su, J., Liu, Z., Wang, J., & Wang, T., (2019). miR-144 reverses cisplatin resistance in cervical cancer via targeting LHX2. *Journal of Cellular Biochemistry, 120*(9), 15018–15026.

Shi, M., Du, L., Liu, D., et al., (2012). Glucocorticoid regulation of a novel HPV–E6–p53–miR-145 pathway modulates invasion and therapy resistance of cervical cancer cells. *The Journal of Pathology, 228*(2), 148–157.

Shiba, Y., Masuda, H., Watanabe, N., Ego, T., Takagaki, K., Ishiyama, K., Ohgi, T., & Yano, J., (2007). Chemical synthesis of a very long oligoribonucleotide with 2-cyanoethoxymethyl (CEM) as the 2'-O-protecting group: Structural identification and biological activity of a synthetic 110mer precursor-microRNA candidate. *Nucleic Acids Research, 35*(10), 3287–3296.

Shu, L., Zhang, Z., & Cai, Y., (2018). MicroRNA-204 inhibits cell migration and invasion in human cervical cancer by regulating transcription factor 12. *Oncology Letters, 15*(1), 161–166.

Slezak-Prochazka, I., Durmus, S., Kroesen, B. J., & Van, D. B. A., (2010). MicroRNAs, macrocontrol: Regulation of miRNA processing. *RNA, 16*(6), 1087–1095.

Song, G., Wang, R., Guo, J., et al., (2015). miR-346 and miR-138 competitively regulate hTERT in GRSF1-and AGO2-dependent manners, respectively. *Scientific Reports, 5*(1), 1–15.

Song, G., Zhang, Y., & Wang, L., (2009). MicroRNA-206 targets notch3, activates apoptosis, and inhibits tumor cell migration and focus formation. *The Journal of Biological Chemistry, 284*(46), 31921–31927.

Song, R., Cong, L., Ni, G., Chen, M., Sun, H., Sun, Y., & Chen, M., (2017). MicroRNA-195 inhibits the behaviour of cervical cancer tumors by directly targeting HDGF. *Oncology Letters, 14*(1), 767–775.

Stavast, C. J., & Erkeland, S. J., (2019). The non-canonical aspects of microRNAs: Many roads to gene regulation. *Cells, 8*(11), 1465. https://doi.org/10.3390/cells8111465.

Su, Z., Yang, H., Zhao, M., Wang, Y., Deng, G., & Chen, R., (2017). MicroRNA-92a promotes cell proliferation in cervical cancer via inhibiting p21 expression and promoting cell cycle progression. *Oncology Research, 25*(1), 137.

Suardi, R. B., Ysrafil, Y., Sesotyosari, S. L., Martien, R., Wardana, T., Astuti, I., & Haryana, S. M., (2020). The effects of combination of mimic miR-155–5p and antagonist miR-324–5p encapsulated chitosan in ovarian cancer SKOV3. *Asian Pacific Journal of Cancer Prevention, 21*(9), 2603–2608.

Svoronos, A. A., Engelman, D. M., & Slack, F. J., (2016). OncomiR or tumor suppressor? The duplicity of microRNAs in cancer. *Cancer Research, 76*(13), 3666–3670.

Tahiri, A., Leivonen, S. K., Lüders, T., et al., (2014). Deregulation of cancer-related miRNAs is a common event in both benign and malignant human breast tumors. *Carcinogenesis, 35*(1), 76–85.

Tan, D., Zhou, C., Han, S., Hou, X., Kang, S., & Zhang, Y., (2018). MicroRNA-378 enhances migration and invasion in cervical cancer by directly targeting autophagy-related protein 12. *Molecular Medicine Reports, 17*(5), 6319–6326.

Tang, T., Wong, H. K., Gu, W., et al., (2013). MicroRNA-182 plays an onco-miRNA role in cervical cancer. *Gynecologic Oncology, 129*(1), 199–208.

Tao, P., Wen, H., Yang, B., Zhang, A., Wu, X., & Li, Q., (2018). miR-144 inhibits growth and metastasis of cervical cancer cells by targeting VEGFA and VEGFC. *Experimental and Therapeutic Medicine, 15*(1), 562–568.

Tili, E., Michaille, J. J., Luo, Z., Volinia, S., Rassenti, L. Z., Kipps, T. J., & Croce, C. M., (2012). The downregulation of miR-125b in chronic lymphocytic leukemias leads to metabolic adaptation of cells to a transformed state. *Blood, 120*(13), 2631–2638.

Tomaić, V., (2016). Functional roles of E6 and E7 oncoproteins in HPV-induced malignancies at diverse anatomical sites. *Cancers, 8*(10), 95.

Urbanek-Trzeciak, M. O., Galka-Marciniak, P., Nawrocka, P. M., et al., (2020). Pan-cancer analysis of somatic mutations in miRNA genes. *EBio Medicine, 61*, 103051.

Van, P. G., Lefever, S., Anckaert, J., et al., (2014). miRBase tracker: Keeping track of microRNA annotation changes. *Database*, bau080.

Van, R. E., Sutherland, L. B., Qi, X., Richardson, J. A., Hill, J., & Olson, E. N., (2007). Control of stress-dependent cardiac growth and gene expression by a microRNA. *Science, 316*(5824), 575–579.

Vasudevan, S., Tong, Y., & Steitz, J. A., (2008). Cell-cycle control of microRNA-mediated translation regulation. *Cell Cycle, 7*(11), 1545–1549.

Vishnoi, A., & Rani, S., (2017). MiRNA biogenesis and regulation of diseases: An overview. *Methods in Molecular Biology, 1509*, 1–10.

Wang, D., Qiu, C., Zhang, H., Wang, J., Cui, Q., & Yin, Y., (2010). Human microRNA oncogenes and tumor suppressors show significantly different biological patterns: From functions to targets. *PLoS One, 5*(9), e13067.

Wang, D., Wang, H., Li, Y., & Li, Q., (2018). MiR-362-3p functions as a tumor suppressor through targeting MCM5 in cervical adenocarcinoma. *Bioscience Reports, 38*(3), BSR20180668.

Wang, F., Li, Y., Zhou, J., et al., (2011). miR-375 is down-regulated in squamous cervical cancer and inhibits cell migration and invasion via targeting transcription factor SP1. *The American Journal of Pathology, 179*(5), 2580–2588.

Wang, H. W., Terinate, P., Gao, Y., & Kalra, K. L., (2011). Investigation of microRNA-146a and microRNA-218 expression in cervical cancer. *The FASEB Journal, 25*(S1), lb316.

Wang, J. Y., & Chen, L. J., (2019). The role of miRNAs in the invasion and metastasis of cervical cancer. *Biosci. Rep., 39*(3). https://doi.org/10.1042/BSR20181377.

Wang, L. Q., Zhang, Y., Yan, H., Liu, K. J., & Zhang, S., (2015). MicroRNA-373 functions as an oncogene and targets YOD1 gene in cervical cancer. *Biochemical and Biophysical Research Communications, 459*(3), 515–520.

Wang, N., Zhou, Y., Zheng, L., & Li, H., (2014). MiR-31 is an independent prognostic factor and functions as an oncomir in cervical cancer via targeting ARID1A. *Gynecologic Oncology, 134*(1), 129–137.

Wang, P., Zhang, L., Zhang, J., & Xu, G., (2022). MicroRNA-124-3p inhibits cell growth and metastasis in cervical cancer by targeting IGF2BP1. *Experimental and Therapeutic Medicine, 23*(3), 233.

Wang, S., Cao, X., Ding, B., et al., (2016). The rs767649 polymorphism in the promoter of miR-155 contributes to the decreased risk for cervical cancer in a Chinese population. *Gene, 595*(1), 109–114.

Wang, S., Zhang, Y., Yuan, S., & Ji, X., (2018). MicroRNA-485 targets MACC1 and inhibits cervical cancer cell proliferation and invasion. *Molecular Medicine Reports, 18*(2), 2407–2416.

Wang, X., Tang, S., Le, S. Y., Lu, R., Rader, J. S., Meyers, C., & Zheng, Z. M., (2008). Aberrant expression of oncogenic and tumor-suppressive microRNAs in cervical cancer is required for cancer cell growth. *PLoS One, 3*(7), e2557.

Wang, X., Wang, H. K., McCoy, J. P., et al., (2009). Oncogenic HPV infection interrupts the expression of tumor-suppressive miR-34a through viral oncoprotein E6. *RNA, 15*(4), 637–647.

Wang, Y., Dong, X., Hu, B., Wang, X. J., Wang, Q., & Wang, W. L., (2016). The effects of micro-429 on inhibition of cervical cancer cells through targeting ZEB1 and CRKL. *Biomedicine and Pharmacotherapy, 80*, 311–321.

Wang, Z., Ren, C., Yang, L., Zhang, X., Liu, J., Zhu, Y., & Jiang, D., (2021). Silencing of circular RNA_0000326 inhibits cervical cancer cell proliferation, migration and invasion by boosting microRNA-338-3p-dependent down-regulation of CDK4. *Aging, 13*(6), 9119–9134.

Wei, H., Zhang, J. J., & Tang, Q. L., (2017). MiR-638 inhibits cervical cancer metastasis through Wnt/β-catenin signaling pathway and correlates with prognosis of cervical cancer patients. *European Review for Medical and Pharmacological Sciences, 21*(24), 5587–5593.

Wei, Q., Li, Y. X., Liu, M., Li, X., & Tang, H., (2012). MiR-17-5p targets TP53INP1 and regulates cell proliferation and apoptosis of cervical cancer cells. *IUBMB Life, 64*(8), 697–704.

Wei, Y. Q., Jiao, X. L., Zhang, S. Y., Xu, Y., Li, S., & Kong, B. H., (2019). MiR-9-5p could promote angiogenesis and radiosensitivity in cervical cancer by targeting SOCS5. *European Review for Medical and Pharmacological Sciences, 23*(17), 7314–7326.

Weiss, C. N., & Ito, K., (2017). A macro view of microRNAs: The discovery of microRNAs and their role in hematopoiesis and hematologic disease. *International Review of Cell and Molecular Biology, 334*, 99–175.

Wen, S. Y., Lin, Y., Yu, Y. Q., et al., (2015). miR-506 acts as a tumor suppressor by directly targeting the hedgehog pathway transcription factor Gli3 in human cervical cancer. *Oncogene, 34*(6), 717–725.

Wu, H., Chen, J., Li, D., Liu, X., Li, L., & Wang, K., (2017). MicroRNA-30e functions as a tumor suppressor in cervical carcinoma cells through targeting GALNT7. *Translational Oncology, 10*(6), 876–885.

Wu, X., Xi, X., Yan, Q., Zhang, Z., Cai, B., Lu, W., & Wan, X., (2013). MicroRNA-361-5p facilitates cervical cancer progression through mediation of epithelial-to-mesenchymal transition. *Medical Oncology, 30*(4), 751.

Xiang, J., & Wu, J., (2010). Feud or friend? The role of the miR-17-92 cluster in tumorigenesis. *Current Genomics, 11*(2), 129–135.

Xie, H., Lee, L., Scicluna, P., Kavak, E., Larsson, C., Sandberg, R., & Lui, W. O., (2015). Novel functions and targets of miR-944 in human cervical cancer cells. *International Journal of Cancer, 136*(5), E230–E241.

Xie, H., Zhao, Y., Caramuta, S., Larsson, C., & Lui, W. O., (2012). miR-205 expression promotes cell proliferation and migration of human cervical cancer cells. *PLoS One, 7*(10), e46990.

Xie, M., Li, M., Vilborg, A., et al., (2013). Mammalian 5′-capped microRNA precursors that generate a single microRNA. *Cell, 155*(7), 1568–1580.

Xie, Q., Lin, S., Zheng, M., Cai, Q., & Tu, Y., (2019). Long noncoding RNA NEAT1 promotes the growth of cervical cancer cells via sponging miR-9-5p. *Biochemistry and Cell Biology = Biochimie et Biologie Cellulaire, 97*(2), 100–108.

Xu, J., Wan, X., Chen, X., Fang, Y., Cheng, X., Xie, X., & Lu, W., (2016). miR-2861 acts as a tumor suppressor via targeting EGFR/AKT2/CCND1 pathway in cervical cancer induced by human papillomavirus virus 16 E6. *Scientific Reports, 6*, 28968.

Xu, L. J., Duan, Y., Wang, P., & Yin, H. Q., (2018). MiR-199b-5p promotes tumor growth and metastasis in cervical cancer by down-regulating KLK10. *Biochemical and Biophysical Research Communications, 503*(2), 556–563.

Yan, S., Li, X., Jin, Q., & Yuan, J., (2016). MicroRNA-145 sensitizes cervical cancer cells to low-dose irradiation by downregulating OCT4 expression. *Experimental and Therapeutic Medicine, 12*(5), 3130–3136.

Yang, C. X., Zhang, S. M., Li, J., et al., (2016). MicroRNA-320 regulates the radiosensitivity of cervical cancer cells C33AR by targeting β-catenin. *Oncology Letters, 12*(6), 4983–4990.

Yang, L., Liu, L., Zhang, X., Zhu, Y., Li, L., Wang, B., Liu, Y., & Ren, C., (2020). miR-96 enhances the proliferation of cervical cancer cells by targeting FOXO1. *Pathology, Research and Practice, 216*(4), 152854.

Yang, M., Chen, J., Su, F., et al., (2011). Microvesicles secreted by macrophages shuttle invasion-potentiating microRNAs into breast cancer cells. *Molecular Cancer, 10*(1), 1–13.

Yang, T., Xue, L., & An, L., (2007). Functional diversity of miRNA in plants. *Plant Science, 172*(3), 423–432.

Yang, Y. K., Xi, W. Y., Xi, R. X., Li, J. Y., Li, Q., & Gao, Y. E., (2015). MicroRNA-494 promotes cervical cancer proliferation through the regulation of PTEN. *Oncology Reports, 33*(5), 2393–2401.

Yang, Y., Ding, L., Hu, Q., et al., (2017). MicroRNA-218 functions as a tumor suppressor in lung cancer by targeting IL-6/STAT3 and negatively correlates with poor prognosis. *Molecular Cancer, 16*(1), 141.

Yang, Y., Liu, Y., Li, G., Li, L., Geng, P., & Song, H., (2018). microRNA-214 suppresses the growth of cervical cancer cells by targeting EZH2. *Oncology Letters, 16*(5), 5679–5686.

Yang, Y., Song, K. L., Chang, H., & Chen, L., (2014). Decreased expression of microRNA-126 is associated with poor prognosis in patients with cervical cancer. *Diagnostic Pathology, 9*, 220.

Ye, C., Hu, Y., & Wang, J., (2019). MicroRNA-377 targets zinc finger E-box-binding homeobox 2 to inhibit cell proliferation and invasion of cervical cancer. *Oncology Research, 27*(2), 183–192.

Ye, H., Yu, X., Xia, J., Tang, X., Tang, L., & Chen, F., (2016). MiR-486-3p targeting ECM1 represses cell proliferation and metastasis in cervical cancer. *Biomedicine and Pharmacotherapy, 80*, 109–114.

Yi, Y., Li, H., Lv, Q., et al., (2016). miR-202 inhibits the progression of human cervical cancer through inhibition of cyclin D1. *Oncotarget, 7*(44), 72067–72075.

Yin, Z. L., Wang, Y. L., Ge, S. F., Guo, T. T., Wang, L., Zheng, X. M., & Liu, J., (2015). Reduced expression of miR-503 is associated with poor prognosis in cervical cancer. *European Review for Medical and Pharmacological Sciences, 19*(21), 4081–4085.

Yu, Y., Zhang, Y., & Zhang, S., (2013). MicroRNA-92 regulates cervical tumorigenesis, and its expression is upregulated by human papillomavirus-16 E6 in cervical cancer cells. *Oncology Letters, 6*(2), 468–474.

Yue, Z., Yun-Shan, Z., & Feng-Xia, X., (2016). miR-205 mediates the inhibition of cervical cancer cell proliferation using Olmesartan. *Journal of the Renin-Angiotensin-Aldosterone System, 17*(3), 1470320316663327.

Zhang, B., Pan, X., Cobb, G. P., & Anderson, T. A., (2007). microRNAs as oncogenes and tumor suppressors. *Developmental Biology, 302*(1), 1–12.

Zhang, H., Zhang, Z., Wang, S., Zhang, S., & Bi, J., (2018). The mechanisms involved in miR-9 regulated apoptosis in cervical cancer by targeting FOXO3. *Biomedicine and Pharmacotherapy, 102*, 626–632.

Zhang, J., Li, Y. H., Liu, H. L., Zhang, Y., Zhang, Q. S., & Li, S. Z., (2018). Correlations of microRNA-21 gene polymorphisms with chemosensitivity and prognosis of cervical cancer. *The American Journal of the Medical Sciences, 356*(6), 544–551.

Zhang, J., Zhao, X., Zhang, J., Zheng, X., & Li, F., (2018). Circular RNA hsa_circ_0023404 exerts an oncogenic role in cervical cancer through regulating miR-136/TFCP2/YAP pathway. *Biochemical and Biophysical Research Communications, 501*(2), 428–433.

Zhang, J., Zheng, F., Yu, G., Yin, Y., & Lu, Q., (2013). miR-196a targets netrin 4 and regulates cell proliferation and migration of cervical cancer cells. *Biochemical and Biophysical Research Communications, 440*(4), 582–588.

Zhang, W., Zhou, J., Zhu, X., & Yuan, H., (2017). MiR-126 reverses drug resistance to TRAIL through inhibiting the expression of c-FLIP in cervical cancer. *Gene, 627*, 420–427.

Zhang, X., & Zhang, H., (2022). Circ_ZFR is linked to paclitaxel resistance in cervical cancer via miR-944 sponging and IL-10 upregulation. *Analytical Cellular Pathology, 4807*287.

Zhang, X., Cai, D., Meng, L., & Wang, B., (2016). MicroRNA-124 inhibits proliferation, invasion, migration and epithelial-mesenchymal transition of cervical carcinoma cells by targeting astrocyte-elevated gene-1. *Oncology Reports, 36*(4), 2321–2328.

Zhang, Y. X., Qin, L. L., & Yang, S. Y., (2016). Down-regulation of miR-664 in cervical cancer is associated with lower overall survival. *European Review for Medical and Pharmacological Sciences, 20*(9), 1740–1744.

Zhao, H., Yan, P., Wang, J., et al., (2019). Clinical significance of tumor miR-21, miR-221, miR-143, and miR-106a as biomarkers in patients with osteosarcoma. *The International Journal of Biological Markers, 34*(2), 184–193.

Zhao, S., Yao, D., Chen, J., Ding, N., & Ren, F., (2015). MiR-20a promotes cervical cancer proliferation and metastasis *in vitro* and *in vivo*. *PLoS One, 10*(3), e0120905.

Zheng, T., Wang, J., Chen, X., & Liu, L., (2010). Role of microRNA in anticancer drug resistance. *International Journal of Cancer, 126*(1), 2–10.

Zheng, W., Liu, Z., Zhang, W., & Hu, X., (2015). miR-31 functions as an oncogene in cervical cancer. *Archives of Gynecology and Obstetrics, 292*(5), 1083–1089.

Zheng, Z. M., & Wang, X., (2011). Regulation of cellular miRNA expression by human papillomaviruses. *Biochimica et Biophysica Acta, 1809*(11, 12), 668–677.

Zhou, C., Shen, L., Mao, L., Wang, B., Li, Y., & Yu, H., (2015). miR-92a is upregulated in cervical cancer and promotes cell proliferation and invasion by targeting FBXW7. *Biochemical and Biophysical Research Communications, 458*(1), 63–69.

Zhou, M., Chen, X., Wu, J., He, X., & Ren, R., (2018). MicroRNA-143 regulates cell migration and invasion by targeting GOLM1 in cervical cancer. *Oncology Letters, 16*(5), 6393–6400.

Zhou, Q., Dong, J., Luo, R., Zhou, X., Wang, J., & Chen, F., (2019). MicroRNA-20a regulates cell proliferation, apoptosis and autophagy by targeting thrombospondin 2 in cervical cancer. *European Journal of Pharmacology, 844*, 102–109.

Zhou, X., Yue, Y., Wang, R., Gong, B., & Duan, Z., (2017). MicroRNA-145 inhibits tumorigenesis and invasion of cervical cancer stem cells. *International Journal of Oncology, 50*(3), 853–862.

Zhu, C., Ding, Y., & Liu, H., (2011). MiR398 and plant stress responses. *Physiologia Plantarum, 143*(1), 1–9.

Zhu, X., Er, K., Mao, C., et al., (2013). miR-203 suppresses tumor growth and angiogenesis by targeting VEGFA in cervical cancer. *Cellular Physiology and Biochemistry, 32*(1), 64–73.

CHAPTER 10

Cervical Cancer and Natural Products: Anticancerous Efficacy and Mechanism

10.1 INTRODUCTION

Cancer of the cervix is the fourth most prominent type of malignancy among women worldwide (Bray et al., 2018), rendering it one of the leading causes of cancer-related deaths. Geographic location influences the incidence and death rate (Urasa & Darj, 2011). According to numerous research, cervical cancer cannot be caused solely by one risk. Apart from HPV, which has been identified as the key risk factor for cervical cancer development, socioeconomic status, venereal diseases, reproductive variables, long-term oral contraceptives, smoking, and obesity have also been identified as risk factors (Mitra & Elangovan, 2021). Furthermore, genetic and epigenetic alterations play a crucial role in the evolution of cervical cancer. Surgery, specifically pelvic lymphadenectomy and radical hysterectomy is the most common treatment for cervical cancer. This type of cancer is also treated with conventional methods like radiotherapy and chemotherapy, nevertheless, all of these treatments have been linked to serious adverse effects like bleeding, organ damage, and the risk of blood clots. Radiotherapy may cause menopause, pain during sexual activity, or infertility, but chemotherapy may cause cytotoxicity throughout the body, not just in tumor cells. Furthermore, cisplatin and other commonly recommended medications for cervical carcinoma can cause serious adverse effects and possibly drug resistance (Alfaro et al., 2021).

Natural compounds have been proven to have the capacity to influence gene expression by targeting diverse components of the genetic and

Cervical Cancer: Signaling Pathways, Molecular Mechanisms, Natural Products, and Therapeutic Approaches. Pratibha Pandey, Fahad Khan, Saher Islam, and Devarajan Thangadurai, (Eds.)

epigenetic machinery in recent years (Chizenga & Abrahamse, 2021). Plant-derived natural compounds have recently been touted as the most promising oncology therapy possibilities. They can selectively kill tumor cells while causing minimal toxicity to normal cells. Chemical variety, structural diversity, innate bioactivity, and negligible side effects are all factors (Mann, 2002; Aung et al., 2017). Natural bioactive compounds such as phenols, flavonoids, terpenoids, and alkaloids, have been recognized as antitumor natural products that can inhibit tumor cell growth, stimulate apoptosis, suppress angiogenesis, reverse multidrug resistance, and so on (Guerra et al., 2018; Lin et al., 2020; Chopra & Dhingra, 2021).

10.2 FLAVONOIDS

Flavonoids are ubiquitous polyphenolic chemicals that are produced as secondary metabolites in plants and are accountable for their color, odor, and biological properties (Ullah et al., 2020). Fruits and vegetables are excellent sources of flavonoids, but they are also prominent in cocoa products, green tea, and red wine. Berries, cherries, plums, and apples are the fruits with a rich content of flavonoids, while tropical fruits have the minimum content (Tungmunnithum et al., 2018; Dias et al., 2021; Shen et al., 2022). However, vegetables like broad beans, onions, olives, spinach, and shallot have the highest quantities of flavonoids. Their structural variability allows them to be classified into different subgroups as flavones, flavanones, flavanols, isoflavones, flavonols, and anthocyanidins depending on their carbon skeletons (C6-C3-C6) tagged with A, B, and C rings (Wang et al., 2018). They are strong antioxidants that protect plants from harmful environmental circumstances. Thus they have received considerable interest and have been explored in a lot of preclinical and clinical investigations to see if they can help with a variety of chronic human diseases (Owona et al., 2020). Several researchers have found that flavonoids have an important role in cancer prevention and treatment due to their diverse therapeutic properties, including antioxidant, anti-inflammatory, anti-hyperlipidemic, anti-aging, and so on. By suppressing different cancer signaling pathways and genes in tumor cells, they can stimulate apoptosis in tumor cells (Rodríguez-García et al., 2019; Khan et al., 2021; Liskova et al., 2021) (Table 10.1).

TABLE 10.1 Antitumor Effects of Flavonoids on Cervical Cancer and Their Associated Molecular Targets

Natural Product	Class	Structure	Cervical Cell Line/ Model	Molecular Targets
Baicalein	Flavones	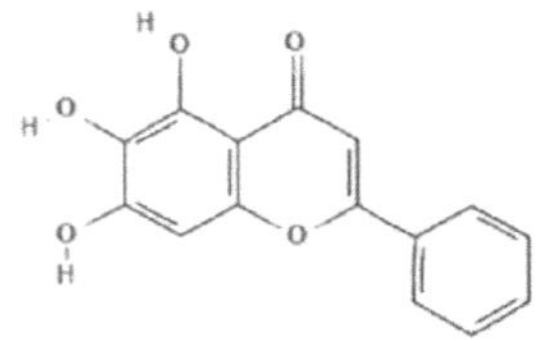	HeLa	Upregulated: Caspase-3, PARP cleavage. Downregulated: caspase-8, cIAP1, cIAP2, FLIP, MMP2 and 9, cyclin D1, COX-2, IL-8, MCP1, Bcl2. Inhibited: NF-κB, ERK1/2
			Xenografts (HeLa cells) female BALB/c mice	Suppressed tumor growth
Wogonin	Flavones	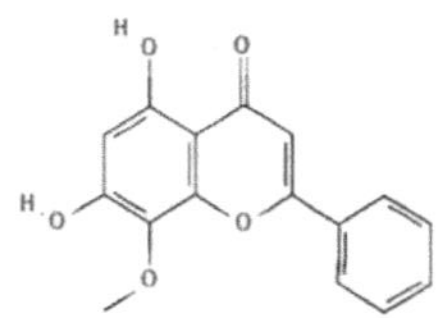	SiHa and CaSki	Upregulated: Bax, p53, pRb; activation of caspase 3 and 9; Cyt c release; PARP cleavage. Downregulated: MMP; Bcl-2, E6, E7
Apigenin	Flavones	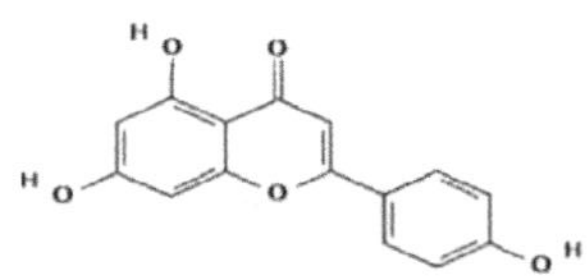	HeLa, SiHa, CaSki, and C33A	Upregulated: ROS, H_2O_2, caspase 3 and 9, Fas, FasL, TNF-α. Downregulated: Bcl-2, Bcl-xl, Cyclin (A, D, E), CDK2/6, MMP. Inhibited: PTEN/PI3K/AKT
			Xenografts (HeLa cells) female BALB/c mice	Suppressed tumor growth via ERβ/Erα downregulation

TABLE 10.1 *(Continued)*

Natural Product	Class	Structure	Cervical Cell Line/ Model	Molecular Targets
Luteolin	Flavones	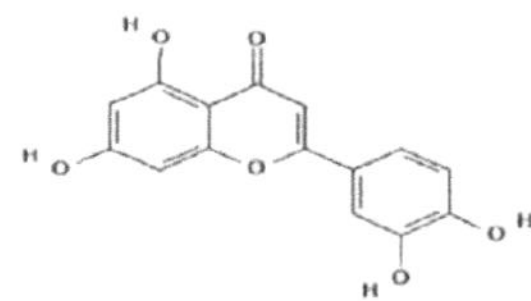	HeLa	Upregulated: p16, JNK. Downregulated: UHRF1, DNMT1, A20, c-IAP1; G2/M phase cell cycle arrest
Naringin	Flavanones	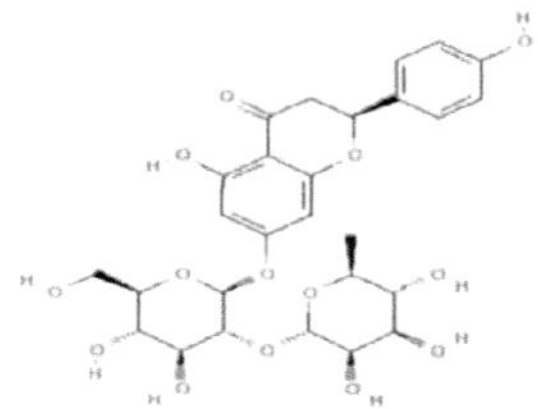	SiHa	Upregulated: p53, Bax, Fas, FADD; triggered caspase 3, 8 and 9
Hesperidin	Flavanones	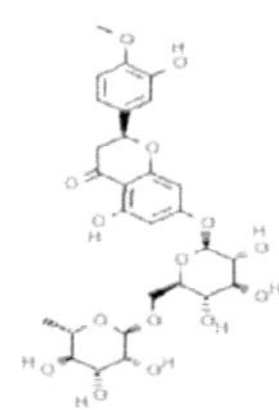	HeLa	Upregulated: AIF, stimulation of caspase 3, Cyt c release. Downregulated: MMP, cyclin D1/E1, CDK2; G0/G1 cell cycle arrest
Silibinin	Flavanones	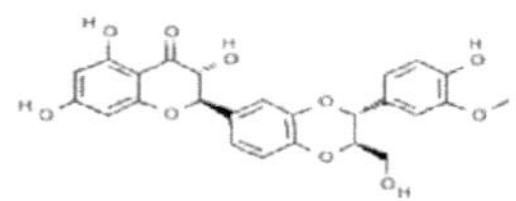	HeLa and SiHa	Upregulated: activation of Drp1 Downregulated: MMP, ATP, ROS, Cdc25C, CDK1, cyclin B1; G2/M cell cycle arrest

TABLE 10.1 *(Continued)*

Natural Product	Class	Structure	Cervical Cell Line/ Model	Molecular Targets
Kaempferol	Flavonols	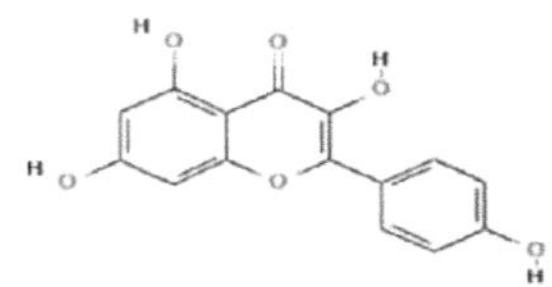	HeLa	Upregulated: Bax, p53. Downregulated: Bcl-2, hTERT. Inhibited: PI3K/AKT
Quercetin	Flavonols	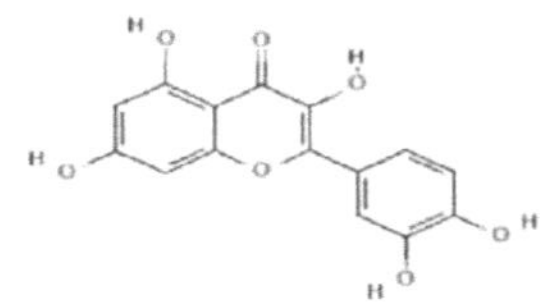	HeLa and SiHa	Upregulated: ROS, Bax, p53, stimulation of caspase 3 and Cyt c release. Downregulated: MMP, Bcl-2, AKT; G2/M cell cycle arrest
Fisetin	Flavonols	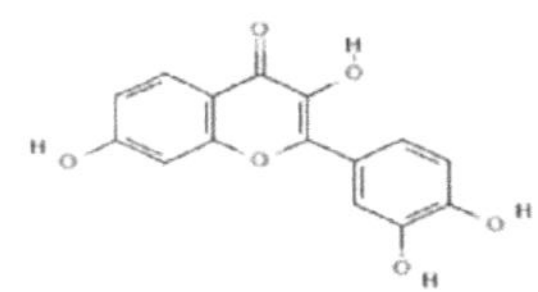	HeLa	Upregulated: Stimulation of caspase-3 and -8, ERK1/2, activation
			Xenografts (HeLa cells) male BALB/c mice	Suppressed tumor growth
Epigallocatechin gallate	Flavanols	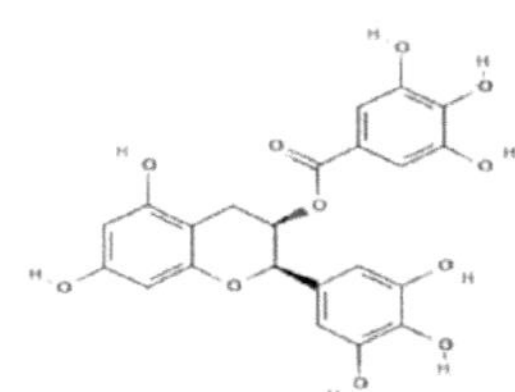	HeLa	Upregulated: ROS, p53, Bax, Cyt c release. Downregulated: Bcl-2, COX-2 Inhibited: AKT and NF-κB

TABLE 10.1 *(Continued)*

Natural Product	Class	Structure	Cervical Cell Line/ Model	Molecular Targets
Genistein	Isoflavones	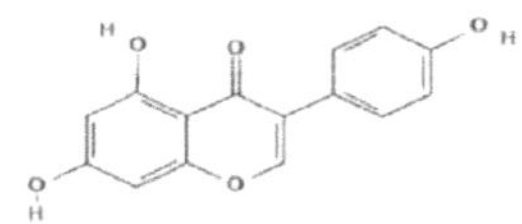	HeLa and CaSki	Upregulated: P38-MAPK, p38-JNK. Downregulated: ERK1/2, AKT
			C57BL/6 cervical cancer cell mice model	Suppressed tumor growth
Formononetin	Isoflavones	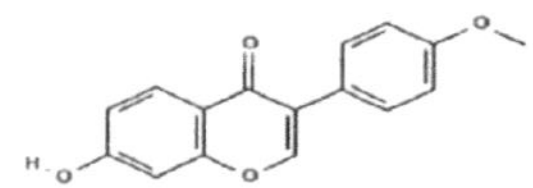	HeLa	Upregulated: ROS, Bax stimulation of caspase 3 and 9 Downregulated: Bcl-2, MMP, MRP1 and MRP2
			Xenografts (HeLa cells) BALB/c nude mice	Suppressed tumor growth
Cyanidin 3-O-glucoside	Anthocyanin	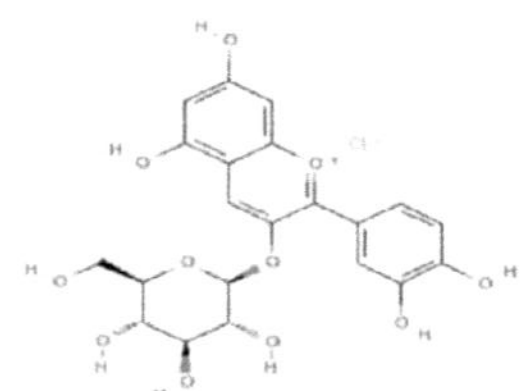	HeLa	Upregulated: p53, Bax, TIMP-1 Downregulated: Bcl-2, cyclin D1; G2/M phase cell arrest. Inhibited: PI3K/AKT/mTOR

10.2.1 BAICALEIN

Baicalein is a substantial active component obtained from the root of *Scutellariae radix* (commonly known as Chinese Huang Qin). The distinctive structural characteristic of bicalein is the presence of di-orthohydroxyl functional group on ring-A and it exhibits a number of therapeutic properties, including the ability to suppress cell migration and proliferation, as well as trigger cell cycle arrest and apoptosis (Verma et al., 2021). Cervical cancer may have a therapeutic target in Cyclin D1. Baicalein suppresses proliferation and induces death in cervical carcinoma cells HeLa and SiHa by inhibiting cyclin D1 overexpression and arresting the cell cycle progression at G0/G1 stage via the Wnt/β-catenin and protein kinase B/glycogen synthase kinase-3 (AKT/GSK-3) signaling pathways (Wu et al., 2018; Xia et al., 2019). Baicalein, on the other hand, inhibited TNF-alpha mediated nuclear movement of p65 by blocking the phosphorylation and breakdown of the inhibitory subunit of NF-kB inhibitory unit (IkB-alpha), caspase 8 stimulation, and enhanced the cleavage of PARP (poly(ADP-ribose polymerase)) expression to stimulate apoptotic cell death in cervical cancer HeLa cells (Li et al., 2016). Furthermore, baicalein inhibited the activation of p38 and extracellular signal-regulated kinases 1/2 (ERK1/2), which lowered the inflammatory cytokines expression such as MCP-1 (monocyte chemoattractant protein 1) and IL-8 (interleukin 8) (Peng et al., 2015). Baicalein also inhibited the growth of cervical cancer cells by inactivating the AKT/mTOR signaling pathway by manipulating the circHIAT1/miR-19a-3p axis (Hu et al., 2021; Lei et al., 2021). Another research concluded that administering 10 mg/kg/d baicalin for four weeks dramatically reduced cervical carcinoma xenograft tumor growth and metastasis *in vivo*. Baicalein was also found to suppress the expression level of long non-coding RNA (lncRNA) in a concentration and time responsive manner and named as BDLNR (baicalein suppressed long non-coding RNA). It firmly connected itself to YBX1 (Y-box binding protein 1), attracted YBX1 to the promoter of PIK3CA, and activated the PI3K/Akt cascade to facilitate the antitumor actions of baicalein in cervical carcinoma (Yu et al., 2018). BDLNR has been proposed as a promising therapeutic target for enhancing baicalein's anticancer impact.

10.2.2 WOGONIN

Wogonin is a natural monoflavonoid derived from the perennial Labiate *Scutellaria baicalensis* Georgi plant. It has been proven in several studies to decrease the proliferation and growth of cancerous cells (Banik et al., 2022). Wogonin suppressed the HPV E6 and E7 expression level and induced cell death in SiHa and CaSki cervical cancer cells via the mitochondria-dependent pathway, lowering MMP (mitochondrial membrane potential), increasing the ratio of pro-apoptotic/antiapoptotic protein level (Bax/Bcl-2), causing cytochrome C leakage, and inducing caspase activation (Kim et al., 2013). Wogonin also suppressed HeLa cell growth by promoting apoptotic cell death and causing cell-cycle arrest at G1 phase through downregulating the expression level of cyclin D1, CDK 4, E2f-1 and pRb, along with upregulating the expression level of CDK inhibitor proteins ($p21^{cip1}$) via p53 mediated pathway (Yang et al., 2009). Wogonin can also improve the efficacy of cisplatin on tumor cell death by ROS-mediated mechanism (He et al., 2012). Thus, these findings suggest that wogonin could be used as a chemotherapeutic agent against cervical cancer.

10.2.3 APIGENIN

Apigenin is a natural flavonoid that can be present in many foods, including fruits and vegetables. *In vivo* and *in vitro* studies revealed its strong antiproliferative potential against several cancer cells (Ahmed et al., 2021). Apigenin 7-glucoside, a derivative of apigenin, possesses anti-oxidant, anti-inflammatory, and antitumor properties. Apigenin 7-glucoside substantially inhibited HeLa cell growth and promote apoptosis via mitochondrial dependent and independent pathways which resulted in the upregulation of several key molecules like ROS, TNF-α, Fas, FasL, FADD (Fas-associated death domain), TNF receptor-associated death domain (TRADD), executioner caspases and, lowering the expression of procaspases and anti-apoptotic proteins in human cervical cancer HeLa cells (Wang et al., 2020). Apigenin 7-glucoside therapy also enhanced p16 (INK4A) expression while decreasing Cyclin A, D, E, CDK2 and CDK6 expression. Furthermore, it suppressed the cervical cancer HeLa cells migration and invasion by inhibiting PTEN/PI3K/AKT cell signaling pathway (Liu et al., 2020). Few research findings revealed that apigenin exhibited selective responsiveness for different cervical tumor cells HeLa, CaSki, SiHa, and C33A, with IC_{50} of 10, 76, 68 and 40 μmol/L, respectively. Apigenin also caused mitochondrial dysfunction, reduced MMP and stopped cervical cancer cells from migrating and invading (Souza et al., 2017). An *in vivo* investigation directed by Zhang et al. (2020) demonstrated that intraperitoneal dosing (100 mg/kg apigenin+1 mg/kg histamine) of apigenin in mice model resulted in decreased cervical tumor growth by modulating histamine-induced aberrant estrogen receptor pathway. Apigenin also activated the PI3K/Akt/mTOR signaling pathway in HeLa cells, causing autophagy and death. As a result, apigenin and its derivatives may help to prevent the onset and disease progression and may be useful in cervical cancer treatment.

10.2.4 LUTEOLIN

Luteolin is a flavonoid present in a wide range of plant, particularly in vegetables, fruits, and medicinal botanicals. Plants high in luteolin have been used to cure a variety of ailments, including hypertension, cancer, and inflammation (Lin et al., 2008; Tuorkey et al., 2016). Luteolin inhibited the growth of HeLa cervical cancer cells in a dose-responsive way, with an IC_{50} of 21.8 mol/L. By decreasing the expression of UHRF1 and DNA methyltransferase 1 (DNMT1) with a decline in overall DNA methylation and upregulating p16 INK4A expression, luteolin triggered cell death and growth arrest at G2/M stage in HeLa cells (Krifa et al., 2013). By blocking TNF-induced NF-kB stimulation, attenuating expression of A20 and c-IAP1, and increasing c-Jun N-terminal kinase (JNK) activity, luteolin increased apoptosis (Shi et al., 2004). It was also shown that luteoloside decreased HeLa cell proliferation through both endogenous and external mechanisms, upregulating Fas expression and activating caspase-8 and -3. To achieve anti-cervical-cancer actions, luteoloside inhibited mTOR and stimulated the p38 mitogen-activated protein kinase (MAPK) signaling cascade at the same time (Shao et al., 2018). Furthermore, luteolin in combination with TNF-related apoptosis-inducing ligand (TRAIL) triggered apoptosis in HeLa cells by upregulating death receptor 5 (DR5) and Bid cleavage, as well as activating caspase-8 (Horinaka et al., 2005).

These findings show that luteolin could be used as promising therapeutics for the treatment of cervical malignancy.

10.2.5 NARINGIN

Naringin is a flavonoid glycoside that may be extracted from citrus fruits like oranges, tangerines, lemons, and limes. It possesses a myriad of therapeutic applications (Ghanbari-Movahed et al., 2021). Naringin inhibits cancer cell survival and multiplication while causing minimal harm to normal tissue cells (Yang et al., 2022). After a 24-hour treatment, the IC_{50} of naringin reported for HeLa, SiHa, and C33A cervical carcinoma cells were 793, 764, and 745 μmol/L, respectively, with a dose-dependent relationship. Naringin activated the CHOP (apoptosis-related protein) and other allied pro-apoptotic proteins by phosphorylating eIF2 and increasing the level of endoplasmic reticulum (ER) stress sensors (PARP1). Importantly, naringin inhibited the β-catenin signaling pathway by lowering the production of β-catenin (Ser576) and GSK-3β (Ser9) proteins and caused apoptosis in cervical cancer cells by elevating the expression of cell-cycle checkpoint proteins $p21^{cip1}$ and $p27^{kip1}$ to induce cell-cycle arrest at G0/G1 phase (Lin et al., 2020). Another study found that naringin triggers apoptosis in HeLa cells via increasing the expression of apoptotic related proteins, including Bax, caspases-3, -8, -9, p53, Fas death receptor, and its adaptor protein FADD through the mitochondrial independent pathway and the mitochondrial route. Exogenous pathway activation was linked to elevated caspase 8 expression, which regulated the death receptor by cleaving Bid into tBid, and interaction between the death receptor and mitochondrial pathways (Ramesh & Alshatwi, 2013). Furthermore, naringin reduced the expression of NF-Bp65, COX-2, and caspase 1 in HeLa cells, causing growth inhibition and apoptosis (Zeng et al., 2014). These findings show that naringin could be used as a new therapeutic agent for cervical cancer treatment.

10.2.6 HESPERIDIN AND ITS ANALOG HESPERETIN

Hesperidin is a citrus flavonoid with antioxidation, anticancer, and anti-angiogenesis properties, as well as the ability to shield mitochondrial membranes from free radical damage and prevent tumor cell motility and invasion (de Oliveira et al., 2020; Pandey & Khan, 2021). With IC_{50} values of 650 μmol/L, hesperetin decreased the number of viable SiHa cells in a concentration- and time-responsive manner. By depolarizing MMP and boosting the expression of Bax, caspase (3, 8, 9), Fas, p53, and FADD, hesperetin triggered cell-cycle arrest at G2/M stage and cell death in SiHa cells via death receptor and mitochondrial pathways (Alshatwi et al., 2013). Hesperidin also decreased HeLa cell growth and triggered death via ER stress and mitochondria-mediated pathways by lowering the expression of cyclin D1, cyclin E1, and CDK2, boosting Cyt c release, and the expression of GADD153/CHOP, AIF (apoptosis-inducing factor), and GRP78 (glucose-regulated protein of 78 kDa) (Wang et al., 2015). Hesperidin has the potential to prevent and treat cervical cancer, opening up new cancer treatment alternatives.

10.2.7 SILIBININ

Silibinin is a substantial active component obtained from the seed and fruit of *Silybum marianum*. It has been utilized to treat various ailments, including liver, gallbladder, and renal disease (Polachi et al., 2016; Boojar et al., 2020). Silibinin suppressed the proliferation of cervical cancer (HeLa and SiHa) cells in a concentration and time-responsive pattern. It activated the Drp1-mediated mitochondrial fission mechanism and lowered ATP, mtDNA copy number, and MMP levels, caused G2/M cell-cycle arrest by lowering CDK1, cyclin B1, and Cdc25C expression (You et al., 2020). Silibinin inhibited the mTOR/p70S6K/4E-BP1 signaling pathway and decreased the aggregation and expression level of hypoxia-inducible factor-1 (HIF-1) and the release of VEGF in HeLa cells, suppressing angiogenesis and promoting death. Furthermore, reducing AKT activation with the PI3K/AKT inhibitor LY294002 improved silibinin's anti-angiogenic efficacy (Garcia-Maceira et al., 2009). Simultaneously, silibinin induced apoptosis in HeLa cells via the mitochondrial and death-inducing pathways, resulting in decreased CDK1 and CDK2 protein expression and an increased Bax/Bcl-2 ratio, accompanied by Cyt c leak and caspase-9 activation, as well as upregulated level of Fas and FasL and caspase 8 activation (Zhang et al., 2012). Silibinin suppresses HeLa cell growth in a dose-dependent manner by boosting caspase-3 and apoptotic targets, as well as enhancing the activation of p53 and JNK. The PUMA (p53-upregulated modulator of apoptosis) pathway, which elevated the ratio of Bax:Bcl-2, lowers MMP, and increases ROS generation, then interferes with mitochondrial function. Then, in HeLa cells, ROS causes autophagy and apoptosis (Fan et al., 2011). Furthermore, in HeLa cells, p53-mediated glutathione (GSH) depletion greatly increased NO cytotoxicity (Fan et al., 2012a, b). It could be a classic candidate for anticancer medication development.

10.2.8 KAEMPFEROL

Kaempferol is one of the most widely distributed aglycone flavonoids. It is a yellow tetrahydroxyflavone with four hydroxy groups situated at positions 3, 5, 7, and 4′. Kaempferol can be found in a wide range of plant parts, including seeds, leaves, fruits, flowers, and even vegetables (Calderón-Montaño et al., 2011; Alam et al., 2020). Cardioprotective, neuroprotective, anti-inflammatory, antidiabetic, antioxidant, antibacterial, antitumor, and anticancer properties have been demonstrated for kaempferol and its glycosylated derivatives (Rajendran et al., 2014). Kaempferol is a possible cancer treatment agent with powerful anticancer, anti-inflammatory, and antioxidant effects, according to emerging data (Imran et al., 2019). By inhibiting MMP and rising intracellular free Ca^{2+} concentration, it hindered SiHa cell growth and proliferation and encouraged SiHa cell death, resulting in shrinkage of spindle shaped SiHa cells and disruption to their microtubule networks (Tu et al., 2016). Kaempferol reduced HeLa cell development in a dose and time responsive manner, with an IC_{50} value of 10.48 μmol/L at 72 hours, but it demonstrated minimal toxicity for normal cells with an IC_{50} value of 707 μmol/L at 72 hours, according to another study. It triggered apoptosis and senescence in HeLa cells by repressing the PI3K/AKT pathway and human telomerase reverse transcriptase (hTERT) transcriptional activity while modulating the p53 pathway (Kashafi et al., 2017). Telomerase is a novel and possibly selective target for cancer treatment. Kaempferol-induced telomerase suppression could be a safe and effective way to treat cervical cancer. Furthermore, overexpression of P-glycoprotein (P-gp) induces chemotherapeutic drug efflux from cells and is one of the key mechanisms associated with multidrug resistance (MDR) in tumor (Kumar & Jaitak, 2019). In MDR human cervical cancer KB-V1 cells, kaempferol significantly reduced P-gp activity and function in a dose-dependent pattern, limit drug efflux, effective sensitivity to anti-cancer drugs (vinblastine and paclitaxel) and cytotoxicity, all of which led to apoptotic induction and MDR reversal (Limtrakul et al., 2005). Because of its safety and low cost, kaempferol could be a good choice for cancer prevention and treatment.

10.2.9 QUERCETIN

Quercetin is a dietary polyphenolic component found in a wide range of vegetables and fruits that possesses anti-allergic, anti-inflammatory, and antitumor properties (Darband et al., 2018; Tang et al., 2020). Through the intrinsic apoptosis pathway, which involves PI3K, MAPK, and Wnt signaling pathway, quercetin can reduce tumor cell proliferation and triggered DNA damage, apoptosis, and cell-cycle arrest (Kedhari Sundaram et al., 2019). Vidya Priyadarsini et al. (2010) demonstrated that quercetin inhibited the growth of HeLa cells by targeting both opposite signaling cascade, p53 and NF-kB. By inhibiting the interaction of the E6/E6AP complex, stimulating p53, and augmenting the transcriptional level of target p21, quercetin triggered apoptosis in HeLa and SiHa cells (Clemente-Soto et al., 2019). Furthermore, by downregulating the expression of AKT and Bcl-2 and blocking the cell cycle at G2/M phase, quercetin enhanced apoptosis and reduced migration of HeLa cells within 18 hours. ROS mediated enhanced Cyt c release, MMP depolarization, and caspase 3 activation, all of which had significant anti-proliferative and pro-apoptotic effects on cervical cancer HeLa cells (Bishayee et al., 2013). Interestingly, combining quercetin with additional chemical agents significantly increased the anticancer activity. Cell viability of SiHa and HeLa cancer cells were reduced with quercetin treatment in a time and dose dependent manner (IC_{50} of 30 μmol/L for HeLa cells after 24 h) and (IC_{50} of 50 μmol/L for SiHa cells after 48 hrs.). Individual exposure with cisplatin or quercetin did not diminish MMP2 protein expression in cervical cancer cells, but their combination dramatically reduced MMP2 expression, inhibiting cervical cancer cell migration and invasion. Moreover, quercetin improved cancerous cell chemosensitivity by suppressing the level of P-gp and METTL3 (methyltransferase-like 3), which are involved in cell growth and apoptotic cell death in HeLa cells (Xu et al., 2021). By downregulating the expression level of the MRP (multidrug resistance-associated protein) and the heat shock protein (Hsp72), quercetin improved the susceptibility of HeLa cells against cisplatin, thus causing cell death and reversing resistance (Jakubowicz-Gil et al., 2005). This research laid the groundwork for the management of cisplatin-resistant cervical cancer patients.

10.2.10 FISETIN

Fisetin is a flavonol prevalent in fruits, vegetables, and nuts with anti-cancer, anti-invasive, anti-angiogenic, cardioprotective, and neuroprotective properties (Kashyap et al., 2018). Fisetin prevented the cell migration and invasion of cervical cancer SiHa cells by inhibiting urokinase-type plasminogen activator (u-PA) production via blocking the activation of p38/MAPK and the nuclear movement of NF-κB. Fisetin's inhibitory effect on u-PA activity and expression was further improved by the administration of the p38 MAPK agonist SB203580 (Chou et al., 2013). Fisetin also suppressed the activity of COX-2, ERK1/2, and prostaglandin E2 (PGE2) synthesis via disrupting the NF-kB/p300 signaling pathway, resulting in HeLa cell death (Liu et al., 2013). Furthermore, in a HeLa cell line administered mice model, fisetin effectively suppressed tumor growth with repression rate of 82.65% and 92.62% without noticeable side effects (Ying et al., 2012). Fisetin coupled with sorafenib was also shown to initiate the DR5-directed death receptor cascade as well as the mitochondria-dependent route in the lab, which led to apoptotic induction in HeLa cells by upregulating the Bax/Bcl-2 ratio and promoting caspase (3 and 8) initiation, MMP disruption, and PARP cleavage (Lin et al., 2016). Fisetin is anticipated to be an anticancerous medication used to treat cervical cancer in humans.

10.2.11 EPIGALLOCATECHIN GALLATE (EGCG)

EGCG is the most bioactive component of green tea, obtained from *Camellia sinensis*, and possesses antiproliferative, antimetastatic, anti-angiogenic, and proapoptotic properties. Antitumoral effects of EGCG include cell cycle arrest in the G1 phase, which ultimately resulted in apoptotic cell death (Singh et al., 2011). Various research has exhibited the crucial role of estrogen in the HPV-positive cervical cancer progression.

Increased expression of aromatase causes enhanced estrogen receptor expression levels, suppression of ER and aromatase, and cancer cell growth suppression (Moody & Laimins, 2010). Furthermore, Qiao et al. (2009) identify various other benefits of EGCG, including reduction of HPV E6/E7 expression, ERα, and aromatase. Sharma et al. (2012) investigated HeLa cells treated with EGCG and found that growth suppression was mediated through apoptosis in a time-dependent way. Similarly, green tea polyphenol E, which is identical to EGCG, has been shown to inhibit cervical cancer cell growth. A study conducted by Zou et al. (2010) examined the effects of these two drugs on the afflicted cells. Differences were discovered between two types of cells, squamous cell carcinoma and adenocarcinoma, respectively. When dealing with adenocarcinoma cells, the inhibition was lower, implying that the type of cells involved in the formation of cervical cancer can influence therapy outcomes.

10.2.12 GENISTEIN

Genistein is a phytoestrogen isoflavone found in soybeans (5.6–276 mg/100 g) and legumes (0.2–0.6 mg/100 g). One of the most frequently explored plant-based estrogens in the Asian diet, which is regarded as the major isoflavone in soy foods (Goh et al., 2022). In a cervical cancer mouse model, oral administration of 20 mg/kg genistein had growth inhibitory and immunomodulatory effects, which further promoted lactate dehydrogenase (LDH) release and lymphocyte differentiation and elevated cytolytic function and IFN-γ secretion, and stimulated protective antitumor immunity (Ghaemi et al., 2012). The AKT signaling pathway is a crucial factor for cell proliferation and apoptosis regulation. By reducing the expression of the AKT/mTOR pathway, p-p70S6K1 and p-4E-BP1, genistein increased the action of cisplatin, resulting in the growth suppression of cervical cancer cells (Sahin et al., 2012). After 48 hours, Kim et al. discovered that genistein reduced the growth of HeLa and CaSki cervical cancer cells with IC_{50} values of 20 and 60 μmol/L, respectively. It suppressed cervical cancer cell proliferation by inhibiting the function of ERK1/2 and triggering p38 MAPK, with AKT and JNK playing a role in genistein-induced cancer cell growth reduction (Kim et al., 2009). By downregulating Bcl-2, VEGF, and TRAF1 (tumor expression necrosis factor-associated receptor factor 1) and increasing apoptosis in HeLa cells, genistein inhibited the estrogen receptor-mediated PI3K/Akt-NF-kB signaling pathway and exerted anticancer effects (Chen et al., 2018). In HeLa cells, genistein caused apoptosis via a p53-dependent mechanism that disrupted the connection between p53 and APE1 and increased p53 intracellular stability (Zhu et al., 2015). Therefore, genistein might possibly be applied to the treatment of cervical cancer.

10.2.13 FORMONONETIN

Formononetin is a 7-hydroxy-40-methoxy natural isoflavone derived from *Pycnanthus angolensis*, chickpea, red clovers, and other plants that exhibited antioxidant, anti-inflammatory, chemopreventive, antibacterial, antiallergic, and cardioprotective properties (Tay et al., 2019). As per the research findings, formononetin inhibits MRP1 and MRP2 via ROS while activating the mitochondrial apoptotic pathway, which resulted in MMP dysfunction, enhanced Bax/Bcl-2 ratio, and caspase 3 and caspase 9 activation. Formononetin, on the other hand, may boost epirubicin cytotoxicity in HeLa cells via caspase 8 apoptotic pathway/the death receptor pathway (Lo & Wang, 2013). Apart from that, formononetin reduced HeLa cell growth with an IC_{50} of 72.112 ± 5.671 μmol/L in a dose-responsive manner. Formononetin is best carried by multiwalled carbon nanotubes, and their conjunction can increase ROS-mediated mitochondrial damage (Guo et al., 2018). Furthermore, in a BALB/c animal model injected with HeLa cells, oral gavage of 10 mg/kg formononetin for 31 days effectively suppressed tumor growth and lowered the production of HIF-1 and VEGF in tumor tissues without serious side effects (Zhang et al., 2019). Furthermore, by blocking the transduction of the PI3K/AKT signal pathway, formononetin (dose of 20 and 40 mg/kg orally for 35 days) stimulated caspase 3 and increased the expression level of Bax, followed by the secretion of Cyt c, and triggered apoptotic cell death in cervical cancer HeLa cells (Jin et al., 2014). It could be a therapeutic option for cervical cancer treatment and management.

10.2.14 ANTHOCYANINS

Anthocyanins are widely distributed in plants which are the most ubiquitous flavonoids. Anthocyanins are the main components of cell vacuoles and are responsible for the changing colors of flowers and fruit with the seasons. Thus, strawberries, grapes, apples, purple cauliflower, and corn, for example, can be blue, red, or purple in color. In nature, about 600 structurally different anthocyanins have been discovered (Liu et al., 2021). The major active component of anthocyanins is cyanidin 3-O-glucoside, which has preventative and therapeutic benefits against various disorders such as cerebral ischemia and Alzheimer's disease (Mattioli et al., 2020). The inhibitory efficacy of individual cisplatin or cyanidin 3-O-glucoside, and their co-administration on HeLa tumor growth were 17.43%, 34.98%, and 63.38%, respectively, as reported by research findings. In HeLa cells, cyanidin 3-O-glucoside exposure elevated Bax, p53 expression, and tissue inhibitor of metalloproteinase-1 (TIMP-1), suppressed cyclin D1 and Bcl-2 expression, and halted the cell cycle at the G1 phase, promoting apoptotic cell death (Li et al., 2021a). Cyanidin 3-O-glucoside significantly increased the susceptibility of HeLa cancer cells against cisplatin. Cisplatin, when combined with cyanidin 3-O-glucoside effectively suppresses the activation of catalase (CAT), SOD, and glutathione peroxidase (GSH-PX) by downregulating the expression of heme oxygenase-1 (HO-1) and NAD(P)H quinone dehydrogenase 1 (NQO1), along with altering the Nrf2 signaling cascade to stimulate oxidative stress-mediated apoptosis in HeLa cancer cells (Li et al., 2021b). It's possible that cyanidin 3-O-glucoside can boost cisplatin's anticancer efficacy and lessen the side effects of treatment in cervical cancer.

10.3 TERPENOIDS

Terpenoids are the most diverse group of natural products, with over 40,000 structures and are frequently used in the cosmetics, perfumes, and pharmaceutical industries (Bergman et al., 2019). Terpenoids comprised of five carbon isoprene subunits that are grouped into subclasses based on their structures, such as hemiterpenoids, monoterpenoids, diterpenoids, sesquiterpenoids, sesterterpenoids, triterpenoids, tetraterpenoids, and polyterpenoids. Each subgroup of terpenoids has its own range of biological features. Terpenoids have antitumor properties because they inhibit cell growth, induce cell death, prevent metastasis and angiogenesis (Tholl, 2015). Many terpenoids influence epigenetic and apoptotic mechanisms by targeting NF-kB, Janus kinases-signal transducer and activated transcription proteins (JAK-STAT), activator protein-1 (AP-1), metalloproteinases (MMPs), DNA topoisomerase I and II, obstructing the endoplasmic reticulum (ER) calcium ATPase pump, and inhibiting DNA topoisomerase I and II, p53 activation and DNA minor groove modulation (Wang et al., 2005) (Table 10.2).

10.3.1 CARVACROL

Numerous aromatic plants, particularly thyme, oregano, and others, produce carvacrol, a monoterpene phenol. It possesses different types of therapeutic and pharmacological properties like antibacterial, anti-inflammatory, antitumor, hepatoprotective, and antispasmodic activities (Suntres et al., 2015; Silva et al., 2018). Carvacrol was also demonstrated to have antiproliferative and apoptotic-inducing effects on the cervical cell lines HeLa and SiHa (Mehdi et al., 2011). Potonjak et al. (2018) observed that carvacrol induces cell cycle arrest and apoptosis in HeLa cancer cells that concomitantly increases caspase-9 activation, PARP cleavage, and ERK activation. A study showed that carvacrol treatment in SiHa cells resulted in suppression of cellular proliferation and cell death induction via p53 and caspase activation along with elevated Bax/Bcl2 ratio (Al-Fatlawi, 2018). Furthermore, carvacrol was found to be cytotoxic against cervical cancer HeLa cells with apoptotic and antiproliferative effects in another investigation (Ahmad & Ansari, 2021).

10.3.2 TANSHINONE IIA

Tanshinone IIA is a diterpenoid naphthoquinone dispersed in *Salvia miltiorrhiza*, a traditional Chinese medicine herb. It contains anti-inflammatory and antioxidant properties, and it is frequently used to prevent and cure cardiovascular disease (Yen et al., 2018). Munagala et al. (2015) reported that tanshinone IIA increased the expression of $p21^{cip1/waf1}$, p53, p130, and pRb and triggered p53-mediated anticancer action by reducing the level of HPV E6 and E7 oncoproteins, resulting in cervical cancer cell growth inhibition. Intraperitoneal injection of 30 mg/kg tanshinone IIA for 8 weeks significantly decreased the expression of the proliferation marker PCNA in tumor tissues and the amount of cervical cancer transplanted tumors in nude mice. Tanshinone IIA also inhibited intracellular

TABLE 10.2 Antitumor Effects of Terpenoids on Cervical Cancer and Their Associated Molecular Targets

Natural Product	Class	Structure	Cervical Cell Line/Model	Molecular Targets
Carvacrol	Monoterpenoids	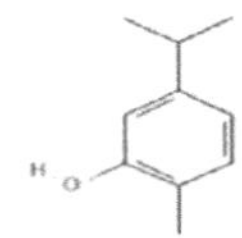	HeLa, SiHa	Upregulated: Bax, LC3β-I/II, stimulation of caspase-3, -8, -9; PARP cleavage. Downregulated: ERK, Bcl-2, E6, E7, G0/G1 phase cell arrest
Tanshinone IIA	Diterpenoids	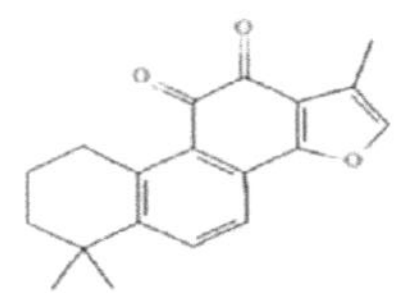	HeLa, SiHa, CaSki, and C33A	Upregulated: p53, Bax, PERK, p130, p21, IRE1, p38, pRb, JNK, stimulation of caspase 3 and 9; PARP cleavage; Cyt c and Ca^{2+} release Downregulated: Bcl-2, E6, E7
			Cervical cancer cell line U14 mice models	Suppressed tumor growth and metastasis
Oridonin	Diterpenoids	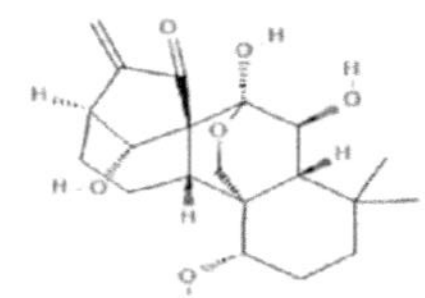	HeLa	Upregulated: Bax, stimulation of caspase 3 and 9; Cyt c release Decreased: Bcl-2, MMP
Betulinic acid	Triterpenoids	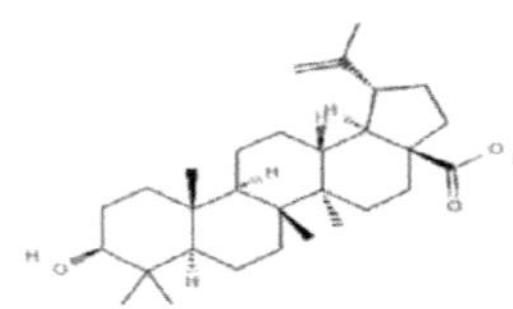	HeLa	Upregulated: ROS, Bad, p27 and p21; stimulation of caspase 9. Downregulated: G0/G1 phase cell arrest. Inhibited: PI3K/AKT

TABLE 10.2 *(Continued)*

Natural Product	Class	Structure	Cervical Cell Line/Model	Molecular Targets
Ginsenoside Rh2	Triterpenoids	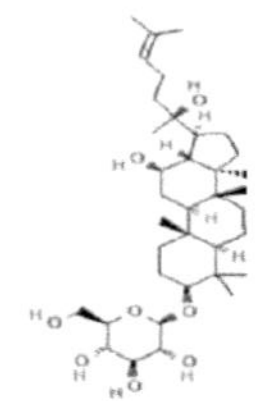	HeLa	Upregulated: ROS, Bax, VDAC1, Cyt c release. Downregulated: MMP

AKT/mTOR and HIF-1 activity, which lowered glycolysis. Moreover, a 40 mg/kg intraperitoneal injection of tanshinone IIA given for 20 days, successfully reduced tumor development and metastasis in U14 cervical cancer mice (Liu et al., 2019). Another research revealed that Tanshinone IIA suppressed the proliferation of HeLa, CaSki, SiHa, and C33A cells in a dose-responsive manner, with IC_{50} values of 6.97, 5.51, 14.47, and 9.89 µmol/L, respectively, and had a stronger growth inhibitory impact than paclitaxel (18.45 µmol/L). Tanshinone IIA exposure also cleaved PARP, elevated the ratio of Bax/Bcl-2 and JNK, secreted Cyt c that interacts with Apaf-1, and phosphorylated p38 to promote ER stress-related apoptosis via IRE1 and PERK-linked pathways. Particularly, Tanshinone IIA has been shown to increase paclitaxel chemosensitivity, indicating that it could be used to combat paclitaxel resistance in cervical cancer cells (Pan et al., 2013). Importantly, tanshinone IIA prevented the invasion and metastasis of cervical cancer stem cells (CSCs) via reducing the stability and transcriptional activity of the YAP gene by preventing the cytoplasmic movement of HuR from the nucleus. It was also discovered that tanshinone IIA not only destroyed the cervical CSCs functionality but also re-established their adriamycin sensitivity (Qin et al., 2018). It has the potential to be a helpful treatment for people with cervical cancer who are resistant to chemotherapy.

10.3.3 BETULINIC ACID

Betulinic acid, a naturally occurring pentacyclic triterpenoid found in white birch bark, is one of the really substantial cancer therapeutic substance, with antitumor, anti-inflammatory, anti-metabolic, and anti-cardiovascular properties (Ríos & Máñez, 2018; Jiang et al., 2021). Through regulation of the PI3K/AKT and mitochondrial pathways, betulinic acid promoted apoptosis in HeLa cells. It suppressed the growth of cervical cancer HeLa cells via the phosphorylation of AKT at specific amino acid residues (Thr308 and Ser473), Bad activation, caspase 9 activation, p27, p21 modulation as well as induction of cell-cycle arrest at the G0/G1 phase (Xu et al., 2017). By directly activating proteasome 1, 2, betulinic acid induced HIF-1 accumulation and suppressed expression of HIF linked genes (VEGF, GLUT1, PDK1) in HeLa cancer cells. Furthermore, betulinic acid suppressed cell proliferation and migration by decreasing Bcl-2 and cyclin D1 expression and increasing Bax gene expression (Rzeski et al., 2006; Kim et al., 2020). At a maximal dose of 500 mg/kg, betulinic acid has been proven to be nontoxic *in vivo* (Sarek et al., 2003). Betulinic acid is predicted to be a possible drug candidate for adjuvant therapy in human cancer therapy in the near future.

10.3.4 GINSENOSIDE Rh2

Ginsenoside Rh2 is a biologically active molecule produced from ginseng that has a variety of health benefits, including immune system stimulation, cardiovascular health enhancement, and anti-stress capabilities (Leung & Wong, 2010). Ginsenoside Rh2 reduced glycolysis and mitochondrial oxidative phosphorylation in HeLa cervix cancer cells while activating the mitochondria-dependent apoptotic pathway. Ginsenoside Rh2 also hindered energy metabolism and promoted cell death in HeLa cells by elevating the level of voltage-dependent anion channel 1 (VDAC1), resulting in MMP depolarization and ROS generation (Liu et al., 2020). VDAC1 is thought to be a novel target of this bioactive compound. Ginsenoside Rh2 suppressed HeLa cell proliferation by targeting the Akt pathway in a dose- and time-dependent manner, as well as preventing HeLa cell migration and invasion by reducing Akt/GSK3β, Snail expression, and EMT (Shi et al., 2018). Thus, ginsenoside Rh2 could be used as a possible drug candidate for adjuvant therapy in human cervical cancer therapy.

10.3.5 ORIDONIN

Oridonin is an active diterpenoid constituent obtained from *Rabdosia rubescens* and having antimicrobial, anti-inflammatory, and anticancer properties (Owona & Schluesener, 2015) Oridonin, an AKT inhibitor, inhibited cancer cell proliferation by inhibiting AKT signaling (Song et al., 2018). Oridonin decreased cell viability in HeLa cells in a dose- and time-dependent manner, with an IC_{50} value of 4.13 μmol/L for 48 h as reported by Hu et al. (2007). Numerous reports have revealed that oridonin caused apoptosis through many molecular mechanisms. In HeLa cell lines, it strongly suppressed the action of constitutively activated PI3K targets including FOXO (forkhead box O protein), GSK3β, and Akt. Exposure of HeLa cells with oridonin stimulated the apoptotic pathway by suppressing Akt kinase signaling, causing MMP loss to promote mitochondrial Cyt c release, resulting in downstream stimulation of caspase 9, caspase 3, and downregulation of survival proteins (XIAP, cIAP1, and survivin), that finally lead to cervical cancer cell death (Zhang et al., 2004). Oridonin mediated ROS generation in HeLa cells causes elevated level of Bax and caspase 8, decreased pro-caspase and Bcl-2 expression, which resulted in apoptosis and autophagy induction in HeLa cells. Oridonin also promoted apoptosis in HeLa cells by suppressing the expression of p-AKT and cellular telomerase FKHRL and GSK3β (Zhang et al., 2011).

10.4 ALKALOIDS

Alkaloids have received much interest since the beginning of herbal therapy because of their undeniable physiological characteristics. From an evolutionary standpoint, different plants used these secondary metabolites to protect themselves from herbivorous predators (Schläger & Dräger, 2016). Alkaloids are a broad collection of molecules that possess cyclic structures and minimum of one basic nitrogen (N) atom. These chemicals are primarily found in plants belonging to the Papaveraceae, Ranunculaceae, Menispermaceae, Leguminosae, and Loganiaceae families. Several alkaloids are well-known as strong chemotherapeutic drugs, including camptothecin, vincristine, vinblastine, berberine, evodiamine, piperine, and matrine (Hashmi et al., 2018) (Table 10.3).

10.4.1 BERBERINE

Berberine is an isoquinoline alkaloid compound derived from the herb, possesses antimicrobial, anti-inflammatory, anti-angiogenic, and antitumor properties. In clinical practice, it is commonly utilized as an antibacterial agent (Song et al., 2020). Berberine decreased HeLa and SiHa cell proliferation in a dose-dependent manner. It activated caspase-3 and lowered cell proliferation and hTERT activity via a mitochondria-mediated mechanism and led to apoptotic cell death. Berberine can also suppress the activity of the transcription factor Activator Protein-1 (AP-1) and the expression of HPV E6/E7 oncoproteins while increasing the expression of p53 and Rb, resulting in an anticancer action against cervical cancer cells (Mahata et al., 2011). Berberine prevented the migration of SiHa cells through lowering MMP2 and u-PA transcriptional activity, which enabled the downregulation of TGF-1 expression and the angiogenic activity of

TABLE 10.3 Antitumor Effects of Alkaloids on Cervical Cancer and Their Associated Molecular Targets

Natural Product	Class	Structure	Cervical Cell Line/ Model	Molecular Targets
Berberine	Alkaloids	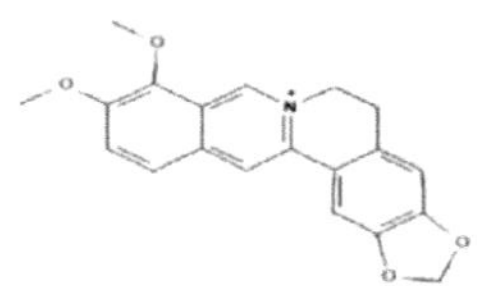	HeLa and SiHa	Upregulated: Bax, Fas, FasL, TNF-α, TRAF-1, p53, pRb, MAPK; DNA fragmentation; stimulation of caspase 3 Downregulated: Bcl-2, E6, E7, c-Fos, c-Jun, AP-1, S phase cell arrest.
Piperine	Alkaloids	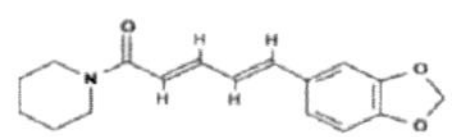	HeLa	Upregulated: ROS; activation of caspase 3 Downregulated: MMP, G2/M phase cell arrest.
Matrine	Alkaloids	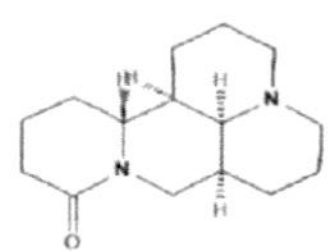	Xenografts (HeLa cells) BALB/c nude mice.	Suppressed tumor growth via p38, MMP2 and 9 downregulation.

SiHa cells. Berberine stimulated the death receptor pathway of apoptosis through elevating level of Fas, FasL, TNF-α, and TRAF-1 in HeLa cells. Consequently, berberine promoted apoptosis in cervical cancer HeLa cells by initiating the mitochondrial route, releasing Cyt c, and considerably enhancing the Bax/Bcl-2 ratio, which halted the cell cycle at the S phase. Berberine also activated the MAPK pathway and boosted p53 expression, implying that p53 could be a therapeutic target for cervical cancer treatment (Lu et al., 2010). Furthermore, N-Mannich bases berberine analogs displayed considerable cytotoxicity in cervical carcinoma HeLa and CaSki cells (Mistry et al., 2017). It suggested that berberine and its analogs might have anticancer properties in cervical cancer cells.

10.4.2 PIPERINE

Piperine is a nitrogen-rich stimulant present in black and long pepper fruits. It exhibits anticancer, antimicrobial, hepatoprotective, antiulcer, and immunomodulatory efficacies in *in vitro* and *in vivo* systems (Haq et al., 2021). Piperine slowed wound healing and blocked the G2/M phase of the cell cycle, inhibiting HeLa cell growth by enhancing ROS generation and nuclear cohesion. Piperine also caused HeLa cell apoptosis by MMP dysruption and activating caspase-3 (Jafri et al., 2019). Piperine has recently been proven to have the ability to reverse drug resistance in human cervical cancer cells. Piperine decreased Mcl-1 expression, phosphorylated AKT, and facilitated paclitaxel-mediated apoptosis in drug-resistant cervical cancer cells (Xie et al., 2019). Piperine also blocked STAT3/NF-kB, inhibiting Bcl-2 signaling and increasing Bid, caspase, and PARP activities, thus improving the chemotherapeutic and antitumor effects of mitomycin C on chemoresistance cervical cancer HeLa and MMC cells (Han et al., 2017). As a result, the combination of these two medications can effectively suppress tumor growth *in vivo* and may be employed to treat human cervical cancer as an anticancer agent.

10.4.3 MATRINE

Matrine is an active ingredient of the Chinese medication *Sophora flavescens*. It has been classified as an anticancer medicine in China due to its wide spectrum of pharmacological effects. For a long time, it has been utilized in therapeutic strategies to treat neuropathic pain, viral hepatitis, heart illness, skin infections, and other ailments (Cai et al., 2020). *S. flavescens* suppresses cervical cancer cell growth and stimulates cell death by inhibiting the AKT/mTOR signaling pathway, lowering the expression of cyclin A, Bcl-2, and MMP2, halting the G2/M phase cell cycle, and increasing Bax and E-calmodulin. Matrine inhibits HeLa cell adhesion and migration by reducing vasodilator-stimulated phosphoprotein (VASP) phosphorylation via repressing protein kinase A (PKA) function (You et al., 2019). Furthermore, intraperitoneal injection of matrine at 50 mg/kg/d for 21 days efficiently suppressed the growth of cervical cancer xenografts in mice inoculated with HeLa cells, with a 58.33% inhibition rate. It also suppresses the cell growth, metastasis, and invasion of cervical cancer cells by modulating the p38 signal pathway, which inhibits the expression activities of extracellular matrix components MMP2 and MMP9 (Zhang et al., 2007; Wu et al., 2017). Matrine could be used as a therapeutic or adjuvant treatment for human cervical cancer.

10.5 PHENOLS

Secondary metabolites in plants having a unique aromatic ring consisting of one or more hydroxyl groups are defined as phenolic compounds. So far, around 8,000 natural phenolic substances have been documented (Jacobo-Velázquez & Cisneros-Zevallos, 2017). Simple phenols, flavonoids, tannins, xanthones, lignins, lignans, and coumarins are examples of phenolic chemicals obtained from plants. These phenolics have been shown to have strong antitumor properties as well as counteract several oxidative stress-linked disorders. Previous research has shown that health-promoting properties of dietary phenols are related to their antioxidant, anti-clastogenic, and anti-inflammatory properties (Floris et al., 2021) (Table 10.4).

10.5.1 CURCUMIN

Curcumin is a phenolic molecule isolated from the rhizome of the herbal plant turmeric of the Zingiberaceae family. It has been used for a very long time as a spice and culinary coloring agent. Previous investigations have demonstrated its safety and effectiveness as a conventional herbal

TABLE 10.4 Antitumor Effects of Phenols on Cervical Cancer and Their Associated Molecular Targets

Natural Product	Class	Structure	Cervical Cell Line/Model	Molecular Targets
Curcumin	Phenols	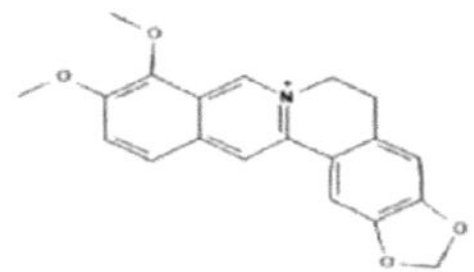	HeLa SiHa and CaSki	Upregulated: AIF; stimulation of caspase 3 and 9; Cyt c release.
				Downregulated: COX-2, iNOS, cyclin D1; Inhibited: Ras/Raf.
			Xenografts (CaSki cells) BALB/c mice	Suppressed tumor growth via VEGF and EGFR downregulation.
Ellagic acid	Phenols	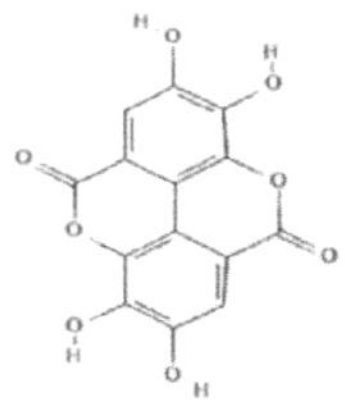	SiHa	Upregulated: Bcl-2, p53, stimulation of caspase 3 and 9.
				Downregulated: Bax; G2 phase cell arrest.
Resveratrol	Phenols	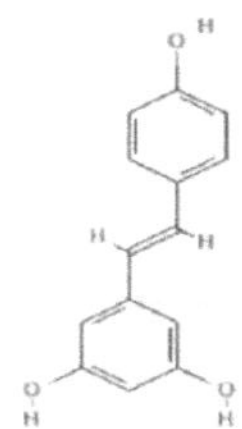	HeLa and CaSki	Upregulated: Bax, p53, p16.
				Downregulated: VEGF, HIF-1α.
				Inhibited: PI3K/AKT, ERK1/2.
			Xenografts (HeLa cells) BALB/c nude mice.	Suppressed tumor growth.

treatment. It also has antitumor properties through a variety of pathways, including cell growth suppression, invasion, metastasis inhibition, and epigenetic modifications (Kotha & Luthria, 2019). Curcumin decreased telomerase activity in HeLa, CaSki, and SiHa cells in a dose-responsive manner, promoted Cyt c release, triggered AIF, and repressed cyclin D1 and Ras proteins, further downregulating downstream targets Ras/Raf and consequently, inducing apoptosis through the mitochondrial pathway. Curcumin also exhibited growth inhibitory and anti-inflammatory properties in cervical cancer cells through downregulating iNOS and COX-2 production as well as activating caspase 3 and 9 (Singh & Singh, 2009). In a mouse model inoculated with cervical cancer CaSki cells, oral dosing of curcumin (500–1,500 mg/kg/d) for 30 days significantly decreased tumor growth (21.03%) and the levels of VEGF and EGFR, thereby inhibiting angiogenesis (Yoysungnoen-Chintana et al., 2014). Curcumin also suppressed HeLa, C33A, CaSki, and ME180 cell growth in a dose and time-dependent manner, and elevated ER-resident unfolded protein response (UPR) sensors (IRE-1a, PERK, ATF6) and their targets (CHOP) in cervical cancer cells. CHOP stimulation augmented Bax/Bcl-2 ratio and ROS generation, resulting in apoptotic cell death in cervical cancer cells (Kim et al., 2016). Curcumin, on the other hand, triggered cell-cycle arrest at the G2/M phase and induced cell autophagy and death via downregulating cyclin B1 and Cdc25. It also induced cellular senescence by upregulating the p53/p21 pathway. Curcumin exposure also decreased P-gp expression and improved the susceptibility of vinblastine drug-resistant KB-V1 cells (Wang et al., 2020). Furthermore, Sajomsang et al. introduced a delivery mechanism for oral curcumin to improve its bioavailability. It has been shown that curcumin-loaded micelles have improved antiproliferative efficacy as compared to free curcumin in HeLa, C33a, and SiHa cancer cell lines. The amount of curcumin-carrying micelles is raised by a factor of six when compared to free curcumin. Curcumin micelles enhance the percentage of HeLa, C33A and SiHa cells that underwent early apoptosis to 30–55% (Sajomsang et al., 2014).

10.5.2 ELLAGIC ACID

Ellagic acid is a naturally occurring phenol molecule abundant in pomegranates, raspberries, and walnuts that possesses potent antitumor, anti-angiogenic, and anti-metastatic properties (Ceci et al., 2018). Ellagic acid suppressed SiHa cell growth in a concentration-dependent manner and also induced apoptosis by modulating the expression of p53, Bax, Bcl-2, and caspase 3/9, and arresting the cell cycle at the G2-phase (Chen et al., 2020). Li et al. (2018) demonstrated that ellagic acid inhibited the activation of the Janus kinase 2 (JAK2)/STAT3 signaling and down-regulated the expression of Cyclin D1, Bcl-xl, and Mcl-1, resulting in G1-phase cell-cycle arrest and apoptotic cell death. Furthermore, ellagic acid suppresses HeLa cell growth and metastasis via inhibiting the AKT/mTOR signaling pathway by elevating insulin-like growth factor-binding protein 7 (IGFBP7) (Guo et al., 2016). A recent study found that treating HeLa cells with ellagic acid, curcumin, or both for 72 hours resulted in an improved anticancer efficacy, indicating that ellagic acid and curcumin have a combinatorial antitumor impact. This combination recovered p53 expression, stimulated ROS production, p21, Bax level and boosted DNA damage in HeLa cells, thereby resulting in apoptotic induction (Kumar et al., 2016). Thus, ellagic acid has the ability to be an excellent drug candidate for cervical cancer treatment.

10.5.3 RESVERATROL

Resveratrol is a polyphenol that can be found in berries, grapes, peanuts, and other plants. It has numerous biological properties that could include cancer treatment and prevention (Risuleo & Mesa, 2019). Resveratrol suppressed HeLa and CaSki cell growth in a dose- and time-dependent manner, by suppressing the expression level of HPV E6 and E7 oncoproteins and increasing p53, Bax, and p16 expression which further accompanied by G1/S phase cell cycle arrest. A study reported that resveratrol repressed cervical cancer cell growth by increased expression of SOCS3 (suppressors of cytokine signaling 3) as well as stimulated STAT3 (PIAS3), limiting STAT3's DNA-binding activity and resulting in STAT3 inactivation (Zhang et al., 2015; Sun et al., 2021). Additionally, resveratrol inhibited the phosphorylation of STAT3 (Tyr705), which inhibited EMT and ECM breakdown (Sun et al., 2020). A study reported that resveratrol triggered apoptosis cell death in HeLa cancer cells by decreasing the expression of hTERT at both mRNA and protein levels, thereby suppressing telomerase activity. Interestingly, by inhibiting the ERK1/2 and PI3K/Akt signaling pathways, resveratrol repressed the production of HIF-1 and VEGF in cervical cancer cells, thereby successfully reversing the angiogenic property produced through HPV E6/E7 oncoproteins (Tang et al., 2007). Another analysis revealed that injecting 10 mg/kg resveratrol intraperitoneally for 28 days substantially slowed the formation of xenograft tumors in nude mice. Resveratrol inhibited cell growth and proliferation of HeLa cells by lowering the expression levels of phospholipid scramblase 1 (PLSCR1). Resveratrol also suppressed HeLa invasion and metastasis by inhibiting MMP9 expression level mediated by NF-kB and AP-1 (Zhao et al., 2019). Resveratrol may have therapeutic promise in the treatment and management of cervical cancer.

10.6 CONCLUSIONS AND PERSPECTIVES

Cervical cancer is the fourth most prevalent disease among women, the most frequently diagnosed cancer in 28 countries, and the primary cause of cancer mortality in 42 nations. Cervical cancer is treated with surgery, radiotherapy, and chemotherapy, but these treatments have side effects and risks, thus a new treatment for cervical cancer using natural bioactive substances is gaining attraction. As a result, it's critical to look into the most recent research on natural products that are beneficial in cervical cancer, as well anticancer mechanism of processes like apoptosis. Despite the fact that natural compounds were successful at inhibiting cervical cancer cells, there are still differences in stability and toxicity. The recent studies of some natural products with diverse effects on cervical cancer were evaluated in the previous section, as well as various mechanisms, concentrations, and experimental models. The latest research of natural compounds with diverse effects on cervical cancer was investigated in the above, as well as various mechanisms, concentrations, and experimental models (Figure 10.1). Natural products may have potential as an alternative therapy for cervical cancer because they have fewer adverse effects. Additional study is needed to identify the most beneficial and least toxic doses for humans before natural products can be used in clinical practice. There is also a need for research into the combinatorial effects of natural products and conventional therapies like surgery, radiation, and chemotherapy for cervical cancer therapeutics. We look forward to more research into identifying compounds with excellent anticancer properties, and we believe that this research will serve as the foundation for developing new cervical cancer treatments.

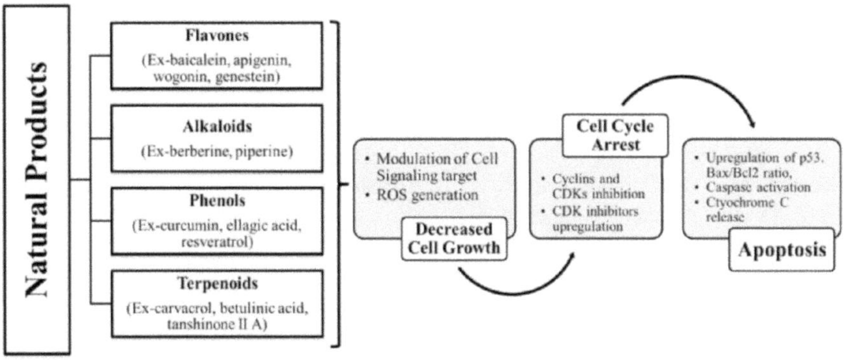

FIGURE 10.1 Mode of action of various classes of anticancerous natural compounds via targeting cell cycle proteins, apoptotic related proteins, and caspase activation in cervical cancer.

KEYWORDS

- **anticancer mechanism**
- **cervical cancer treatments**
- **cervix**
- **chemotherapy**
- **cycle proteins**
- **radiation**
- **radiotherapy**

REFERENCES

Ahmad, A., & Ansari, I. A., (2021). Carvacrol exhibits chemopreventive potential against cervical cancer cells via caspase-dependent apoptosis and abrogation of cell cycle progression. *Anticancer Agents in Medicinal Chemistry, 21*(16), 2224–2235.

Ahmed, S. A., Parama, D., Daimari, E., et al., (2021). Rationalizing the therapeutic potential of apigenin against cancer. *Life Sciences, 267*, 118814.

Alam, W., Khan, H., Shah, M. A., Cauli, O., & Saso, L., (2020). Kaempferol as a dietary anti-inflammatory agent: Current therapeutic standing. *Molecules, 25*(18), 4073.

Alfaro, K., Maza, M., Cremer, M., Masch, R., & Soler, M., (2021). Removing global barriers to cervical cancer prevention and moving towards elimination. *Nature Reviews Cancer, 21*(10), 607–608.

Al-Fatlawi, A. A. Y., (2018). Anti-proliferative and pro-apoptotic activity of carvacrol on human cancer cells. *Int. J. Pharm. Res., 10*, 174–180.

Alshatwi, A. A., Ramesh, E., Periasamy, V. S., & Subash-Babu, P., (2013). The apoptotic effect of hesperetin on human cervical cancer cells is mediated through cell cycle arrest, death receptor, and mitochondrial pathways. *Fundamental and Clinical Pharmacology, 27*(6), 581–592.

Aung, T. N., Qu, Z., Kortschak, R. D., & Adelson, D. L., (2017). Understanding the effectiveness of natural compound mixtures in cancer through their molecular mode of action. *Int. J. Mol. Sci., 18*(3), 656.

Banik, K., Khatoon, E., Harsha, C., et al., (2022). Wogonin and its analogs for the prevention and treatment of cancer: A systematic review. *Phytotherapy Research, 36*(5), 1854–1883.

Bergman, M. E., Davis, B., & Phillips, M. A., (2019). Medically useful plant terpenoids: Biosynthesis, occurrence, and mechanism of action. *Molecules, 24*(21), 3961.

Bishayee, K., Ghosh, S., Mukherjee, A., Sadhukhan, R., Mondal, J., & Khuda-Bukhsh, A. R., (2013). Quercetin induces cytochrome-c release and ROS accumulation to promote apoptosis and arrest the cell cycle in G2/M, in cervical carcinoma: Signal cascade and drug-DNA interaction. *Cell Proliferation, 46*(2), 153–163.

Boojar, M. M. A., Boojar, M. M. A., & Golmohammad, S., (2020). Overview of silibinin antitumor effects. *Journal of Herbal Medicine, 23*, 100375.

Bray, F., Ferlay, J., Soerjomataram, I., Siegel, R. L., Torre, L. A., & Jemal, A., (2018). Global cancer statistics 2018: GLOBOCAN estimates of incidence and mortality worldwide for 36 cancers in 185 countries. *CA: A Cancer Journal for Clinicians, 68*(6), 394–424.

Cai, X. H., Zhang, H. Y., & Xie, B., (2020). Matrine-family alkaloids: Versatile precursors for bioactive modifications. *Medicinal Chemistry, 16*(4), 431–453.

Calderón-Montaño, J. M., Burgos-Morón, E., Pérez-Guerrero, C., & López-Lázaro, M., (2011). A review on the dietary flavonoid kaempferol. *Mini Reviews in Medicinal Chemistry, 11*(4), 298–344.

Ceci, C., Lacal, P. M., Tentori, L., De Martino, M. G., Miano, R., & Graziani, G., (2018). Experimental evidence of the antitumor, antimetastatic and antiangiogenic activity of ellagic acid. *Nutrients, 10*(11), 1756.

Chen, H. H., Chen, S. P., Zheng, Q. L., Nie, S. P., Li, W. J., Hu, X. J., & Xie, M. Y., (2018). Genistein promotes proliferation of human cervical cancer cells through estrogen receptor-mediated PI3K/Akt-NF-κB pathway. *Journal of Cancer, 9*(2), 288–295.

Chen, W., Shen, X., Ma, L., Chen, R., Yuan, Q., Zheng, Y., Li, C., & Peng, G., (2020). Phenolic compounds from *Polygonum chinense* induce growth inhibition and apoptosis of cervical cancer SiHa cells. *BioMed Research International*, 8868508.

Chizenga, E. P., & Abrahamse, H., (2021). Biological therapy with complementary and alternative medicine in innocuous integrative oncology: A case of cervical cancer. *Pharmaceutics, 13*(5), 626.

Chopra, B., & Dhingra, A. K., (2021). Natural products: A lead for drug discovery and development. *Phytotherapy Research, 35*(9), 4660–4702.

Chou, R. H., Hsieh, S. C., Yu, Y. L., Huang, M. H., Huang, Y. C., & Hsieh, Y. H., (2013). Fisetin inhibits migration and invasion of human cervical cancer cells by down-regulating urokinase plasminogen activator expression through suppressing the p38 MAPK-dependent NF-κB signaling pathway. *PLoS One, 8*(8), e71983.

Clemente-Soto, A. F., Salas-Vidal, E., Milan-Pacheco, C., Sánchez-Carranza, J. N., Peralta-Zaragoza, O., & González-Maya, L., (2019). Quercetin induces G2 phase arrest and apoptosis with the activation of p53 in an E6 expression-independent manner in HPV-positive human cervical cancer-derived cells. *Molecular Medicine Reports, 19*(3), 2097–2106.

Darband, S. G., Kaviani, M., Yousefi, B., et al., (2018). Quercetin: A functional dietary flavonoid with potential chemo-preventive properties in colorectal cancer. *Journal of Cellular Physiology, 233*(9), 6544–6560.

De Oliveira, J. M. P. F., Santos, C., & Fernandes, E., (2020). Therapeutic potential of hesperidin and its aglycone hesperetin: Cell cycle regulation and apoptosis induction in cancer models. *Phytomedicine, 73*, 152887.

Dias, M. C., Pinto, D. C., & Silva, A., (2021). Plant flavonoids: Chemical characteristics and biological activity. *Molecules, 26*(17), 5377.

Fan, S., Li, L., & Chen, S., (2011). Silibinin induced-autophagic and apoptotic death is associated with an increase in reactive oxygen and nitrogen species in HeLa cells. *Free Radical Research, 45*(11, 12), 1307–1324.

Fan, S., Qi, M., Yu, Y., et al., (2012a). P53 activation plays a crucial role in silibinin induced ROS generation via PUMA and JNK. *Free Radical Research, 46*(3), 310–319.

Fan, S., Yu, Y., Qi, M., et al., (2012b). P53-mediated GSH depletion enhanced the cytotoxicity of NO in silibinin-treated human cervical carcinoma HeLa cells. *Free Radical Research, 46*(9), 1082–1092.

Floris, B., Galloni, P., Conte, V., & Sabuzi, F., (2021). Tailored functionalization of natural phenols to improve biological activity. *Biomolecules, 11*(9), 1325.

Garcia-Maceira, P., & Mateo, J., (2009). Silibinin inhibits hypoxia-inducible factor-1α and mTOR/p70S6K/4E-BP1 signaling pathway in human cervical and hepatoma cancer cells: Implications for anticancer therapy. *Oncogene, 28*(3), 313–324.

Ghaemi, A., Soleimanjahi, H., Razeghi, S., Gorji, A., Tabaraei, A., Moradi, A., Alizadeh, A., & Vakili, M. A., (2012). Genistein induces a protective immunomodulatory effect in a mouse model of cervical cancer. *Iranian Journal of Immunology, 9*(2), 119–127.

Ghanbari-Movahed, M., Jackson, G., Farzaei, M. H., & Bishayee, A., (2021). A systematic review of the preventive and therapeutic effects of naringin against human malignancies. *Frontiers in Pharmacology, 12*, 250.

Goh, Y. X., Jalil, J., Lam, K. W., Husain, K., & Premakumar, C. M., (2022). Genistein: A review on its anti-inflammatory properties. *Frontiers in Pharmacology, 13*, 820969.

Guerra, A. R., Duarte, M. F., & Duarte, I. F., (2018). Targeting tumor metabolism with plant-derived natural products: Emerging trends in cancer therapy. *Journal of Agricultural and Food Chemistry, 66*(41), 10663–10685.

Guo, B., Liao, C., Liu, X., & Yi, J., (2018). Preliminary study on conjugation of formononetin with multiwalled carbon nanotubes for inducing apoptosis via ROS production in HeLa cells. *Drug Design, Development and Therapy, 12*, 2815–2826.

Guo, H., Zhang, D., & Fu, Q., (2016). Inhibition of cervical cancer by promoting IGFBP7 expression using ellagic acid from pomegranate peel. *Medical Science Monitor, 22*, 4881–4886.

Han, S. Z., Liu, H. X., Yang, L. Q., Cui, L. D., & Xu, Y., (2017). Piperine (PP) enhanced mitomycin-C (MMC) therapy of human cervical cancer through suppressing Bcl-2 signaling pathway via inactivating STAT3/NF-κB. *Biomedicine and Pharmacotherapy, 96*, 1403–1410.

Haq, I. U., Imran, M., Nadeem, M., Tufail, T., Gondal, T. A., & Mubarak, M. S., (2021). Piperine: A review of its biological effects. *Phytotherapy Research, 35*(2), 680–700.

Hashmi, M. A., Khan, A., Farooq, U., & Khan, S., (2018). Alkaloids as cyclooxygenase inhibitors in anticancer drug discovery. *Current Protein and Peptide Science, 19*(3), 292–301.

He, F., Wang, Q., Zheng, X. L., et al., (2012). Wogonin potentiates cisplatin-induced cancer cell apoptosis through the accumulation of intracellular reactive oxygen species. *Oncology Reports, 28*(2), 601–605.

Horinaka, M., Yoshida, T., Shiraishi, T., et al., (2005). The combination of TRAIL and luteolin enhances apoptosis in human cervical cancer HeLa cells. *Biochemical and Riophysical Research Communications, 333*(3), 833–838.

Hu, H. Z., Yang, Y. B., Xu, X. D., et al., (2007). Oridonin induces apoptosis via PI3K/Akt pathway in cervical carcinoma HeLa cell line 1. *Acta Pharmacologica Sinica, 28*(11), 1819–1826.

Hu, J., Wang, R., Liu, Y., Zhou, J., Shen, K., & Dai, Y., (2021). Baicalein represses cervical cancer cell growth, cell cycle progression and promotes apoptosis via blocking AKT/mTOR pathway by the regulation of circHIAT1/miR-19a-3p axis. *OncoTargets and Therapy, 14*, 905–916.

Imran, M., Salehi, B., Sharifi-Rad, J., et al., (2019). Kaempferol: A key emphasis to its anticancer potential. *Molecules, 24*(12), 2277.

Jacobo-Velázquez, D. A., & Cisneros-Zevallos, L., (2017). Recent advances in plant phenolics. *Molecules, 22*(8), 1249.

Jafri, A., Siddiqui, S., Rais, J., Ahmad, M. S., Kumar, S., Jafar, T., Afzal, M., & Arshad, M., (2019). Induction of apoptosis by piperine in human cervical adenocarcinoma via ROS mediated mitochondrial pathway and caspase-3 activation. *EXCLI Journal, 18*, 154–164.

Jakubowicz-Gil, J., Paduch, R., Piersiak, T., Głowniak, K., Gawron, A., & Kandefer-Szerszeń, M., (2005). The effect of quercetin on pro-apoptotic activity of cisplatin in HeLa cells. *Biochemical Pharmacology, 69*(9), 1343–1350.

Jiang, W., Li, X., Dong, S., & Zhou, W., (2021). Betulinic acid in the treatment of tumor diseases: Application and research progress. *Biomedicine and Pharmacotherapy, 142*, 111990.

Jin, Y. M., Xu, T. M., Zhao, Y. H., Wang, Y. C., & Cui, M. H., (2014). *In vitro* and *in vivo* anticancer activity of formononetin on human cervical cancer cell line HeLa. *Tumor Biology, 35*(3), 2279–2284.

Kashafi, E., Moradzadeh, M., Mohamadkhani, A., & Erfanian, S., (2017). Kaempferol increases apoptosis in human cervical cancer HeLa cells via PI3K/AKT and telomerase pathways. *Biomedicine and Pharmacotherapy, 89*, 573–577.

Kashyap, D., Sharma, A., Sak, K., Tuli, H. S., Buttar, H. S., & Bishayee, A., (2018). Fisetin: A bioactive phytochemical with potential for cancer prevention and pharmacotherapy. *Life Sciences, 194*, 75–87.

Kedhari, S. M., Raina, R., Afroze, N., Bajbouj, K., Hamad, M., Haque, S., & Hussain, A., (2019). Quercetin modulates signaling pathways and induces apoptosis in cervical cancer cells. *Bioscience Reports, 39*(8), BSR20190720.

Khan, A. U., Dagur, H. S., Khan, M., Malik, N., Alam, M., & Mushtaque, M., (2021). Therapeutic role of flavonoids and flavones in cancer prevention: Current trends and future perspectives. *European Journal of Medicinal Chemistry Reports, 3*, 100010.

Kim, B., Kim, H. S., Jung, E. J., Lee, J. Y., Tsang, B., Lim, J. M., & Song, Y. S., (2016). Curcumin induces ER stress-mediated apoptosis through selective generation of reactive oxygen species in cervical cancer cells. *Molecular Carcinogenesis, 55*(5), 918–928.

Kim, H. J., Cho, H. S., Ban, H. S., & Nakamura, H., (2020). Suppression of HIF-1α accumulation by betulinic acid through proteasome activation in hypoxic cervical cancer. *Biochemical and Biophysical Research Communications, 523*(3), 726–732.

Kim, M. S., Bak, Y., Park, Y. S., et al., (2013). Wogonin induces apoptosis by suppressing E6 and E7 expressions and activating intrinsic signaling pathways in HPV-16 cervical cancer cells. *Cell Biology and Toxicology, 29*(4), 259–272.

Kim, S. H., Kim, S. H., Kim, Y. B., Jeon, Y. T., Lee, S. C., & Song, Y. S., (2009). Genistein inhibits cell growth by modulating various mitogen-activated protein kinases and AKT in cervical cancer cells. *Annals of the New York Academy of Sciences, 1171*, 495–500. https://doi.org/10.1111/j.1749-6632.2009.04899.x.

Kotha, R. R., & Luthria, D. L., (2019). Curcumin: Biological, pharmaceutical, nutraceutical, and analytical aspects. *Molecules, 24*(16), 2930.

Krifa, M., Alhosin, M., Muller, C. D., et al., (2013). *Limoniastrum guyonianum* aqueous gall extract induces apoptosis in human cervical cancer cells involving p16INK4A re-expression related to UHRF1 and DNMT1 down-regulation. *Journal of Experimental and Clinical Cancer Research, 32*(1), 1–10.

Kumar, A., & Jaitak, V., (2019). Natural products as multidrug resistance modulators in cancer. *European Journal of Medicinal Chemistry, 176*, 268–291.

Kumar, D., Basu, S., Parija, L., Rout, D., Manna, S., Dandapat, J., & Debata, P. R., (2016). Curcumin and ellagic acid synergistically induce ROS generation, DNA damage, p53 accumulation and apoptosis in HeLa cervical carcinoma cells. *Biomedicine and Pharmacotherapy, 81*, 31–37.

Lei, H., Shi, J., Teng, Y., Song, C., Zou, L., Ye, F., & Zhang, H., (2021). Baicalein modulates the radiosensitivity of cervical cancer cells *in vitro* via miR-183 and the JAK2/STAT3 signaling pathway. *Advances in Clinical and Experimental Medicine, 30*(7), 727–736.

Leung, K. W., & Wong, A. S. T., (2010). Pharmacology of ginsenosides: A literature review. *Chinese Medicine, 5*(1), 1–7.

Li, J., Ma, J., Wang, K. S., et al., (2016). Baicalein inhibits TNF-α-induced NF-κB activation and expression of NF-κB-regulated target gene products. *Oncology Reports, 36*(5), 2771–2776.

Li, L. W., Na, C., Tian, S. Y., Chen, J., Ma, R., Gao, Y., & Lou, G., (2018). Ellagic acid induces HeLa cell apoptosis via regulating signal transducer and activator of transcription 3 signaling. *Experimental and Therapeutic Medicine, 16*(1), 29–36.

Li, X., Mu, J., Lin, Y., Zhao, J., & Meng, X., (2021b). Combination of cyanidin-3-O-glucoside and cisplatin induces oxidative stress and apoptosis in HeLa cells by reducing the activity of endogenous antioxidants, increasing bax/bcl-2 mRNA expression ratio, and downregulating Nrf2 expression. *Journal of Food Biochemistry, 45*(7), e13806.

Li, X., Zhao, J., Yan, T., Mu, J., Lin, Y., Chen, J., Deng, H., & Meng, X., (2021a). Cyanidin-3-O-glucoside and cisplatin inhibit proliferation and downregulate the PI3K/AKT/mTOR pathway in cervical cancer cells. *Journal of Food Science, 86*(6), 2700–2712.

Limtrakul, P., Khantamat, O., & Pintha, K., (2005). Inhibition of P-glycoprotein function and expression by kaempferol and quercetin. *Journal of Chemotherapy, 17*(1), 86–95.

Lin, M. T., Lin, C. L., Lin, T. Y., et al., (2016). Synergistic effect of fisetin combined with sorafenib in human cervical cancer HeLa cells through activation of death receptor-5 mediated caspase-8/caspase-3 and the mitochondria-dependent apoptotic pathway. *Tumor Biology, 37*(5), 6987–6996.

Lin, R., Hu, X., Chen, S., Shi, Q., & Chen, H., (2020). Naringin induces endoplasmic reticulum stress-mediated apoptosis, inhibits β-catenin pathway and arrests the cell cycle in cervical cancer cells. *Acta Biochimica Polonica, 67*(2), 181–188.

Lin, S. R., Chang, C. H., Hsu, C. F., et al., (2020). Natural compounds as potential adjuvants to cancer therapy: Preclinical evidence. *British Journal of Pharmacology, 177*(6), 1409–1423.

Lin, Y., Shi, R., Wang, X., & Shen, H. M., (2008). Luteolin, a flavonoid with potential for cancer prevention and therapy. *Current Cancer Drug Targets, 8*(7), 634–646.

Liskova, A., Samec, M., Koklesova, L., et al., (2021). Flavonoids as an effective sensitizer for anticancer therapy: Insights into multi-faceted mechanisms and applicability towards individualized patient profiles. *EPMA Journal, 12*(2), 155–176.

Liu, J., Zhou, H., Song, L., Yang, Z., Qiu, M., Wang, J., & Shi, S., (2021). Anthocyanins: Promising natural products with diverse pharmacological activities. *Molecules, 26*(13), 3807.

Liu, M. M., Ma, R. H., Ni, Z. J., Thakur, K., Cespedes-Acuña, C. L., Jiang, L., & Wei, Z. J., (2020). Apigenin 7-O-glucoside promotes cell apoptosis through the PTEN/PI3K/AKT pathway and inhibits cell migration in cervical cancer HeLa cells. *Food and Chemical Toxicology, 146*,111843.

Liu, Y., Wang, J., Qiao, J., Liu, S., Wang, S., Zhao, D., Bai, X., & Liu, M., (2020). Ginsenoside Rh2 inhibits HeLa cell energy metabolism and induces apoptosis by upregulating voltage-dependent anion channel 1. *International Journal of Molecular Medicine, 46*(5), 1695–1706.

Liu, Z., Zhu, W., Kong, X., Chen, X., Sun, X., Zhang, W., & Zhang, R., (2019). Tanshinone IIA inhibits glucose metabolism leading to apoptosis in cervical cancer. *Oncology Reports, 42*(5), 1893–1903.

Lo, Y. L., & Wang, W., (2013). Formononetin potentiates epirubicin-induced apoptosis via ROS production in HeLa cells *in vitro*. *Chemico-Biological Interactions, 205*(3), 188–197.

Lu, B., Hu, M., Liu, K., & Peng, J., (2010). Cytotoxicity of berberine on human cervical carcinoma HeLa cells through mitochondria, death receptor and MAPK pathways, and in-silico drug-target prediction. *Toxicology in vitro, 24*(6), 1482–1490.

Mahata, S., Bharti, A. C., Shukla, S., Tyagi, A., Husain, S. A., & Das, B. C., (2011). Berberine modulates AP-1 activity to suppress HPV transcription and downstream signaling to induce growth arrest and apoptosis in cervical cancer cells. *Molecular Cancer, 10*, 39.

Mann, J., (2002). Natural products in cancer chemotherapy: Past, present and future. *Nature Reviews Cancer, 2*(2), 143–148.

Mattioli, R., Francioso, A., Mosca, L., & Silva, P., (2020). Anthocyanins: A comprehensive review of their chemical properties and health effects on cardiovascular and neurodegenerative diseases. *Molecules, 25*(17), 3809.

Mehdi, S. J., Ahmad, A., Irshad, M., Manzoor, N., & Rizvi, M. M. A., (2011). Cytotoxic effect of carvacrol on human cervical cancer cells. *Biol. Med., 3*(2), 307–312.

Mistry, B. M., Shin, H. S., Keum, Y. S., et al., (2017). Synthesis and evaluation of antioxidant and cytotoxicity of the N-mannich base of berberine bearing benzothiazole moieties. *Anticancer Agents in Medicinal Chemistry, 17*(12), 1652–1660.

Mitra, T., & Elangovan, S., (2021). Cervical cancer development, chemoresistance, and therapy: A snapshot of involvement of microRNA. *Molecular and Cellular Biochemistry, 476*(12), 4363–4385.

Moody, C. A., & Laimins, L. A., (2010). Human papillomavirus oncoproteins: Pathways to transformation. *Nature Reviews Cancer, 10*(8), 550–560.

Munagala, R., Aqil, F., Jeyabalan, J., & Gupta, R. C., (2015). Tanshinone IIA inhibits viral oncogene expression leading to apoptosis and inhibition of cervical cancer. *Cancer Letters, 356*(2 Pt B), 536–546.

Owona, B. A., & Schluesener, H. J., (2015). Molecular insight in the multifunctional effects of oridonin. *Drugs in R and D, 15*(3), 233–244.

Owona, B. A., Abia, W. A., & Moundipa, P. F., (2020). Natural compounds flavonoids as modulators of inflammasomes in chronic diseases. *International Immunopharmacology, 84*, 106498.

Pan, T. L., Wang, P. W., Hung, Y. C., Huang, C. H., & Rau, K. M., (2013). Proteomic analysis reveals tanshinone IIA enhances apoptosis of advanced cervix carcinoma CaSki cells through mitochondria intrinsic and endoplasmic reticulum stress pathways. *Proteomics, 13*(23, 24), 3411–3423.

Pandey, P., & Khan, F., (2021). A mechanistic review of the anticancer potential of hesperidin, a natural flavonoid from citrus fruits. *Nutrition Research, 92*, 21–31.

Peng, Y., Guo, C., Yang, Y., Li, F., Zhang, Y., Jiang, B., & Li, Q., (2015). Baicalein induces apoptosis of human cervical cancer HeLa cells *in vitro*. *Molecular Medicine Reports, 11*(3), 2129–2134.

Polachi, N., Bai, G., Li, T., et al., (2016). Modulatory effects of silibinin in various cell signaling pathways against liver disorders and cancer – a comprehensive review. *European Journal of Medicinal Chemistry, 123*, 577–595.

Potočnjak, I., Gobin, I., & Domitrović, R., (2018). Carvacrol induces cytotoxicity in human cervical cancer cells but causes cisplatin resistance: Involvement of MEK-ERK activation. *Phytotherapy Research, 32*(6), 1090–1097.

Qiao, Y., Cao, J., Xie, L., & Shi, X., (2009). Cell growth inhibition and gene expression regulation by (-)-epigallocatechin-3-gallate in human cervical cancer cells. *Arch Pharm Res., 32*(9), 1309–1315.

Qin, J., Shi, H., Xu, Y., Zhao, F., & Wang, Q., (2018). Tanshinone IIA inhibits cervix carcinoma stem cells migration and invasion via inhibiting YAP transcriptional activity. *Biomedicine and Pharmacotherapy, 105*, 758–765.

Rajendran, P., Rengarajan, T., Nandakumar, N., Palaniswami, R., Nishigaki, Y., & Nishigaki, I., (2014). Kaempferol, a potential cytostatic and cure for inflammatory disorders. *European Journal of Medicinal Chemistry, 86*, 103–112.

Ramesh, E., & Alshatwi, A. A., (2013). Naringin induces death receptor and mitochondria-mediated apoptosis in human cervical cancer (SiHa) cells. *Food and Chemical Toxicology, 51*, 97–105.

Ríos, J. L., & Máñez, S., (2018). New pharmacological opportunities for betulinic acid. *Planta Medica, 84*(1), 8–19. https://doi.org/10.1055/s-0043-123472.

Risuleo, G., & Mesa, C. L., (2019). Resveratrol: Biological activities and potential use in health and disease. *Nutraceuticals in Veterinary Medicine*, 215–226.

Rodríguez-García, C., Sánchez-Quesada, C., & Gaforio, J. J., (2019). Dietary flavonoids as cancer chemopreventive agents: An updated review of human studies. *Antioxidants, 8*(5), 137.

Rzeski, W., Stepulak, A., Szymański, M., Sifringer, M., Kaczor, J., Wejksza, K., Zdzisińska, B., & Kandefer-Szerszeń, M., (2006). Betulinic acid decreases expression of bcl-2 and cyclin D1, inhibits proliferation, migration and induces apoptosis in cancer cells. *Naunyn-Schmiedeberg's Archives of Pharmacology, 374*(1), 11–20.

Sahin, K., Tuzcu, M., Basak, N., Caglayan, B., Kilic, U., Sahin, F., & Kucuk, O., (2012). Sensitization of cervical cancer cells to cisplatin by genistein: The role of NFκB and Akt/mTOR signaling pathways. *Journal of Oncology, 461*562.

Sajomsang, W., Gonil, P., Saesoo, S., Ruktanonchai, U. R., Srinuanchai, W., & Puttipipatkhachorn, S., (2014). Synthesis and anticervical cancer activity of novel pH responsive micelles for oral curcumin delivery. *International Journal of Pharmaceutics, 477*(1, 2), 261–272.

Sarek, J., Klinot, J., Dzubák, P., et al., (2003). New Lupane derived compounds with pro-apoptotic activity in cancer cells: Synthesis and structure-activity relationships. *Journal of Medicinal Chemistry, 46*(25), 5402–5415.

Schläger, S., & Dräger, B., (2016). Exploiting plant alkaloids. *Current Opinion in Biotechnology, 37*, 155–164.

Shao, J., Wang, C., Li, L., Liang, H., Dai, J., Ling, X., & Tang, H., (2018). Luteoloside inhibits proliferation and promotes intrinsic and extrinsic pathway-mediated apoptosis involving MAPK and mTOR signaling pathways in human cervical cancer cells. *International Journal of Molecular Sciences, 19*(6), 1664.

Sharma, C., Nusri, Q., Begum, S., Javed, E., Rizvi, T. A., & Hussain, A., (2012). (-)-Epigallocatechin-3-gallate induces apoptosis and inhibits invasion and migration of human cervical cancer cells. *Asian Pacific Journal of Cancer Prevention, 13*(9), 4815–4822.

Shen, N., Wang, T., Gan, Q., Liu, S., Wang, L., & Jin, B., (2022). Plant flavonoids: Classification, distribution, biosynthesis, and antioxidant activity. *Food Chemistry, 1325*31.

Shi, R. X., Ong, C. N., & Shen, H. M., (2004). Luteolin sensitizes tumor necrosis factor-α-induced apoptosis in human tumor cells. *Oncogene, 23*(46), 7712–7721.

Shi, X., Yang, J., & Wei, G., (2018). Ginsenoside 20(S)-Rh2 exerts anticancer activity through the Akt/GSK3β signaling pathway in human cervical cancer cells. *Molecular Medicine Reports, 17*(3), 4811–4816.

Silva, E. R., De Carvalho, F. O., Teixeira, L., et al., (2018). Pharmacological effects of carvacrol in *in vitro* studies: A review. *Current Pharmaceutical Design, 24*(29), 3454–3465.

Singh, B. N., Shankar, S., & Srivastava, R. K., (2011). Green tea catechin, epigallocatechin-3-gallate (EGCG): Mechanisms, perspectives and clinical applications. *Biochemical Pharmacology, 82*(12), 1807–1821.

Singh, M., & Singh, N., (2009). Molecular mechanism of curcumin induced cytotoxicity in human cervical carcinoma cells. *Molecular and Cellular Biochemistry, 325*(1, 2), 107–119.

Song, D., Hao, J., & Fan, D., (2020). Biological properties and clinical applications of berberine. *Frontiers of Medicine, 14*(5), 564–582.

Song, M., Liu, X., Liu, K., et al., (2018). Targeting AKT with oridonin inhibits growth of esophageal squamous cell carcinoma *in vitro* and patient-derived xenografts *in vivo*. *Molecular Cancer Therapeutics, 17*(7), 1540–1553.

Souza, R. P., Bonfim-Mendonça, P. S., Gimenes, F., et al., (2017). Oxidative stress triggered by apigenin induces apoptosis in a comprehensive panel of human cervical cancer-derived cell lines. *Oxidative Medicine and Cellular Longevity, 1512*745.

Sun, X., Fu, P., Xie, L., et al., (2021). Resveratrol inhibits the progression of cervical cancer by suppressing the transcription and expression of HPV E6 and E7 genes. *International Journal of Molecular Medicine, 47*(1), 335–345.

Sun, X., Xu, Q., Zeng, L., et al., (2020). Resveratrol suppresses the growth and metastatic potential of cervical cancer by inhibiting STAT3^{Tyr705} phosphorylation. *Cancer Medicine, 9*(22), 8685–8700.

Suntres, Z. E., Coccimiglio, J., & Alipour, M., (2015). The bioactivity and toxicological actions of carvacrol. *Critical Reviews in Food Science and Nutrition, 55*(3), 304–318.

Tang, S. M., Deng, X. T., Zhou, J., Li, Q. P., Ge, X. X., & Miao, L., (2020). Pharmacological basis and new insights of quercetin action in respect to its anticancer effects. *Biomedicine and Pharmacotherapy, 121*, 109604.

Tang, X., Zhang, Q., Nishitani, J., Brown, J., Shi, S., & Le, A. D., (2007). Overexpression of human papillomavirus type 16 oncoproteins enhances hypoxia-inducible factor 1α protein accumulation and vascular endothelial growth factor expression in human cervical carcinoma cells. *Clinical Cancer Research, 13*(9), 2568–2576.

Tay, K. C., Tan, L. T., Chan, C. K., et al., (2019). Formononetin: A review of its anticancer potentials and mechanisms. *Frontiers in Pharmacology, 10*, 820.

Tholl, D., (2015). Biosynthesis and biological functions of terpenoids in plants. *Advances in Biochemical Engineering/Biotechnology, 148*, 63–106.

Tu, L. Y., Bai, H. H., Cai, J. Y., & Deng, S. P., (2016). The mechanism of kaempferol induced apoptosis and inhibited proliferation in human cervical cancer SiHa cell: From macro to nano. *Scanning, 38*(6), 644–653.

Tungmunnithum, D., Thongboonyou, A., Pholboon, A., & Yangsabai, A., (2018). Flavonoids and other phenolic compounds from medicinal plants for pharmaceutical and medical aspects: An overview. *Medicines, 5*(3), 93.

Tuorkey, M. J., (2016). Molecular targets of luteolin in cancer. *European Journal of Cancer Prevention, 25*(1), 65.

Ullah, A., Munir, S., Badshah, S. L., et al., (2020). Important flavonoids and their role as a therapeutic agent. *Molecules, 25*(22), 5243.

Urasa, M., & Darj, E., (2011). Knowledge of cervical cancer and screening practices of nurses at a regional hospital in Tanzania. *African Health Sciences, 11*(1), 48–57.

Verma, E., Kumar, A., Daimary, U. D., et al., (2021). Potential of baicalein in the prevention and treatment of cancer: A scientometric analyses-based review. *Journal of Functional Foods, 86*, 104660.

Vidya, P. R., Senthil, M. R., Maitreyi, S., Ramalingam, K., Karunagaran, D., & Nagini, S., (2010). The flavonoid quercetin induces cell cycle arrest and mitochondria-mediated apoptosis in human cervical cancer (HeLa) cells through p53 induction and NF-κB inhibition. *European Journal of Pharmacology, 649*(1–3), 84–91.

Wang, G., Tang, W., & Bidigare, R. R., (2005). Terpenoids as therapeutic drugs and pharmaceutical agents. In: *Natural Products* (pp. 197–227). Humana Press.

Wang, T. Y., Li, Q., & Bi, K. S., (2018). Bioactive flavonoids in medicinal plants: Structure, activity and biological fate. *Asian Journal of Pharmaceutical Sciences, 13*(1), 12–23.

Wang, T., Wu, X., Al Rudaisat, M., Song, Y., & Cheng, H., (2020). Curcumin induces G2/M arrest and triggers autophagy, ROS generation and cell senescence in cervical cancer cells. *Journal of Cancer, 11*(22), 6704–6715.

Wang, W., Yue, R. F., Jin, Z., He, L. M., Shen, R., Du, D., & Tang, Y. Z., (2020). Efficiency comparison of apigenin-7-O-glucoside and trolox in antioxidative stress and anti-inflammatory properties. *The Journal of Pharmacy and Pharmacology, 72*(11), 1645–1656.

Wang, Y., Yu, H., Zhang, J., Gao, J., Ge, X., & Lou, G., (2015). Hesperidin inhibits HeLa cell proliferation through apoptosis mediated by endoplasmic reticulum stress pathways and cell cycle arrest. *BMC Cancer, 15*(1), 1–11.

Wu, X., Yang, Z., Dang, H., Peng, H., & Dai, Z., (2018). Baicalein inhibits the proliferation of cervical cancer cells through the GSK3β-dependent pathway. *Oncology Research, 26*(4), 645–653.

Wu, X., Zhou, J., Cai, D., & Li, M., (2017). Matrine inhibits the metastatic properties of human cervical cancer cells via downregulating the p38 signaling pathway. *Oncology Reports, 38*(2), 1312–1320.

Xia, X., Xia, J., Yang, H., Li, Y., Liu, S., Cao, Y., Tang, L., & Yu, X., (2019). Baicalein blocked cervical carcinoma cell proliferation by targeting CCND1 via Wnt/β-catenin signaling pathway. *Artificial Cells, Nanomedicine, and Biotechnology, 47*(1), 2729–2736.

Xie, Z., Wei, Y., Xu, J., Lei, J., & Yu, J., (2019). Alkaloids from *Piper nigrum* synergistically enhanced the effect of paclitaxel against paclitaxel-resistant cervical cancer cells through the downregulation of Mcl-1. *Journal of Agricultural and Food Chemistry, 67*(18), 5159–5168.

Xu, T., Pang, Q., Wang, Y., & Yan, X., (2017). Betulinic acid induces apoptosis by regulating PI3K/Akt signaling and mitochondrial pathways in human cervical cancer cells. *International Journal of Molecular Medicine, 40*(6), 1669–1678.

Xu, W., Xie, S., Chen, X., Pan, S., Qian, H., & Zhu, X., (2021). Effects of quercetin on the efficacy of various chemotherapeutic drugs in cervical cancer cells. *Drug Design, Development and Therapy, 15*, 577–588.

Yang, L., Zhang, H. W., Hu, R., et al., (2009). Wogonin induces G1 phase arrest through inhibiting Cdk4 and cyclin D1 concomitant with an elevation in p21Cip1 in human cervical carcinoma HeLa cells. *Biochemistry and Cell Biology = Biochimie et Biologie Cellulaire, 87*(6), 933–942.

Yang, Y., Trevethan, M., Wang, S., & Zhao, L., (2022). Beneficial effects of citrus flavanones naringin and naringenin and their food sources on lipid metabolism: An update on bioavailability, pharmacokinetics, and mechanisms. *The Journal of Nutritional Biochemistry, 108967*.

Yen, J. H., Huang, S. T., Huang, H. S., Fong, Y. C., Wu, Y. Y., Chiang, J. H., & Su, Y. C., (2018). HGK-sestrin 2 signaling-mediated autophagy contributes to the antitumor efficacy of tanshinone IIA in human osteosarcoma cells. *Cell Death and Disease, 9*(10), 1003.

Ying, T. H., Yang, S. F., Tsai, S. J., Hsieh, S. C., Huang, Y. C., Bau, D. T., & Hsieh, Y. H., (2012). Fisetin induces apoptosis in human cervical cancer HeLa cells through ERK1/2-mediated activation of caspase-8-/caspase-3-dependent pathway. *Archives of Toxicology, 86*(2), 263–273.

You, L., Yang, C., Du, Y., et al., (2019). Matrine exerts hepatotoxic effects via the ROS-dependent mitochondrial apoptosis pathway and inhibition of Nrf2-mediated antioxidant response. *Oxidative Medicine and Cellular Longevity, 1045*345.

You, Y., He, Q., Lu, H., et al., (2020). Silibinin induces G2/M cell cycle arrest by activating Drp1-dependent mitochondrial fission in cervical cancer. *Frontiers in Pharmacology, 11*, 271.

Yoysungnoen-Chintana, P., Bhattarakosol, P., & Patumraj, S., (2014). Antitumor and antiangiogenic activities of curcumin in cervical cancer xenografts in nude mice. *BioMed Research International*, 817972.

Yu, X., Yang, Y., Li, Y., Cao, Y., Tang, L., Chen, F., & Xia, J., (2018). Baicalein inhibits cervical cancer progression via downregulating long noncoding RNA BDLNR and its downstream PI3K/Akt pathway. *The International Journal of Biochemistry and Cell Biology, 94*, 107–118.

Zeng, L., Zhen, Y., Chen, Y., et al., (2014). Naringin inhibits growth and induces apoptosis by a mechanism dependent on reduced activation of NF-κB/COX-2-caspase-1 pathway in HeLa cervical cancer cells. *International Journal of Oncology, 45*(5), 1929–1936.

Zhang, C. L., Wu, L. J., Tashiro, S., Onodera, S., & Ikejima, T., (2004). Oridonin induced A375-S2 cell apoptosis via bax-regulated caspase pathway activation, dependent on the cytochrome c/caspase-9 apoptosome. *Journal of Asian Natural Products Research, 6*(2), 127–138.

Zhang, E., Zhang, Y., Fan, Z., Cheng, L., Han, S., & Che, H., (2020). Apigenin inhibits histamine-induced cervical cancer tumor growth by regulating estrogen receptor expression. *Molecules, 25*(8), 1960.

Zhang, L., Wang, T., Wen, X., Wei, Y., Peng, X., Li, H., & Wei, L., (2007). Effect of matrine on HeLa cell adhesion and migration. *European Journal of Pharmacology, 563*(1–3), 69–76.

Zhang, P., Yang, B., Yao, Y. Y., et al., (2015). PIAS3, SHP2 and SOCS3 expression patterns in cervical cancers: Relevance with activation and resveratrol-caused inactivation of STAT3 signaling. *Gynecologic Oncology, 139*(3), 529–535.

Zhang, Y. H., Wu, Y. L., Tashiro, S., Onodera, S., & Ikejima, T., (2011). Reactive oxygen species contribute to oridonin-induced apoptosis and autophagy in human cervical carcinoma HeLa cells. *Acta Pharmacologica Sinica, 32*(10), 1266–1275.

Zhang, Y., Chen, C., & Zhang, J., (2019). Effects and significance of formononetin on expression levels of HIF-1α and VEGF in mouse cervical cancer tissue. *Oncology Letters, 18*(3), 2248–2253.

Zhang, Y., Ge, Y., Chen, Y., Li, Q., Chen, J., Dong, Y., & Shi, W., (2012). Cellular and molecular mechanisms of silibinin induces cell-cycle arrest and apoptosis on HeLa cells. *Cell Biochemistry and Function, 30*(3), 243–248.

Zhao, Y., Yuan, X., Li, X., & Zhang, Y., (2019). Resveratrol significantly inhibits the occurrence and development of cervical cancer by regulating phospholipid scramblase 1. *Journal of Cellular Biochemistry, 120*(2), 1527–1531.

Zhu, J., Zhang, C., Qing, Y., Cheng, Y., Jiang, X., Li, M., Yang, Z., & Wang, D., (2015). Genistein induces apoptosis by stabilizing intracellular p53 protein through an APE1-mediated pathway. *Free Radical Biology and Medicine, 86*, 209–218.

Zou, C., Liu, H., Feugang, J. M., Hao, Z., Chow, H. H., & Garcia, F., (2010). Green tea compound in chemoprevention of cervical cancer. *International Journal of Gynecological Cancer, 20*(4), 617–624.

CHAPTER 11

Therapeutic Approaches for Cervical Cancer Management

11.1 INTRODUCTION

Historically, cervical cancer (locally advanced) was treated using external beam radiation. In 1999, a novel therapeutic method for advanced cervical cancer treatment was introduced. On the basis of five phase III randomized clinical trials, the National Cancer Institute (NCI) validated the use of cisplatin-based chemotherapy in combination with radiotherapy as standard care for cervical cancer (locally advanced) (Franco et al., 1999). A new therapeutic approach was introduced in 1999 for advanced cervical cancer treatment. NCI (National Cancer Institute) validated the use of cisplatin-based chemotherapy, along with radiotherapy as standard care for cervical cancer (locally advanced) (The National Cancer Institute Clinical Announcement on Cervical Cancer, 1999) on the basis of five phase III randomized clinical trials. Chemotherapy has always been considered standard approach for the cervical cancer management (Movva et al., 2009). However, the efficacy of chemotherapeutic drugs is limited with their severe undesirable side effects, lack of specificity, poor biodistribution. Commonly used chemotherapeutic drugs for cervical cancer treatments include paclitaxel, cisplatin, and methotrexate (Pfaendler & Tewari, 2016). Although these drugs disrupt numerous biological functions and apoptosis of cancerous cells via binding to DNA of cells, yet they pose severe abnormalities such as induction of neurotoxicity and renal failure. A third of cervical cancer patients (both recurrent and metastatic stages) responded to platinum-based chemotherapy, however, the responses were

Cervical Cancer: Signaling Pathways, Molecular Mechanisms, Natural Products, and Therapeutic Approaches. Pratibha Pandey, Fahad Khan, Saher Islam, and Devarajan Thangadurai, (Eds.)

either partial or short-lived. These critical issues associated with chemotherapeutic drugs have further compelled researchers to elucidate better potent ways for the management of cervical cancer. This further highlights the urgency to enhance our understanding about the progression of cervical cancer and to elucidate molecular targets with better therapeutic potential. Thus, potent biological and targeted therapeutic approaches, including natural products and immunecheckpoint inhibitors have been summarized in Tables 11.1 and 11.2.

It has been very evident that cervical cancer has been an HPV-related malignancy (Petry, 2014). Viral oncoproteins, including E6 and E7 has been associated with degradation of several tumor suppressor proteins such as p53 and pRb leading to abrogation of cellular onco-suppressive pathways and uncontrolled cell growth (Pal & Kundu, 2020). These oncoproteins has also been reported to deregulate the expression of cellular adherence proteins and telomerase (hTERT), gene apoptotic machinery, and differentiation of cervical epithelial cells leading to angiogenesis (Ibeanu, 2011; Liontos et al., 2019). It has been clearly stated that E7 increases the transcriptional activity of HIF1α (VEGF inducer) and augment VEGF splice variants expression. Furthermore, enhanced VEGF expression adversely affected the survival rate of cervical cancer patients undergoing radiotherapy treatment. Cervical cancer pathogenesis has also been linked to EGFR-activated pathways. Overexpressed EGFR has been found in the majority of newly diagnosed cervical malignancies and has been identified as a poor prognostic marker for cancer patient survival, as well as a predictor of poor response to radiotherapy and cytotoxic medicines (Schrevel et al., 2011). Inhibition of the EGFR gene appears to be a viable therapeutic target.

11.2 VEGF/VEGFR-DIRECTED THERAPY

In several solid tumors, antiangiogenic therapy that targets the VEGF and associated pathways has led to substantial improvements. The expression of VEGF has been linked to poor prognosis and early relapse in cervical cancer (Fujimoto et al., 2004). Bevacizumab is an anti-VEGF-A human recombinant monoclonal antibody (Ig-G1 immunoglobulin) that suppresses signal transduction via VEGFR-1- and VEGFR-2-mediated pathways by downregulating VEGF-A. A phase II study found that the bevacizumab was considerably well tolerated in metastatic carcinoma, that resulted in improved progression-free survival (PFS) and overall survival

TABLE 11.1 Therapies Targeting Signaling Pathways Elements in Cervical Cancer

Therapeutic Agents	Target	Cell Signaling Pathway	Mode of Action	References
Trematinib + GSK2141795	MEK	MAPK	Inhibit MEK activity upon binding with it	Miller et al. (2014)
Sorafenib + Cisplatin/ Radiotherapy	Raf kinase	MAPK	ATP site inhibition (competitive inhibition)	Manzo-Merino et al. (2014)
Wortamannin + Radiotherapy/ Chemotherapy	p110	PI3K	ATP site inhibition (irreversible competitor)	Chen et al. (2013)
CT-1040	MEK	MAPK	Reduces pMAPK expression level	Meng et al. (2020)
PD98059 + Doxorubicin and Cisplatin	MEK	MAPK	Inhibits kinase protein	Yeh et al. (2002)
LY294002	P110	PI3K	ATP site inhibition (reversible competitor)	Fuhrman et al. (2008)
Indole-3 carbinol	Akt	PI3K	ATP site inhibition (irreversible competitor) and apoptosis induction	Scarinci et al. (2010)
Genistein + Radiotherapy	Akt	PI3K	Inhibits phosphorylation of AKt at Ser473	Kim et al. (2009)
MK-2206	Akt	PI3K	Inhibits Akt allosterically	Cherrin et al. (2010)
Everolimus	Bcl2 and CCND1 mRNA	PI3K	Reduced expression level of CCND1 mRNA and BCL2	Yilmaz et al. (2016)
Temsirolimus + Topotecan	mTOR	PI3K	Promotes complex formation with FK506 binding protein 12	Temkin et al. (2010)
Nimotuzumab + Gemcitabine/ Cisplatin, Paclitaxel/Carboplatin, Brachytherapy	EGFR	EGF	Prevents binding of ligand	Lorente et al. (2019)
Cetuximab + Cisplatin, Paclitaxel/ Topotecan	EGFR	EGF	Prevents binding of ligand	McLachlan et al. (2017)

TABLE 11.1 *(Continued)*

Therapeutic Agents	Target	Cell Signaling Pathway	Mode of Action	References
Lapatinib	EGFR	EGF	Inhibits tyrosine kinase activity	Monk et al. (2010)
Matuzumab + Platinum	EGFR	EGF	Prevents binding of ligand	Blohmer et al. (2005)
Erlotinib + Radiotherapy/ Cisplatin	EGFR	EGF	Blocked EGFR-CREB/GRβ-IL-6 axis and overcomes the paclitaxel-resistant cancer stem cells in MUC1 +ve cervical cancer cells	Lv et al. (2019)
Gefitinib	PTEN	PI3K/Akt	PTEN targeting via mRNA-221 targets leading to reduced sensitivity	Du et al. (2016)
Pazopanib + Chemotherapy/ Lapatinib	VEGF tyrosine kinase	VEGF	Potent antiangiogenic drug	Schutz et al. (2011)
Bevacizumab + Capecitabine/ Flurouracil/Cisplatin/Topotecan/ Radiotherapy	VEGFR-A	VEGF	Prevents binding of ligand and enhanced survival rate	Pfaendler et al. (2018)
Recombinant human TRAIL + Radiation	Death receptor 4/5	Apoptosis	Direct binding with DR (as agonist)	Tan et al. (2012)
Retinoids	EGF, FasL/Fas	Apoptosis	Deregulated EGF pathway and FasL induction	DiSilvestro e al. (1999); Gariglio et al. (2009)
Luteolin + rhTRAIL	DR5	Apoptosis	Bid cleavage induction and activation of caspase-8	Wang et al. (2014)
N101-2	Akt/PI3K, FasL/Fas	Extrinsic apoptosis, Akt/ PI3K	Apoptosis induction and cell cycle growth arrest at G1 phase	Kim et al. (2012)

TABLE 11.1 *(Continued)*

Therapeutic Agents	Target	Cell Signaling Pathway	Mode of Action	References
Avenanthramide 2p	Beta-catenin	Beta-catenin/ Wnt	Induction of beta-catenin degradation and inhibition of nuclear accumulation	Tripathi et al. (2018)
Arsenic trioxide	E6	Multiple signaling pathways	Inhibited cell growth and HPV oncogene expression	Wang et al. (2014)

TABLE 11.2 Immunotherapies to Treat Cervical Cancer

Immunotherapy	Precise Target	Therapeutic Component	Phase of Cervical Carcinoma	Outcomes	References
Vaccines	HPV-16 E7 fusion protein	ADXS11-001 (bacterial)	Advanced/ persistent/recurrent	Substantial clinical efficacy with demonstrated longer survival, tumor response and stabilization of relapse disease compared to present chemotherapeutic drug, cisplatin.	Petit et al. (2014); Basu et al. (2018)
	HPV16 E6/E7 peptide	TA-HPV (viral)	Progressive	Vaccination was well tolerated, and 13.8–37.5% of participants produced cytotoxic T cells selective for HPV, and 27.6–37.5% of patients displayed HPV-mediated responses with a promising therapeutic benefit.	Borysiewicz et al. (1996); Kaufmann et al. (2002)
		SGN-00101	High-grade CIN	Regression of an induced lesion that was connected with an immune response, indicating increased immunogenicity	Roman et al. (2007)
	HPV-16 E7 HLA-A2[a] restricted peptide	ZYC101a	High-grade CIN	All patients reported good compliance, and CIN 2/3 resolution was supported in women under the age of 25.	Garcia et al. (2004)
	Plasmid targeting HPV-16/18 E6 and E7	VGX-3100	CIN2/3 associated with HPV-16/ HPV-18	The first therapeutic vaccine to demonstrate effectiveness against CIN2/3 linked to HPV-16 and -18. Erythema was much more prevalent in the VGX-3100 group (78%) than in the control group (57%).	Trimble et al. (2015)
Immune checkpoint inhibitors (ICIs)	PD-1/PD-L1b	Pembrolizumab	PD-L1 positive tumors	Effective antitumor activity is present, and the toxicity profile has improved.	Frenel et al. (2017); Browne et al. (2020)
		Nivolumab	Advanced/recurrent	Warrants additional research as no fresh safety indicators were found in the patients examined.	Naumann et al. (2019)
		Cemiplimab	Recurrent/ metastatic	Demonstrated therapeutic efficacy and a tolerability similar to that seen with other PD-1 inhibitors in patients who were resistant to or intolerable to platinum and taxane doublets.	Rischin et al. (2020)

TABLE 11.2 *(Continued)*

Immunotherapy	Precise Target	Therapeutic Component	Phase of Cervical Carcinoma	Outcomes	References
		Balstilimab	Recurrent/ metastatic	Demonstrated in controllable safety and considerable and long-lasting therapeutic activity	O'Malley et al. (2021)
	CTLA4c	Ipilimumab	Metastatic/locally advanced/recurrent	Did not cause a substantial response in the patient's tumor.	Lheureux et al. (2018)
		Following chemoradiation (CRT): Ipilimumab	Metastatic/locally advanced/recurrent	Expression of the PD-1 significantly increased on T-cell subsets following CRT and were sustained or increased following ipilimumab treatment. This treatment significantly expanded central and effector memory T-cell populations.	Da Silva et al. (2021)
Adoptive T cell therapy (ACT)	Tumor-infiltrating lymphocytes (TILs)	LN-145 TIL	Recurrent/ persistent/ metastatic	Acceptable safety and efficacy profile, and results in 44% objective response rate and 89% disease control rate in patients previously treated for cervical cancer.	Jazaeri et al. (2019)
		LN-145 TIL + IL-2	Recurrent/ persistent/ metastatic	No results yet.	Mauricio et al. (2021)
		Young TIL	Metastatic squamous cell carcinoma and adenocarcinoma	Objective tumor responses in 3/9 patients with durable complete regression. HPV reactivity of infused T cells correlated positively with clinical responses and remained significant even 1 month after treatment.	Stevanovi´c et al. (2015)

[a]Human leukocyte antigen serotype

[b]Programmed cell death protein (ligand) 1

[c]Cytotoxic T-lymphocyte-associated protein

Source: Reproduced with permission from Burmeister et al. (2022); Copyright © Elsevier (2022).

(OS) rate (Monk et al., 2009). A Gynecologic Oncology Group (GOG) 240 study compared the use of a combination of topotecan, cisplatin, paclitaxel chemotherapeutic drugs with or without therapeutic antibody bevacizumab. This research reported a substantial improvement in PFS and OS when bevacizumab was combined to current chemotherapy in patients with relapsed or chronic illness (Tewari et al., 2014). Tumor-related angiogenesis results in a disrupted vasculature, which limits the drug delivery to tumor cells. Antiangiogenic drugs have been demonstrated to 'normalize' tumor vasculature, improving oxygen and drug delivery to the tumor microenvironment (Jain, 2005). These data demonstrated partly illustrate why the combination of bevacizumab with chemotherapy produces better results. In 2014, the findings of GOG 240 resulted in the authorization of bevacizumab as a first-line treatment for advanced cervical carcinoma by the US Food and Drug Administration. Despite the fact that there was no considerable difference in the overall health-related quality-of-life between the bevacizumab and non-bevacizumab in the GOG 240 study. In addition to this, three detrimental effects were significantly more common with the addition of bevacizumab that are linked to hypertension, gastrointestinal, and venous thrombotic systems. The cost-benefit assessment is a critical consideration when deciding on a therapy in the real world. The projected total cost of bevacizumab therapy is almost 13.2 times that of chemotherapeutics alone, and this treatment is unaffordable to most patients with cervical carcinoma in developing nations, where the major portion of cancer patients reside (Minion et al., 2015). The two tyrosine kinase antagonists, sunitinib and pazopanib, did not show substantial improvement in PFS or OS response rates in advanced-grade cervical cancer. These two inhibitors mainly target mediators of angiogenesis, such as VEFGR, PDGFR, c-KIT, FLT-3. Brivanib, a VEGFR and FGFR inhibitor, is now being studied for its potential function in advanced and metastatic stage carcinoma (Mackay et al., 2010).

11.3 EGFR/HER2 THERAPY

The epidermal growth factor receptor (EGFR) protein is expressed at moderate to high levels in cervical cancer (Scambia et al., 1998). However, investigations of gefitinib and erlotinib as single therapeutics in the management of recurrent cervical cancer have demonstrated poor results (Goncalves et al., 2008; Schilder et al., 2009). Cetuximab, an anti-EGFR monoclonal antibody, was also tested in this context, however, many studies with and without cytotoxic chemotherapy found no significant effect (Kurtz et al., 2009; Farley et al., 2011; Santin et al., 2011). In a phase II investigation, a HER2 inhibitor, lapatinib, was compared to pazopanib and failed to show benefit as a single agent. Because the combination of lapatinib (a HER2 inhibitor) and pazopanib (a VEGFR inhibitor) generated significant cytotoxicity, thus enrollment in this phase of the research was stopped early (Monk et al., 2009). A recent analysis of genetic profiling of cervical cancer samples and patient-derived xenograft (PDX) models found that co-administration of trastuzumab and lapatinib effectively suppressed tumor growth in the HER2-model of cervical cancer patients as compared to the control group (Oh et al., 2015). However, hardly one out of every nine individuals had a HER2-amplified malignancy, demanding further investigations to confirm these findings.

11.4 IMMUNOTHERAPY IN CERVICAL CANCER

Cervical cancer displays immense complexity at various levels including cellular, epigenetic, and genetic levels, limiting conventional therapeutic approaches. Due to the development of multiple drug resistance, nonspecificity, dosage limitations, and adverse side effects, previously administered cancer therapy is limited in its long-term efficacy. Furthermore, because to leftover malignant cells and tumor metastases, illness relapse is still a regular occurrence. As a result, better cervical cancer treatment is required. The complex link between tumors and the immune response led to the development of immunotherapy (Abbott & Ustoyev, 2019). Immunotherapy is an appealing treatment approach because viral antigens from high-risk human papillomavirus (HPV) infections in cervical cancer are quickly recognized as foreign matter.

Cancer immunotherapy works by stimulating and enhancing the immune system to develop antitumor responses that attack and kill cancerous cells while protecting healthy cells. Immune checkpoint therapy, which includes the use of PD-1, CTLA-4, and CAR T cells, has shifted the scales in favor of the immune system in the battle against cancer cells. The capacity of tumor cells to elude immune detection and destruction, allowing them to develop resistant in the host, limits cancer immunotherapy (Zhang & Chen, 2018; Pandey et al., 2022). As a result, modern anticancer immunotherapy focuses on cytokine-mediated cell treatment.

Immunotherapy has rejuvenated the tumor immunology field and revolutionized nanomedicine. By removing nonspecific targeting and its accompanying negative effects, nanotherapeutics can improve cervical cancer immunotherapy efficacy. Nanovectors with different surface properties, materials, and sizes induce a prolonged and controlled release of therapeutic drugs at the site of action, bypassing biological barriers. Nanomaterials for gene and drug delivery in cancer therapy should be smaller than 100 nm in order for the therapeutic complex to reach the draining lymphatic system successfully. Following that, due to increased permeability and retention of leaky vasculature and defective lymphatic drainage within the tumor microenvironment, the complex accumulates within the solid tumor (Nam et al., 2021). Although several immunotherapeutic treatments have shown promising clinical results, their efficacies may vary, depending on which patients they benefit. Enhancement of cytokines and activation of anticancer effector cells are required for cancer immunotherapy to be successful. MDR (multiple drug resistance), non-specificity, unpleasant side effects, and dose constraints have all restricted the success of previously used cancer therapy techniques. Immunotherapy using viral antigens from high-risk HPV infections in cervical cancer appears to be an appealing therapeutic strategy (Stern, 2021).

The immune system is stimulated to attack cancerous cells while leaving healthy cells alone, resulting in an antitumor response. Immune checkpoint therapy, which comprises PD-1, CAR (chimeric antigen receptor) T cells, and CTLA-4, has increased the immune system's ability to battle cancer cells. Tumor cells' capacity to avoid immune detection and clearance limits cancer immunotherapy, allowing them to develop resistance in the host. As a result, modern anticancer immunotherapy focuses mostly on cell-mediated cytokine therapy, which boosts the formation and activation of T cells, cytotoxic T lymphocytes, and CD8+/CD4+ cells, resulting in tumor eradication (Eiben et al., 2002). As evidenced by the increased occurrence of HPV-associated cancers in people taking immunosuppressive medicines or suffering from AIDS, cell-mediated immunity is anticipated to be crucial in preventing tumor growth. An infiltration of CD8+ T cells is also a characteristic of malignant tumors. This chapter emphasizes how an efficient vaccination that mounts a cellular immune response against HPV-related proteins could help eliminate or prevent HPV-expressing tumors, such as cervical carcinomas. The goal of therapeutic vaccination against HPV-induced carcinomas is to cause immune system cellular components to recognize and attack HPV-infected cells, including malignant tissue. Many alternative vaccination techniques can be used to modify the immune response to HPV-infected cells. The use of cytokines in cancer therapy has been limited due to side effects of therapeutic medications such as myelo suppression, metabolic deregulations, and serum sickness (Peralta-Zaragoza et al., 2012). By removing non-specific targeting and its associated side effects, nanotherapeutics improved the immunotherapeutic efficacy of cervical cancer therapeutic drugs. Nano-vectors of varied sizes, surfaces, and materials elicited a controlled and sustained release of therapeutic compounds at the site of action, thereby bypassing biological barriers. Nanotherapy in cancer treatment is based on the relationship between the cancerous cells and immune system. Nanocarriers not only helps in vectoring the therapeutic agents but also work synergistically with its payload, thereby reversing immunosuppression and enhancing the immunogenic effects. Systemic/targeted drug delivery systems such as liposomes, nanoparticles, hydrogels, dendrimers, and localized drug delivery systems such as cervical patches, films, rings, and other localized drug delivery systems are safer than traditional chemotherapy, as evidenced by several drug delivery systems currently undergoing clinical trials (Aggarwal et al., 2018; Ghosh et al., 2022).

11.5 IMMUNE CHECKPOINT BLOCKADE THERAPIES IN CERVICAL CANCER

Checkpoint immunity inhibitors aid to restore the antitumor immune response by inhibiting the physiological mechanisms used by cancer cells to elude immunological identification. By leveraging the patient's own immune system and priming it to spot and destroy tumors, checkpoint inhibition immunotherapy, which has had tremendous success in cancer treatment, offers the potential to overcome immune escape in CC (Hargadon et al., 2018). Pembrolizumab, a PD-1/PD-L1 inhibitor that has proven clinical efficacy and hence been granted fast approval by the FDA, gives support to this belief (Passiglia et al., 2018). On the other hand, oncologic outcomes following monotherapy with these biologics have been generally moderate and unpredictable, which can be attributable to various tumor response resistance mechanisms. As a result, the use of medicines that boost immune responses through checkpoint-independent activation will increase the release of T cell inhibition by checkpoint inhibitors, resulting in stronger and longer-lasting clinical responses (Chitsike & Duerksen-Hughes, 2020). A number of powerful checkpoint inhibitors, such as atezolizumab, durvalumab, avelumab, ipilimumab, pembrolizumab, and nivolumab, have been authorized by the US FDA for the treatment of various malignancies. These IC inhibitors primarily target CTLA-4 or PD-1 receptors, which let the immune system to recognize aberrant proteins, preventing tumor-mediated immune suppression and tumor cell death. CTLA-4 (surface antigen) is found on T cells and suppresses T cell activation when triggered, leading to immune response breakdown. Several malignant T cell variations can up-regulate CTLA-4 expression in the TME (tumor microenvironment), allowing them to avoid immune system detection and destruction. As a result of the reduced antigen presentation by viral oncoproteins, anti-CTLA-4 therapy has emerged as a potent therapeutic method for cervical cancer management (Menderes et al., 2016). Ipilimumab (IgG1 m Ab) is an anti-CTLA-4 ICI (immune checkpoint inhibitor) that binds to CTLA-4 receptors and blocks immune response downregulation, proving to be a tolerable, safe, and effective treatment for cervical cancer. Ipilimumab has also been demonstrated to be beneficial against malignant cervical cells by blocking CTLA-4 receptors, according to Lheureux et al. (2018). When administered in combination with tremelimumab (another IgG1 mAb), durvalumab (another IgG1 mAb) showed great anticancer potential against cervical cancer via preventing the interaction of PD-1 with CD80 and PD-L1 molecules (Dyer et al., 2021). Most of these research, including continuing ones, are now limited to recurrence, persisting, and metastatic disease, which affects only a small percentage of cervical cancer patients. There are various future directions to which more attention should be paid. First, the most recent evidence suggests that PD-1/PD-L1 inhibitors can be used as a neoadjuvant therapy in lung cancer. Studies with a small sample size can be undertaken for patients diagnosed with primary-stage malignancy to study PD-1/PD-L1 inhibitors in conjunction with surgical intervention or to limit postoperative relapse. Second, PD-1/PD-L1 inhibitors may be a beneficial treatment for patients with localized advanced cervical carcinoma who are not susceptible to CCRT or who experience a short-term relapse after the first treatment, and we look forward to further investigation into this population. Third, determining if PD-1/PD-L1 antagonists can improve therapeutic success in tumors with elevated levels of PD-L1 prior to the start of CCRT will give researchers a better understanding of the inhibitors' impact in patients with locally advanced cervical cancer. Finally, because PD-L1 expression is linked to HPV status, more research is required to determine the association between HPV prevalence and the effectiveness of PD-1/PD-L1 antagonists in cancer patients (Liu et al., 2019).

ICIs that target PD-L1/PD-1 have also revolutionized the treatment of a variety of cancers, including cervical cancer. The cell's IR (immune response) is regulated by PD-1 (surface protein), which promotes T cell death and suppresses T cell inflammatory activity within lymph nodes. In the KEYNOTE-158 (NCT02628067) trial, the anti-cancer potential of pembrolizumab medication targeting PD-1 in cervical cancer patients was boosted in cervical cancer cells when given with chemotherapy. In the Phase Ib PROLOG study, atezolizumab (IgG1 isotype PD-L1) inhibited PD-1 activity in cervical cancer cells (NCT02914470) (Enwere et al., 2017). Gradalis® (Vigil™) and atezolizumab in combination showed antiangiogenic therapy, improved immunotherapy efficacy, and boosted intratumoral T cell infiltration in gynecological malignancies in a Phase II trial. Nivolumab inhibited the interaction of PD-1 and PD-L1 thereby allowing an effective immune response and was assessed in cervical cancer during Phase II study NRG-GY002 (Orbegoso et al., 2018).

Adoptive cell therapies that target tumor neoantigens with T cells can produce other effective immune anticancer responses. Adoptive T cell treatment, which uses endogenous TILs (tumor infiltrating lymphocytes) collected directly from patients with malignant tumors, as well as genetically modified T cells such T-cell receptor T cells and chimeric antigen receptor (CAR) T cells, are examples of such therapies (Moreno et al., 2021). TILs are associated with a greater tumor specificity and a substantially improved clinical result in cervical cancer. T cells that have been adopted have shown to have a higher rate of tumor regression than lymphocytes that have been vaccinated. In cervical cancer, TILs have primarily focused on viral antigens such as HPV-16's E6 and E7 antigens (Zhu et al., 2022). TILs also have a number of drawbacks, including difficulty in extracting and growing them from various tumor types, MHC down regulation, and poor T cell localization. These constraints, however, were circumvented by genetically altering T cells. Lymphocytes from the patient's peripheral blood were genetically altered to have both α- and β-chain T-cell receptors, allowing them to recognize specific MHC antigens (Gooden et al., 2011).

11.6 PARP (POLY(ADP-RIBOSE) POLYMERASE) INHIBITORS THERAPY

PARP is a constitutively produced key enzyme that plays an important regulatory role in replication, base excision DNA repair, transcription, and cellular differentiation. Its suppression has been found to be synthetic harmful with homologous recombination DNA repair abnormalities. A study designed to investigate the combined effect of veliparib (PARP inhibitor) and cytotoxic drug cisplatin in advanced stage cervical cancer patients (Thaker et al., 2017). On day 1, cisplatin and paclitaxel were given, followed by dose escalation of veliparib (twice daily) for seven days. Veliparib was given at a maximum dose of 400 mg twice daily. Two patients (6.9%) achieved a complete response and eight patients (27.6%) had a mild reaction out of 29 patients with quantifiable symptoms. In addition, 12 patients (41.4%) had illness that was stable. Despite the fact that phase I trials have shown potential activity, additional research is needed to identify the exact significance of this class of medications, especially dose and scheduling.

11.7 ANTIBODY-DRUG CONJUGATE-BASED THERAPY

In various tumors, cytotoxic drugs have been coupled to antibodies that specifically target receptors on cancer cells, which are normally highly toxic on their own. Tisotumab–vedotin, an antibody-drug complex, has been investigated in individuals with recurrent and metastatic cervical cancer. This combination uses a linker to connect a human immunoglobulin to tissue factor, which is significantly expressed in a number of tumors, including cervical cancer, and a microtubule-disrupting drug, MMAE. In a phase II study, 34 participants with advanced disease who had failed standard treatment were included in an expansion cohort (Vergote et al., 2017). In this resistant patient group, the response rate was 32%, with a mean reaction time of 8.3 months in verified responders. However, 53% of treated patients reported ocular toxicity, notably conjunctivitis, and keratitis. Additional procedures such as rigorous dose control, lubricating eye drops, ocular cooling, and steroid drops were used to alleviate this beyond the first 15 patients. The findings have been updated, and this appears to be a promising therapeutic option for patients with advanced stage cervical carcinoma (Figures 11.1 and 11.2).

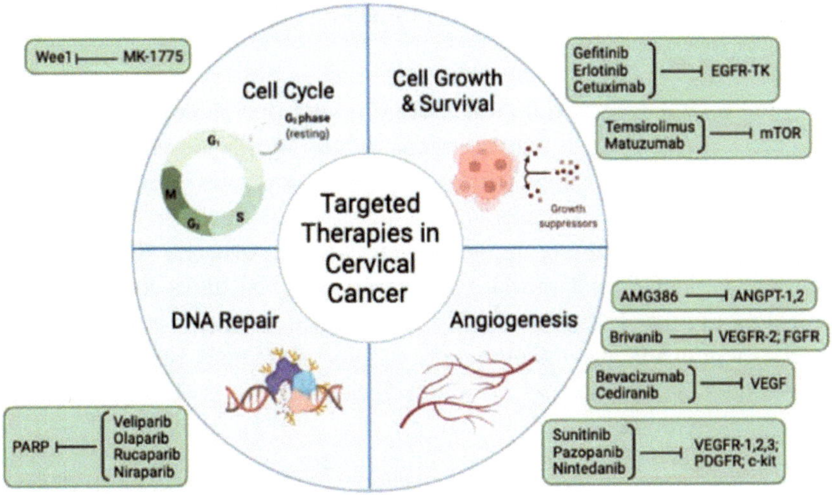

FIGURE 11.1 Therapeutic agents targeting biological pathways and their main molecular targets in various stages of cervical cancer.

Source: Reproduced with permission from Burmeister et al. (2022); Copyright © Elsevier (2022).

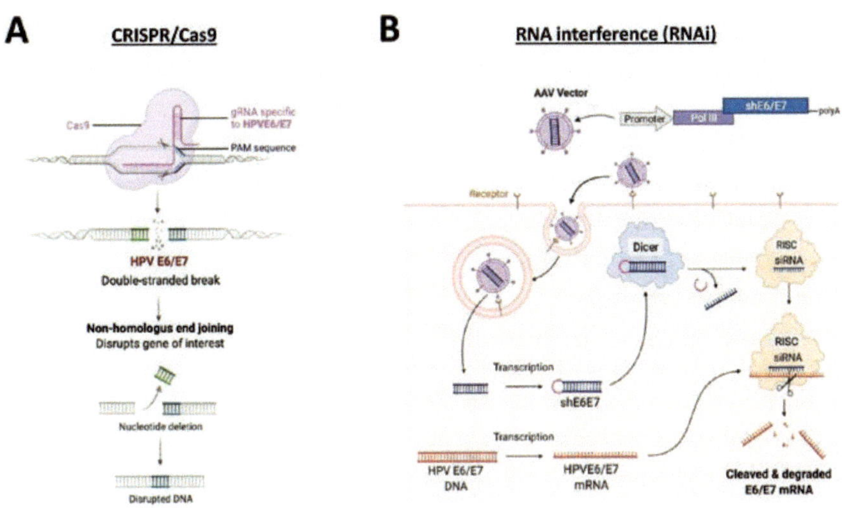

FIGURE 11.2 Schematic diagram showing mechanisms by which HPV E6 and E7 can be targeted in cervical cancer by **(A)** CRISPR/Cas9; and **(B)** RNA interference (RNAi).

Abbreviations PAM: protospacer-adjacent motif; AAV: adeno-associated virus.

Source: Reproduced with permission from Burmeister et al. (2022); Copyright © Elsevier (2022).

11.8 NECESSITY FOR COST-EFFECTIVE THERAPEUTIC STRATEGIES

Cervical cancer ranks second in morbidity and prevalence behind breast cancer in lower Human Development Index (HDI) nations; however, it is the most frequently diagnosed cancer in 28 countries and the common cause of cancer-related deaths in 42 countries specifically in Sub-Saharan Africa and Southeast Asia. In North America and Australia/New Zealand, regional incidence and mortality rates are 7 to 10 times lower than in low-HDI regions (Bray et al., 2018). Cervical cancer is a disease that primarily impacts low-income regions. As previously stated, the cost of adding bevacizumab to cytotoxic chemotherapy is 13 times that of cytotoxic chemotherapy alone (Minion et al., 2015). Even though a cost-effective analysis of immune-based therapy for cervical cancer has yet to be completed, it is clear that these treatments will be out of reach for a large section of the population. Thus, there is a critical need for low-cost therapy solutions that would improve the treatment outcomes in cervical cancer patients.

KEYWORDS

- **cervical cancer**
- **cervical carcinoma**
- **cost-effective analysis**
- **immune-based therapy**
- **low-cost therapy**
- **protospacer-adjacent motif**

REFERENCES

Abbott, M., & Ustoyev, Y., (2019). Cancer and the immune system: The history and background of immunotherapy. *Seminars in Oncology Nursing, 35*(5), 150923.

Aggarwal, U., Goyal, A. K., & Rath, G., (2018). Development of drug targeting and delivery in cervical cancer. *Current Cancer Drug Targets, 18*(8), 792–806.

Basu, P., Mehta, A., Jain, M., Gupta, S., Nagarkar, R. V., John, S., & Petit, R., (2018). A randomized phase 2 study of ADXS11-001 *Listeria monocytogenes*-listeriolysin O immunotherapy with or without cisplatin in treatment of advanced cervical cancer. *Int. J. Gynecol. Cancer., 28*(4), 764–772. https://doi.org/10.1097/IGC.0000000000001235.

Blohmer, J., Gore, M., Kuemmel, S., et al., (2005). Phase II study to determine response rate, pharmacokinetics (PK), pharmacodynamics (PD), safety, and tolerability of treatment with the humanized anti-epidermal growth factor receptor (EGFR) monoclonal antibody EMD 72000 (matuzumab) in patients with recurrent cervical cancer. *Journal of Clinical Oncology, 23*(16), 2534–2534.

Borysiewicz, L. K., Fiander, A., Nimako, M., et al., (1996). A recombinant vaccinia virus encoding human papillomavirus types 16 and 18, E6 and E7 proteins as immunotherapy for cervical cancer. *Lancet, 347.*

Bray, F., Ferlay, J., Soerjomataram, I., Siegel, R. L., Torre, L. A., & Jemal, A., (2018). Global cancer statistics 2018: GLOBOCAN estimates of incidence and mortality worldwide for 36 cancers in 185 countries. *CA: A Cancer Journal for Clinicians, 68*(6), 394–424.

Browne, I., Fennelly, D. W., Crown, J., & Murray, H., (2020). The efficacy and safety of pembrolizumab in advanced cervical cancer – a real world treatment study in an Irish healthcare setting. *J. Clin. Oncol., 38*(15). https://doi.org/10.1200/ jco.2020.38.15_suppl. e18007.

Burmeister, C. A., Khan, S. F., Schäfer, G., Mbatani, N., Adams, T., Moodley, J., & Prince, S., (2022). Cervical cancer therapies: Current challenges and future perspectives. *Tumor Virus Research, 13*, 38.

Chen, Y. J., Cheng, Y. J., Hung, A. C., Wu, Y. C., Hou, M. F., Tyan, Y. C., & Yuan, S. S. F., (2013). The synthetic flavonoid WYC02–9 inhibits cervical cancer cell migration/ invasion and angiogenesis via MAPK14 signaling. *Gynecologic Oncology, 131*(3), 734–743.

Cherrin, C., Haskell, K., Howell, B., et al., (2010). An allosteric Akt inhibitor effectively blocks Akt signaling and tumor growth with only transient effects on glucose and insulin levels *in vivo. Cancer Biology and Therapy, 9*(7), 493–503.

Chesters, P. M., & McCance, D. J., (1989). Human papillomavirus types 6 and 16 in cooperation with Ha-ras transform secondary rat embryo fibroblasts. *The Journal of General Virology, 70* (2), 353–365.

Chitsike, L., & Duerksen-Hughes, P., (2020). The potential of immune checkpoint blockade in cervical cancer: Can combinatorial regimens maximize response? A review of the literature. *Current Treatment Options in Oncology, 21*(12), 1–21.

Da Silva, D. M., Enserro, D. M., Mayadev, J. S., et al., (2021). Immune activation in patients with locally advanced cervical cancer treated with ipilimumab following definitive chemoradiation (GOG-9929). *Clinical Cancer Research, 26*(21), 5621–5630.

DiSilvestro, P. A., Lightfoot, S. A., & Benbrook, D. M., (1999). Ki-67 expression in a cervical cancer organotypic model correlates with growth and EGF-R expression. *Journal of Lower Genital Tract Disease, 3*(2), 111–115.

Du, J., Wang, L., Li, C., et al., (2016). MicroRNA-221 targets PTEN to reduce the sensitivity of cervical cancer cells to gefitinib through the PI3K/Akt signaling pathway. *Tumor Biology, 37*(3), 3939–3947.

Dyer, B. A., Feng, C. H., Eskander, R., et al., (2021). Current status of clinical trials for cervical and uterine cancer using immunotherapy combined with radiation. *International Journal of Radiation Oncology, Biology, Physics, 109*(2), 396–412.

Eiben, G. L., Velders, M. P., & Kast, W. M., (2002). The cell-mediated immune response to human papillomavirus-induced cervical cancer: Implications for immunotherapy. *Advances in Cancer Research, 86*, 113–148.

Enwere, E. K., Kornaga, E. N., Dean, M., et al., (2017). Expression of PD-L1 and presence of CD8-positive T cells in pre-treatment specimens of locally advanced cervical cancer. *Modern Pathology, 30*(4), 577–586.

Farley, J., Sill, M. W., Birrer, M., et al., (2011). Phase II study of cisplatin plus cetuximab in advanced, recurrent, and previously treated cancers of the cervix and evaluation of epidermal growth factor receptor immunohistochemical expression: A gynecologic oncology group study. *Gynecologic Oncology, 121*(2), 303–308.

Franco, E. L., Rohan, T. E., & Villa, L. L., (1999). Epidemiologic evidence and human papillomavirus infection as a necessary cause of cervical cancer. *Journal of the National Cancer Institute, 91*(6), 506–511.

Frenel, J. S., Tourneau, L. C., O'Neil, B., et al., (2017). Safety and efficacy of pembrolizumab in advanced, programmed death ligand 1-positive cervical cancer: Results from the phase IB KEYNOTE-028 trial. *J. Clin. Oncol., 35*(36), 4035–4041. https://doi.org/10.1200/JCO.2017.74.5471.

Fuhrman, C. B., Kilgore, J., LaCoursiere, Y. D., Lee, C. M., Milash, B. A., Soisson, A. P., & Zempolich, K. A., (2008). Radiosensitization of cervical cancer cells via double-strand DNA break repair inhibition. *Gynecologic Oncology, 110*(1), 93–98.

Fujimoto, J., Toyoki, H., Sato, E., Sakaguchi, H., & Tamaya, T., (2004). Clinical implication of expression of vascular endothelial growth factor-C in metastatic lymph nodes of uterine cervical cancers. *British Journal of Cancer, 91*(3), 466–469.

Gao, W., Li, J. Z., Chan, J. Y., Ho, W. K., & Wong, T. S., (2012). mTOR pathway and mTOR inhibitors in head and neck cancer. *ISRN Otolaryngology, 2012*, 953089.

Garcia, F., Petry, K. U., Muderspach, L., et al., (2004). ZYC101a for treatment of high-grade cervical intraepithelial neoplasia: A randomized controlled trial. *Obstet. Gynecol., 103*(2), 317–326. https://doi.org/10.1097/01.

Gariglio, P., Gutiérrez, J., Cortés, E., & Vázquez, J., (2009). The role of retinoid deficiency and estrogens as cofactors in cervical cancer. *Archives of Medical Research, 40*(6), 449–465.

Ghosh, S., Jayaram, P., Kabekkodu, S. P., & Satyamoorthy, K., (2022). Targeted drug delivery in cervical cancer: Current perspectives. *European Journal of Pharmacology*, 174751.

Goncalves, A., Fabbro, M., Lhommé, C., Gladieff, L., Extra, J. M., Floquet, A., Chaigneau, L., Carrasco, A. T., & Viens, P., (2008). A phase II trial to evaluate gefitinib as second- or third-line treatment in patients with recurring locoregionally advanced or metastatic cervical cancer. *Gynecologic Oncology, 108*(1), 42–46.

Gooden, M., Lampen, M., Jordanova, E. S., et al., (2011). HLA-E expression by gynecological cancers restrains tumor-infiltrating CD8+ T lymphocytes. *Proceedings of the National Academy of Sciences of United States of America, 108*(26), 10656–10661.

Hargadon, K. M., Johnson, C. E., & Williams, C. J., (2018). Immune checkpoint blockade therapy for cancer: An overview of FDA-approved immune checkpoint inhibitors. *International Immunopharmacology, 62*, 29–39.

Ibeanu, O. A., (2011). Molecular pathogenesis of cervical cancer. *Cancer Biology and Therapy, 11*(3), 295–306.

Jain, R. K., (2005). Normalization of tumor vasculature: An emerging concept in antiangiogenic therapy. *Science, 307*(5706), 58–62.

Jazaeri, A. A., Zsiros, E., Amaria, R. N., et al., (2019). Safety and efficacy of adoptive cell transfer using autologous tumor infiltrating lymphocytes (LN-145) for treatment of recurrent, metastatic, or persistent cervical carcinoma. *J. Clin. Oncol., 37*(15). https://doi.org/10.1200/ jco.2019.37.15_suppl.2538.

Kaufmann, A. M., Stern, P. L., Rankin, E. M., et al., (2002). Safety and immunogenicity of TA HPV, a recombinant vaccinia virus expressing modified human papillomavirus (HPV)-16 and HPV-18 E6 and E7 genes, in women with progressive cervical cancer. *Clinical Cancer Research, 8*(12), 3676–3685.

Kim, J. H., Kang, J. W., Kim, M. S., et al., (2012). The apoptotic effects of the flavonoid N101-2 in human cervical cancer cells. *Toxicology in Vitro, 26*(1), 67–73.

Kim, S. H., Kim, S. H., Lee, S. C., & Song, Y. S., (2009). Involvement of both extrinsic and intrinsic apoptotic pathways in apoptosis induced by genistein in human cervical cancer cells. *Annals of the New York Academy of Sciences, 1171*(1), 196–201.

Kurtz, J. E., Hardy-Bessard, A. C., Deslandres, M., et al., (2009). Cetuximab, topotecan and cisplatin for the treatment of advanced cervical cancer: A phase II GINECO trial. *Gynecologic Oncology, 113*(1), 16–20.

Lheureux, S., Butler, M. O., Clarke, B., et al., (2018). Association of ipilimumab with safety and antitumor activity in women with metastatic or recurrent human papillomavirus–related cervical carcinoma. *JAMA Oncology, 4*(7), e173776. https://doi.org/10.1001/jamaoncol.2017.3776.

Liontos, M., Kyriazoglou, A., Dimitriadis, I., Dimopoulos, M. A., & Bamias, A., (2019). Systemic therapy in cervical cancer: 30 years in review. *Critical Reviews in Oncology/Hematology, 137*, 9–17.

Liu, Y., Wu, L., Tong, R., et al., (2019). PD-1/PD-L1 inhibitors in cervical cancer. *Frontiers in Pharmacology, 65.*

Lorente, R. R., Alfonso, S., Sanchez, Y., Viada, C., Ortiz, R., & Troche, M., (2019). Nimotuzumab in advanced cervical cancer: Safety and efficacy profile. *International Journal of Oncology Research, 2*, 16.

Lv, Y., Cang, W., Li, Q., et al., (2019). Erlotinib overcomes paclitaxel-resistant cancer stem cells by blocking the EGFR-CREB/GRβ-IL-6 axis in MUC1-positive cervical cancer. *Oncogenesis, 8*(12), 1–12.

Mackay, H. J., Tinker, A., Winquist, E., et al., (2010). A phase II study of sunitinib in patients with locally advanced or metastatic cervical carcinoma: NCIC CTG trial IND.184. *Gynecologic Oncology, 116*(2), 163–167.

Manzo-Merino, J., Contreras-Paredes, A., Vázquez-Ulloa, E., Rocha-Zavaleta, L., Fuentes-Gonzalez, A. M., & Lizano, M., (2014). The role of signaling pathways in cervical cancer and molecular therapeutic targets. *Archives of Medical Research, 45*(7), 525–539.

Mauricio, D., Zeybek, B., Tymon-Rosario, J., Harold, J., & Santin, A. D., (2021). Immunotherapy in cervical cancer. *Curr. Oncol. Rep., 23*(7), 3557. https://doi.org/10.1007/s11912-021-01052-8.

McLachlan, J., Boussios, S., Okines, A., et al., (2017). The impact of systemic therapy beyond first-line treatment for advanced cervical cancer. *Clinical Oncology, 29*(3), 153–160.

Menderes, G., Hicks, C., Black, J. D., Schwab, C. L., & Santin, A. D., (2016). Immune checkpoint inhibitors in gynecologic cancers with lessons learned from non-gynecologic cancers. *Expert Opinion on Biological Therapy, 16*(8), 989–1004.

Meng, T., Zhao, D., Ye, H., Feng, Y., Wang, H., & Zhang, Y., (2020). Construction of an ultrasensitive electrochemical sensing platform for microRNA-21 based on interface impedance spectroscopy. *Journal of Colloid and Interface Science, 578*, 164–170.

Miller, J. W., Plescia, M., & Ekwueme, D. U., (2014). Public health national approach to reducing breast and cervical cancer disparities. *Cancer, 120*(S16), 2537–2539.

Minion, L. E., Bai, J., Monk, B. J., et al., (2015). A Markov model to evaluate cost-effectiveness of antiangiogenesis therapy using bevacizumab in advanced cervical cancer. *Gynecologic Oncology, 137*(3), 490–496.

Monk, B. J., Mas, L. L., Zarba, J. J., et al., (2010). Phase II, open-label study of pazopanib or lapatinib monotherapy compared with pazopanib plus lapatinib combination therapy in patients with advanced and recurrent cervical cancer. *Journal of Clinical Oncology, 28*(22), 3562–3569.

Monk, B. J., Sill, M. W., Burger, R. A., Gray, H. J., Buekers, T. E., & Roman, L. D., (2009). Phase II trial of bevacizumab in the treatment of persistent or recurrent squamous cell carcinoma of the cervix: A gynecologic oncology group study. *Journal of Clinical Oncology, 27*(7), 1069–1074.

Moreno, V., Hernandez, T., De Miguel, M., Doger, B., & Calvo, E., (2021). Adoptive cell therapy for solid tumors: Chimeric antigen receptor T cells and beyond. *Current Opinion in Pharmacology, 59*, 70–84.

Movva, S., Rodriguez, L., Arias-Pulido, H., & Verschraegen, C., (2009). Novel chemotherapy approaches for cervical cancer. *Cancer, 115*(14), 3166–3180.

Nam, J. K., Kim, J. H., Park, M. S., Kim, E. H., Kim, J., & Lee, Y. J., (2021). Radiation-induced fibrotic tumor microenvironment regulates anti-tumor immune response. *Cancers, 13*(20), 5232.

Naumann, R. W., Hollebecque, A., Meyer, T., et al., (2019). Safety and efficacy of nivolumab monotherapy in recurrent or metastatic cervical, vaginal, or vulvar carcinoma: Results from the phase I/II CheckMate 358 trial. *Journal of Clinical Oncology, 37*(31), 2825–2834.

O'Malley, D. M., Oaknin, A., Monk, A. B., et al., (2021). Phase II study of the safety and efficacy of the anti-PD-1 antibody balstilimab in patients with recurrent and/or metastatic cervical cancer. *Gynecol. Oncol., 163*, 274–280. https://doi.org/10.1016/j.ygyno.2021.08.018.

Oh, D. Y., Kim, S., Choi, Y. L., et al., (2015). HER2 as a novel therapeutic target for cervical cancer. *Oncotarget, 6*(34), 36219–36230.

Orbegoso, C., Murali, K., & Banerjee, S., (2018). The current status of immunotherapy for cervical cancer. *Reports of Practical Oncology and Radiotherapy, 23*(6), 580–588.

Pal, A., & Kundu, R., (2020). Human papillomavirus E6 and E7: The cervical cancer hallmarks and targets for therapy. *Frontiers in Microbiology*, 3116.

Pandey, P., Khan, F., Qari, H. A., Upadhyay, T. K., Alkhateeb, A. F., & Oves, M., (2022). Revolutionization in cancer therapeutics via targeting major immune checkpoints PD-1, PD-L1 and CTLA-4. *Pharmaceuticals, 15*(3), 335.

Passiglia, F., Galvano, A., Rizzo, S., Incorvaia, L., Listi, A., Bazan, V., & Russo, A., (2018). Looking for the best immune-checkpoint inhibitor in pre-treated NSCLC patients: An indirect comparison between nivolumab, pembrolizumab and atezolizumab. *International Journal of Cancer, 142*(6), 1277–1284.

Peralta-Zaragoza, O., Bermúdez-Morales, V. H., Pérez-Plasencia, C., Salazar-León, J., Gómez-Cerón, C., & Madrid-Marina, V., (2012). Targeted treatments for cervical cancer: A review. *OncoTargets and Therapy, 5*, 315.

Petit, P. G., Mehta, A., Jain, M., et al., (2014). ADXS11-001 immunotherapy targeting HPV-E7: Final results from a phase II study in Indian women with recurrent cervical cancer. *J. Immuno. Ther. Canc., 2*, 201. https://doi.org/10.1186/2051-1426-2-s3-p92.

Petry, K. U., (2014). HPV and cervical cancer. *Scandinavian Journal of Clinical and Laboratory Investigation, 74*(244), 59–62.

Pfaendler, K. S., & Tewari, K. S., (2016). Changing paradigms in the systemic treatment of advanced cervical cancer. *American Journal of Obstetrics and Gynecology, 214*(1), 22–30.

Pfaendler, K. S., Liu, M. C., & Tewari, K. S., (2018). Bevacizumab in cervical cancer: 5 years after. *The Cancer Journal, 24*(4), 187–192.

Rischin, D., Gil-Martin, M., Gonzalez-Martin, A., et al., (2020). PD-1 blockade in recurrent or metastatic cervical cancer: Data from cemiplimab phase I expansion cohorts and characterization of PD-L1 expression in cervical cancer. *Gynecol. Oncol., 159*(2), 322–328. https://doi.org/ 10.1016/j.ygyno.2020.08.026.

Roman, L. D., Wilczynski, S., Muderspach, L. I., et al., (2007). A phase II study of Hsp-7 (SGN-00101) in women with high-grade cervical intraepithelial neoplasia. *Gynecol. Oncol., 2007*. https://doi.org/10.1016/j. ygyno.2007.05.038.

Santin, A. D., Sill, M. W., McMeekin, D. S., et al., (2011). Phase II trial of cetuximab in the treatment of persistent or recurrent squamous or non-squamous cell carcinoma of the cervix: A gynecologic oncology group study. *Gynecologic Oncology, 122*(3), 495–500.

Scambia, G., Ferrandina, G., Distefano, M., D'Agostino, G., Benedetti-Panici, P., & Mancuso, S., (1998). Epidermal growth factor receptor (EGFR) is not related to the prognosis of cervical cancer. *Cancer Letters, 123*(2), 135–139.

Scarinci, I. C., Garcia, F. A., Kobetz, E., et al., (2010). Cervical cancer prevention: New tools and old barriers. *Cancer, 116*(11), 2531–2542.

Schilder, R. J., Sill, M. W., Lee, Y. C., & Mannel, R., (2009). A phase II trial of erlotinib in recurrent squamous cell carcinoma of the cervix: A gynecologic oncology group study. *International Journal of Gynecological Cancer, 19*(5), 929–933.

Schrevel, M., Gorter, A., Kolkman-Uljee, S. M., Trimbos, J. B. M. Z., Fleuren, G. J., & Jordanova, E. S., (2011). Molecular mechanisms of epidermal growth factor receptor overexpression in patients with cervical cancer. *Modern Pathology, 24*(5), 720–728.

Schutz, F. A., Choueiri, T. K., & Sternberg, C. N., (2011). Pazopanib: Clinical development of a potent antiangiogenic drug. *Critical Reviews in Oncology/Hematology, 77*(3), 163–171.

Stern, P. L., (2021). Harnessing immunity for therapy in human papillomavirus driven cancers. *Tumor Virus Research, 11*, 200212.

Stevanović, S., Draper, L. M., Langhan, M. M., et al., (2015). Complete regression of metastatic cervical cancer after treatment with human papillomavirus-targeted tumor-infiltrating T cells. *J. Clin. Oncol., 33*(14), 1543–1550. https://doi.org/10.1200/JCO.2014.58.9093.

Tan, M. J., White, E. A., Sowa, M. E., Harper, J. W., Aster, J. C., & Howley, P. M., (2012). Cutaneous β-human papillomavirus E6 proteins bind mastermind-like coactivators and repress notch signaling. *Proceedings of the National Academy of Sciences of the United States of America, 109*(23), E1473–E1480.

Temkin, S. M., Yamada, S. D., & Fleming, G. F., (2010). A phase I study of weekly temsirolimus and topotecan in the treatment of advanced and/or recurrent gynecologic malignancies. *Gynecologic Oncology, 117*(3), 473–476.

Tewari, K. S., Sill, M. W., Long, H. J., et al., (2014). Improved survival with bevacizumab in advanced cervical cancer. *The New England Journal of Medicine, 370*(8), 734–743.

Thaker, P. H., Salani, R., Brady, W. E., et al., (2017). A phase I trial of paclitaxel, cisplatin, and veliparib in the treatment of persistent or recurrent carcinoma of the cervix: An NRG oncology study (NCT#01281852). *Annals of Oncology, 28*(3), 505–511.

Trimble, C. L., Morrow, M. P., Kraynyak, K. A., et al., (2015). Safety, efficacy, and immunogenicity of VGX-3100, a therapeutic synthetic DNA vaccine targeting human papillomavirus 16 and 18 E6 and E7 proteins for cervical intraepithelial neoplasia 2/3: A randomized, double-blind, placebo-controlled phase 2b trial. *Lancet, 386*, 2078–2088.

Tripathi, V., Singh, A., & Ashraf, M., (2018). Avenanthramides of oats: Medicinal importance and future perspectives. *Pharmacognosy Reviews, 12*(23).

Vergote, I., Dean, E., Lassen, U., et al., (2017). A phase IIa study of tisotumab vedotin (HuMax®-TF-ADC) in patients with relapsed, recurrent and/or metastatic cervical cancer. *Annals of Oncology, 28*, 330, 331.

Wang, H., Gao, P., & Zheng, J., (2014). Arsenic trioxide inhibits cell proliferation and human papillomavirus oncogene expression in cervical cancer cells. *Biochemical and Biophysical Research Communications, 451*(4), 556–561.

Wang, X. G., Jandl, T., Dadachova, E., & Revskaya, E., (2014). Effect of naive and radiolabeled rhTRAIL on the cervical cancer xenografts in mice. *Therapeutic Delivery, 5*(2), 139–147.

Yeh, L. S., Hung, Y. C., Shen, Y. Y., Kao, C. H., Lin, C. C., & Lee, C. C., (2002). Detecting para-aortic lymph nodal metastasis by positron emission tomography of 18F-fluorodeoxyglucose in advanced cervical cancer with negative magnetic resonance imaging findings. *Oncology Reports, 9*(6), 1289–1292.

Yilmaz, A., Alp, E., Onen, H. I., & Menevse, S., (2016). Reduced BCL2 and CCND1 mRNA expression in human cervical cancer HeLa cells treated with a combination of everolimus and paclitaxel. *Contemporary Oncology, 20*(1), 28.

Zhang, H., & Chen, J., (2018). Current status and future directions of cancer immunotherapy. *Journal of Cancer, 9*(10), 1773.

Zhu, Y., Zhou, J., Zhu, L., Hu, W., Liu, B., & Xie, L., (2022). Adoptive tumor infiltrating lymphocytes cell therapy for cervical cancer. *Human Vaccines and Immunotherapeutics*, 1–11.

Index

β

β-catenin
  accumulation, 37–39
  associated cell adherence, 37
  phosphorylation, 36, 38
β-chain T-cell receptors, 269

A

Aberrant
  gene transcription, 19
  miRNAs expression, 193, 194
Activation-induced cytodine deaminase (AID), 139
Activator protein-1 (AP-1), 51, 144, 145, 162, 232, 237, 244
Acute
  lymphoblastic leukemia, 96
  myeloid leukemia, 93
Adenocarcinoma, 75, 163, 229
Akt
  kinase signaling, 236
  phosphorylation, 71, 73, 76, 109
Alkaloids, 237, 238
Aneuploidies, 11
Angiogenesis, 11, 20, 21, 37, 40, 49, 52, 72, 77, 94, 138, 162, 216, 225, 231, 242, 258, 264
  mediators, 264
Angiogenic
  phenotype, 144, 145
  property, 244
Anthocyanidins, 216
Anthocyanins, 230
Antiangiogenic, 225, 228, 237, 242, 258, 269
  drugs, 264
Anti-apoptotic
  genes, 138
  properties, 136
  protein, 164, 222
Antibacterial, 226, 230, 232, 237
Antibody-drug complex, 270
Anticancer
  mechanism, 244, 245
  medication development, 226
  properties, 226, 236, 239, 244
Anticancerous medication, 228
Anti-cardiovascular properties, 235
Anti-estrogenic potential, 126
Antigen receptors, 136
Anti-inflammatory, 137, 138, 222, 226, 227, 230, 232, 235–237, 240, 242
Antimetastatic, 228
  properties, 242
Antioxidant, 216, 222, 226, 230, 232, 240
  properties, 232
Antiproliferative
  efficacy, 141, 242
  potential, 222
Antispasmodic activities, 232
Antitumor
  baicalein actions, 221
  properties, 222, 227, 231, 237, 240, 242
  therapeutics, 184
Apigenin, 222, 223
  7-glucoside therapy, 222
Apoptosis, 11, 18, 20, 34, 35, 37, 40, 49, 50, 52, 53, 55, 71, 72, 74, 77, 78, 91, 117, 118, 125–129, 138, 144, 154, 157, 163, 164, 177, 178, 180, 182, 183, 194, 197, 216, 221–227, 229–232, 235–237, 239, 242–244, 257
  inducing factor (AIF) & pathways, 117, 225, 242
  suppression, 20
Apoptotic
  inducers, 125
  inducing effects, 232
  induction, 127–129, 227, 228, 243
  pathway inhibition, 164

related proteins, 224, 245
signal transduction, 127
Arachidonic acid, 20
Aromatase, 229
Aromatic plants, 232
Asymmetric cytoskeletal assembly, 36
Atelocollagen, 195, 196
Autophagy induction, 237

B

Bacillus Calmette-Guérin, 64
Baicalein, 221
suppressed long non-coding RNA (BDLNR), 221
Base excision DNA repair, 270
Bax gene expression, 236
B-cell
activating factor (BAFF), 136
chronic lymphoid leukemia (BCLL), 93
lymphoid cancer, 138
Berberine, 237, 239
Beta-catenin expression, 39, 40
Betulinic acid, 235, 236
Bevacizumab, 258
therapy, 264
Biobank-stored animal, 176
Biomarkers, 41
Black non-Hispanic women, 4
Blood-brain barrier (BBB), 196
Bone cancer, 35
Breast cancer, 2, 6, 18, 35, 37, 52, 72, 79, 80, 179, 272

C

Caenorhabditis elegans worm, 177
Camellia sinensis, 228
Camptothecin, 237
Cancer
biomarkers, 184
cell, 13, 34, 37, 39, 40, 53, 54, 62, 76, 125, 129, 160, 162, 163, 178, 182, 183, 194, 195, 197, 222, 227, 229, 231, 232, 235, 236, 239, 240, 242–244, 265–267, 269, 270
differentiation, 35
lines, 39, 55, 76, 99, 164
metastasis, 182
motility, 37
proliferation, 229
detection, 5
development, 54, 100, 137, 139, 141, 162
genome atlas research network, 97
immunotherapy, 265, 266
prevention, 5, 216, 227
progression, 10, 35, 37, 52, 53, 72, 73, 118, 142, 163, 178, 183
stimulation, 54
proliferation, 180
related genes, 54
stem cells (CSCs), 40, 235
stemness, 37
therapy, 158, 236, 265–267
tissues, 39, 40, 97, 183, 184, 193
treatment
agent, 226
alternatives, 225
Cancerous cell chemosensitivity, 227
Canonical NF-kB signaling pathway activation, 137
Carboxy-terminal
domain, 157
module, 157
Carcinogenesis, 2, 13, 17, 20, 35, 37, 41, 52, 72, 75, 92, 117, 135, 140, 142, 155, 158–163, 197, 198
Carcinomas, 12, 13, 35, 37, 41, 53, 93, 98, 138, 160, 162, 266
Cardioprotective properties, 230
Cardiovascular
disease, 232
health enhancement, 236
Carvacrol treatment, 232
Casein kinases, 37
CaSki cervical cancer cell lines, 98
Caspase-9 activation, 117, 225, 232
Catalase (CAT), 231
Catalytic
activity, 156, 162
functions, 71
Catenin-independent pathway, 36
Caveolin-1 (Cav-1), 20, 21
Cell
communication, 91, 183

cycle
progression, 19, 20, 34, 74, 128, 180, 221
regulation, 17, 20, 139
regulatory proteins, 163
cycling proliferation, 193
death, 18, 42, 99, 125, 127–129, 139, 161, 162, 179, 193, 194, 221–223, 225–228, 230–232, 236, 237, 240, 242, 243, 268, 269
differentiation, 35, 98
growth suppression, 229, 242
mediated cytokine therapy, 266
migration, 36, 49, 98, 109, 162, 221, 227, 228, 236
proliferation, 11, 19–21, 36, 37, 40, 49, 52, 72, 74, 77, 91, 94, 100, 126, 136, 138, 157, 164, 178, 179, 182, 197, 223, 227, 229, 235–237
vacuoles, 230
Cellular
apoptosis protein inhibitor, 127
differentiation, 37, 92, 270
inhibitor of apoptosis protein (cIAP), 127
metabolism, 162
onco-suppressive pathways, 258
pathways, 49
proliferation, 140, 141, 160, 161, 183, 232
signaling pathways activation, 49
Centrosome duplication factors, 11
Cervarix
/Gardasil vaccine, 64
plus adjuvant, 64, 65
Cervical
advanced squamous intraepithelial lesions, 76
cancer, 1–6, 8, 9, 11–13, 17, 19, 21, 22, 33–35, 37–41, 43, 49, 53–56, 59, 62–65, 71, 75–78, 80, 91, 97–101, 109, 110, 117, 118, 125–127, 135, 140–145, 153, 160–165, 175, 182–185, 191, 193–195, 197–199, 215, 217, 221–233, 235–245, 257–259, 262, 264–272
development, 5, 9, 11, 13, 53, 54, 139, 143, 144, 161, 163, 165, 194, 215
initiation, 100, 141, 163
management, 33, 35, 145, 163, 198, 244, 257, 258, 268
patients, 17, 34, 39, 41, 55, 62, 76, 125, 143, 161, 257, 258, 265, 268–270, 272
prognostic biomarker, 184
progression, 12, 35, 38, 39, 41, 54, 55, 75, 118, 142, 143, 163–165, 228
regulatory effects, 184
samples, 54, 55, 75, 265
screening, 3–5, 41
squamous cell carcinomas (CCSCC), 78, 80
therapeutics, 244
tissue samples, 100, 164
transplanted tumors, 232
treatment, 5, 194, 198, 199, 223, 224, 230, 239, 243–245, 257, 265
xenografts, 240
carcinogenesis, 17, 21, 35, 37, 182, 193
carcinoma, 1, 2, 5, 8, 22, 97, 100, 109, 142, 143, 180, 183, 184, 193, 198, 199, 215, 221, 224, 239, 264, 266, 268, 270, 272
epithelium, 19, 54, 98, 141
intraepithelial neoplasia (CIN), 9, 13, 19, 62, 100, 143, 160, 161
lesions progression, 143
malignancies, 3, 77, 99, 100, 224, 258
neoplasms, 182
squamous cervical carcinoma (CSCC), 77
tumorigenesis, 13, 164
Cervix, 1, 6–10, 20, 54, 75–77, 141, 142, 184, 215, 236, 245
cancer-derived cells, 77
Checkpoint
immunity inhibitors, 267
independent activation, 267
inhibition immunotherapy, 267
Chemoattractant proteins, 137
Chemokines, 49, 50, 137, 139, 141, 144
Chemo-radiotherapy, 6
Chemo-sensitivity, 197
Chemotherapeutic
agent, 41, 222
drug, 41, 43, 237, 257, 258, 264
efflux, 226

resistance, 77
response, 194
Chemotherapy, 33, 41, 43, 76, 194, 215, 235, 244, 245, 257, 264, 267, 269, 272
Chimeric antigen receptor (CAR), 265, 266, 269
Chlamydia trachomatis, 21, 22
Chromatin acetylation, 129
Chromosomal rearrangements, 10, 179
Chronic
inflammation, 138, 140, 141
inflammatory disorders, 137
leukemia treatment, 33
lymphocytic leukemia, 178
Cisplatin, 76–78, 161, 194, 195, 215, 222, 227–229, 231, 257, 264, 270
based chemotherapy, 257
resistance, 195
resistant
cells, 195
cervical cancer patients, 228
sensitivity, 194
c-Jun N-terminal kinase (JNK), 36, 41, 223, 225, 229, 235
Clear cell renal cell carcinomas, 39
Clinical
development, 196
investigations, 216
Clinicopathological factors, 184
Clonal progression of tumor, 139
Cocoa products, 216
Colorectal cancer, 2, 35, 52, 72
Commercial HPV vaccine Gardasil-9, 3
Complex genetic disorder, 178
Comprehensive gene expression profiling studies, 155
Conventional
contraceptives, 21
treatment methods, 33, 43
Convergent extension movements, 36
Cost-benefit assessment, 264
Cost-effective analysis, 272
Coumarins, 240
Cross-linking pathway, 145
C-terminal transactivation domain, 155
Culinary coloring agent, 240
Cullin 5 (CUL5), 182
Curcumin, 240, 242
micelles, 242
Cyanidin 3-O-glucoside, 231
Cycle proteins, 245
Cyclic adenosine monophosphate-responsive element (CRE), 144
Cyclin
D1, 38, 40, 92, 139, 164, 221, 222, 225, 231, 235, 242, 243
dependent kinase (CDK) & protein kinase inhibitors (CKIs), 11, 19, 22
Cycloheximide therapy, 128
Cyclooxygenase-2 (COX-2), 144, 20, 38, 144, 162, 224, 228, 242
promoter activity, 144
Cystic fibrosis transmembrane conductance regulator (CFTR), 143
Cytohistological assays, 13
Cytokine, 49, 50, 52, 54, 71, 74, 137–141, 144, 153, 156, 157, 162, 266, 267
independent cell growth, 159
mediated cell treatment & senescence, 129, 265
signaling, 158
Cytological screening, 1, 2, 22
Cytoplasmic
catenin expression, 36
HuR movement, 235
inactive GSK3 immunoreactivity, 39
region, 143, 156
tyrosine kinase Src, 153
Cytotoxic
chemotherapy, 265, 272
drugs, 270
medicines, 258
T-lymphocytes, 266
Cytotoxicity, 215, 226, 227, 230, 239, 265

D

Death receptor 5 (DR5), 125, 223, 228
Delta-like, 91
Dendrimers, 267
Dendritic cell, 50, 62
Deoxyribonucleic acid (DNA)
binding, 135, 136, 139, 142, 143
activity, 157, 243

domains, 135
efficacy, 142, 143
methylation, 35, 223
methyltransferase 1 (DNMT1), 223
minor groove modulation, 232
replication, 13, 19
proteins, 19
Dephosphorylation, 71, 155, 158
Diagnosis, 17, 21, 41, 54, 184, 197–199
Diagnostic biomarkers, 41, 43
Dickkopf, 36
Dimerization process, 135
Di-orthohydroxyl functional group, 221
Disease progression, 54, 138, 143, 164, 223
Disheveled, 36, 38
Diterpenoid naphthoquinone, 232
Dosage limitations, 265
Dose
responsive manner, 230, 235, 242
veliparib escalation, 270
Double-stranded RNA, 196, 197
Downregulated Wnt7A expression, 39
Downstream signaling, 49, 144, 145
pathways, 49
Drosophila, 101
Drp1-mediated mitochondrial fission mechanism, 225
Drug-mediated regulation, 93

E

E2F transcription factor, 11, 19
E5
expressing human keratinocytes, 125
mediated tumorigenic actions, 12
oncoprotein, 17, 20, 21, 144
promoted COX-2 expression, 144
E6/E7-notch mediated cellular transformation, 101
E7
co-expression mediated apoptotic induction, 128
expressing human keratinocytes, 128
oncoprotein, 11, 12, 17, 19, 101, 128, 129, 141, 144, 161–165, 193, 232, 237, 243, 244
E-cadherin expression, 40
E-calmodulin, 240
Electron transport chain (ETC), 155
Ellagic acid, 242, 243
Embryonic development, 35, 40, 153, 177
Endometrial cancer, 72, 79
Endometrium, 73, 75
cancers, 75
Endoplasmic reticulum (ER), 95, 224, 225, 229, 232, 235, 242
Endothelin-1 (ET-1), 20
Enhanced immunogenic responses, 64
Epidermal growth factor (EGF), 11, 20, 77, 91, 95, 126, 144, 153, 264
receptor (EGFR), 11, 20, 21, 35, 138, 144, 153, 242, 258, 264
Epigallocatechin gallate (EGCG), 228, 229
Epigenetic
alterations, 215
machinery, 216
modifications, 155, 242
Escherichia coli, 54
Ethnic minorities, 3
Evodiamine, 237
Exogenous pathway activation, 224
Exosomes, 179, 183
Extra domain A (EDA), 62
Extracellular
matrix formation, 20
miRNAs, 179
signal-regulated kinases 1/2 (ERK1/2), 221, 228, 229, 243
Ezrin, 156

F

Fas
associated death domain (FADD), 118, 127, 222, 224, 225
degradation, 127
like ICE (FLICE), 118
induction, 126
ligand, 126
Fisetin, 228
Flavanones, 216
Flavonoids, 216, 217, 226, 230, 240
Flavonols, 216
Food and Drug Administration (FDA), 3, 73, 267, 268

Forkhead box
  O protein (FOXO), 236
  protein M1 (FOXM1), 40
Formalin-fixed paraffin-embedded tissue blocks, 176
Formononetin, 230
Furin-like protease enzyme, 91

G

G1-phase cell-cycle arrest, 243
Gallbladder, 225
Ganoderic acid derivatives, 125
Gardasil plus adjuvant, 64, 65
Gastric
  adenocarcinoma, 159
  cancer, 52, 72
  carcinoma proliferation enhancing transcript 1 (GHET1), 41
    downregulation, 41
  tumor-initiating cells, 180
Gefitinib, 77
Gene
  cluster cistronic expression, 177
  expressions, 135, 138
Genetic
  /drug screening, 101
  alterations, 33, 34, 37, 97
  mutations/deletions, 73
  polymorphisms, 158
  variations, 97, 159, 180
Genistein-induced cancer cell growth, 229
Genital keratinocyte immortalization, 17
Genomic
  amplifications, 179
  stability, 178
Genotoxic stimuli, 129
Geographic
  disparities, 2, 4, 21
  location, 215
Ginsenoside Rh2, 236
Glioblastoma, 160
Glucose-regulated protein of 78 (GRP78), 225
Glutathione (GSH), 226, 231
  peroxidase, 231
Glycogen synthase kinase-3, 37, 221
Glycosyltransferases, 92
G-protein-coupled receptors, 20
Granular lymphocytic leukemia, 159
Growth factor receptor, 74, 75
Gynecologic oncology group (GOG), 264
Gynecological
  carcinomas, 125
  tumors, 53

H

Hairpin precursors, 177
Healthcare system, 5
Health-related quality-of-life, 264
HeLa cell lines, 236
Helicobacter pylori, 2
Hematological
  carcinomas, 159
  malignancies, 110
Hematopoiesis, 153
Hematopoietic malignancies, 94
Heme oxygenase-1 (HO-1), 231
Hepatitis
  B/C viruses, 2
  B-related hepatocellular carcinoma, 159
Hepatoprotective, 232, 239
Hesperidin, 224, 225
Heterochromatin
  formation, 155
  protein 1, 155
Heterodimers, 91, 95, 135, 154, 162
Heterogeneity, 109, 110
High-grade
  ovarian epithelial carcinoma, 159
  precursors, 13
  squamous intraepithelial neoplasia, 140
High-risk HPV (HR-HPV), 127, 139, 140, 161
High-throughput genotyping research analysis, 75
Histamine-induced aberrant estrogen receptor pathway, 223
Histocompatibility genes, 140
Histone
  deacetylase (HDAC), 129, 157
  modifications, 155
HIV infection, 22

Hodgkin lymphomas, 93
Homeostasis, 35, 40, 117
Homodimers, 136, 154
Homologous recombination DNA repair
  abnormalities, 270
Human
  biological samples, 176
  cancers, 73, 75, 79, 80
  carcinomas, 6, 39
  development index (HDI), 272
  disorders pathogenesis, 178
  foreskin keratinocytes (HFKs), 99
  leukemias, 179
  malignancies, 179
  mucosa, 9
  neuroblastoma cells, 53
  osteosarcoma cells, 197
  papillomavirus (HPV), 1–4, 6, 8–14, 17–22, 39–41, 53–55, 62–64, 75–79, 97–99, 101, 109, 125–129, 137, 139–144, 160–165, 193, 194, 215, 222, 228, 229, 232, 237, 243, 244, 258, 265–267, 269, 271
    E6 oncoprotein, 141, 161
    inactive malignancies, 77
    induced carcinogenesis, 78
    infection, 8–10, 19, 39, 41, 53, 54, 75, 137, 140, 141, 160–162, 193, 266
    mediated cervical cancer, 64
    oncoproteins, 9, 98, 99, 141, 164, 165
    positive cervical cancer tissue, 55
    related proteins, 266
  telomerase reverse transcriptase (hTERT), 101, 183, 226, 237, 243, 258
Hydrogels, 267
Hypermethylation, 159, 165, 166
Hypoxia-inducible factor-1 (HIF-1), 63, 94, 225, 230, 235, 243

I

Imiquimod, 64
Immature primary transcripts, 175
Immortalization, 101, 118, 140
Immortalized
  human keratinocyte cell line, 98
  rodent fibroblasts, 128
Immune
  checkpoint
    inhibitor (ICI), 258, 268
    therapy, 265, 266
  compromised animals, 78
  response (IR), 62–64, 135, 139, 140, 179, 265–269
  system cellular components, 267
  therapy, 272
Immunization, 3, 5
  teenage children, 3
Immunogenic
  DNA vaccines properties, 64
  effects, 267
Immunohistochemical
  analysis, 76
  investigation, 72
  studies, 72
Immunomodulatory efficacies, 239
Immunosuppression, 34, 137, 162, 267
Immunosuppressive
  cytokines, 52, 53
  medicines, 266
Immunotherapeutic
  agents, 65
  efficacy, 267
  treatments, 266
Immunotherapy, 265, 266
  development, 265
In situ hybridization, 184
In vitro maturation, 62
Inducible nitric oxide synthase (iNOS), 53, 55, 242
Inflammatory
  autoimmune illnesses, 52
  bowel disease, 136
  cells employment, 137
  cytokines, 50, 51, 136–138, 221
  immune response generation, 136
  response generation, 141
Insertional mutation, 140
Insulin-like growth factor-binding protein 7, 243
Integrin β6 expression, 54
Intercellular communications, 179
Interferon (IFN), 140
  regulatory factor 3 (IRF3), 51

stimulated
regulatory elements, 51
response elements (ISREs), 161
γ (IFN-γ), 141, 164, 229
secretion, 229
Intergenic sequences, 175
Interleukins, 49, 153
International regulatory agencies, 64
Intracellular
death domain, 127
E2F-1 accumulation, 129
mediators, 37
Intraepithelial neoplasia, 54
Intraperitoneal injection, 232
Intrinsic
cellular pathway, 196
pathways activation, 125
Invasive cervical cancer, 13, 41, 54, 140, 193
Ipilimumab, 268
Isoflavones, 216
Isoform-selective PI3K inhibitors, 73

J

Janus kinases (JAKs), 153, 155–159
2 (JAK2), 154–156, 158, 159, 243

K

Kaempferol, 226, 227
induced telomerase suppression, 226
Keratinocyte, 11, 20, 93, 98–100, 109, 125–128, 161
differentiation, 98, 99
models, 99
Kinase
inhibitors, 33
inhibitory region (KIR), 157

L

Lactate dehydrogenase (LDH), 229
Lapatinib, 265
Leguminosae, 237
Ligand-dependent notch activation, 97
Lipid kinases, 71, 80
Lipopolysaccharides (LPS)
induced
TLR4 activation, 52, 53
tumor cell growth, 52
related proinflammatory cytokines, 62
Liposomes, 267
Liver cancer, 52
Localized drug delivery systems, 267
Loganiaceae families, 237
Long
control region (LCR), 13, 139, 140
non-coding RNA (LncRNA), 72, 97, 98, 221
protective duration, 13
Low-cost therapy, 272
Lubricating eye drops, 270
Lung
cancer, 2, 37, 52, 72, 73, 268
metastasis suppression, 197
tumorigenesis, 182
Luteolin, 223
Lymph angiogenesis, 20
Lymphatic system, 266
Lymphocyte differentiation, 229

M

M1-polarization, 137
Macrophage
cells, 137, 141
colony-stimulating factor, 53
Malignant
cervical lesions transformation, 162
melanomas, 93
Mammalian
immune system, 49
rapamycin target, 72, 74, 80, 94
sterile 20-like kinase (MST2), 182
target of rapamycin (mTOR), 41, 55, 71–80, 183, 194, 221, 223, 225, 229, 235, 240, 243
Matrine, 237, 239, 240
Matrix metalloproteinase 2 (MMP2), 38, 53, 94, 227, 237, 240
Medicinal
botanicals, 223
drugs targeting Wnt signaling, 41
Membrane receptors, 37, 91
Menispermaceae, 237
Messenger RNA (mRNA), 39, 50, 55, 62, 127, 175–178, 183, 196, 243

Metabolic
  deregulations, 267
  diseases, 177
  pathway, 72, 177
    regulation, 177
Metalloproteinases (MMPs), 94, 232
Metastasis, 21, 35, 36, 41, 49, 52, 75, 77, 94, 109, 138, 141, 143, 144, 160, 163, 177, 180–182, 184, 194–197, 221, 231, 235, 240, 242–244
  inhibition, 180, 242
  inhibitors, 180
Metastatic
  ability, 197
  carcinoma, 258
  disease, 268
  stage carcinoma, 264
Methotrexate, 257
Methyltransferase-like 3, 227
MicroRNA (miRNAs), 12, 72, 94, 175–185, 191, 193–199
  administration, 196
  dysregulation, 178
  expression patterns & profiles, 184, 198, 199
  mediated translational repression, 177
  precursor genes, 178
  production, 12
  regulation, 178
  related gene regulation, 176
Microtubule-disrupting drug, 270
Minichromosome maintenance complex II (MCM2), 19
MiR-499a-5p transfection enhanced migration, 195
Mitochondria, 117, 155, 222, 225, 228, 236, 237
  dependent apoptotic pathway, 222, 236
  mediated mechanism & pathways, 225, 237
Mitochondrial
  dysfunction, 223
  independent pathway, 224
  mediated pathways, 125
  membrane, 224
    potential (MMP), 109, 125, 197, 222, 223, 225–228, 230, 236, 239
  pathways, 224, 225, 235
  pro-apoptotic events, 117
Mitogen activated protein kinase (MAPK), 51, 62, 126, 144, 180, 193, 223, 227–229, 239
Mitogenesis, 20
Mitomycin C, 129, 239
  resistance, 195
Modern anticancer immunotherapy, 265, 266
Moesin, 156
Molecular
  interactions, 101
  mechanisms, 198, 236
  pathways, 136
Monophosphoryl lipid A, 64
Monoterpene phenol, 232
Monotherapy, 267
Mortality, 1, 3–6, 21, 22, 244, 272
  discrepancy, 6
Mucosal epithelium, 98
Multidrug resistance (MDR), 38, 216, 226, 227, 266
Multiple
  drug resistance, 265, 266
  host cell biological pathways, 75
  myeloma (MM), 72
Murine epidermis, 93
Mutant
  IkB repressor molecule, 140
  oncoproteins, 33
Myelo suppression, 267
Myeloid differentiation factor 88 (MyD88), 50, 51
  independent pathways, 50

N

NAD(P)H quinone dehydrogenase 1 (NQO1), 231
Nanocarriers, 267
Nanoparticles, 164, 267
Nanotherapeutics, 266, 267
Nanotherapy, 267
Nano-vectors, 267
Naringin, 224
Nasopharyngeal cancer, 35

National Cancer Institute (NCI), 2, 257
Natural
  bioactive
    compounds, 216
    substances, 244
  compounds, 215
  monoflavonoid, 222
  phenolic substances, 240
Neoplastic phenotype, 11
Neuroprotective properties, 228
Neutralization antibodies, 64
Next-generation sequencing technology, 198
Nitric oxide (NO), 49, 52, 55, 226
Nitrogen-rich stimulant, 239
Nivolumab, 268, 269
N-Mannich bases berberine analogs, 239
Non-cancerous tissue samples, 163
Non-canonical
  pathway, 36, 51
  Wnt signaling, 36, 41
Non-coding region (NCR), 13
Non-small cell lung cancer (NSCLC), 73, 80, 159, 160
Normal tissue homeostasis, 52
Notch
  intracellular domain (NICD), 92, 96, 98
  receptor, 91–93, 95, 96, 110
    mutations, 97
  signaling, 91–99, 101, 109, 110
Notch1 cytoplasmic localization, 100
Novel
  anticancer agents, 53
  immunotherapeutic agents, 64
  metabolic system, 179
  public health problem, 22
  therapeutic approaches, 34
Nuclear
  factor kappa B (NF-kB), 33, 51, 52, 55, 62, 92, 135–140, 142–144, 221, 223, 227, 228, 230, 231, 239, 244
    activity suppression, 140
    dimers, 136
    expression, 139, 142, 143
    interrelated pathways, 140
    ligand receptor activator, 136
    nuclear translocation, 51
    proteins activation, 139
    signaling pathway, 138, 144, 230
    transcription factor, 141
    transfer & movement, 140, 228
  localization, 96, 141, 143
  transcription factors, 135
  translocation, 62, 135, 142, 159, 162
Nucleic acid-based
  agents, 196
  medications, 195
  pharmaceutical delivery techniques, 196
Nucleus transportation, 135

O

Oncogenic
  HPV variants, 3
  miRNAs (OncomiR), 178–180, 182, 195
    inhibition, 182
Oncogenicity, 11
Oncolytic adenovirus, 99
Oncoproteins, 11, 13, 93, 99, 141, 160, 161, 163, 165, 193, 258, 268
Open reading frames (ORF), 13, 193
Oral administration, 229
Organotypic raft experiments, 98
Oridonin, 236, 237
Oridonin mediated ROS generation, 237
Osteosarcoma, 35, 197
  spontaneous lung metastasis model, 197
Ovarian cancer, 52, 72, 80, 159, 165
Overall survival (OS), 34, 127, 161, 258, 264
Overexpressed oncogenic proteins, 194

P

Paclitaxel
  chemosensitivity, 235
  mediated apoptosis, 239
  resistance acquisition, 194
  resistant miRNA, 194
Pancreatic cancer, 52, 79, 160
Pap smear-based screening, 13
Papaveraceae, 237
Papillomatosis, 11
Papillomaviridae family, 12
Papillomavirus particles, 9
Pathogenic viruses, 127

Pathological angiogenesis, 20
Patient-derived xenograft (PDX), 265
Pazopanib, 264, 265
Pelvic lymphadenectomy, 215
Pembrolizumab, 268, 269
Persistent cervical inflammation, 54
Personalized medicine, 182
P-glycoprotein (P-gp), 226, 227, 242
Pharmaceutical industries, 231
Pharmacological
  effects, 240
  properties, 232
Phenolic compounds, 240
Phenols, 241
Phosphatase and tensin homolog (PTEN), 71, 73, 74, 76, 97, 179, 222
Phosphatidylinositol-3 kinase (PI3K), 35, 72, 80
Phosphoinositide-3-kinase catalytic subunit delta (PIK3CD), 183
Phospholipid scramblase 1 (PLSCR1), 244
Phosphoprotein phosphatase 2A (PP2A), 39, 40, 76, 77, 109
Phosphorylation, 19, 20, 51, 71, 73, 76, 109, 143, 144, 153–157, 159–161, 164, 221, 235, 236, 240, 243
Phosphotyrosine residues, 156
Physiological stress, 138
Phytoestrogen isoflavone, 229
Piperine, 237, 239
Planar cell polarity (PCP), 36
Plasma membrane, 71, 74, 80
Platelet-derived growth factor (PDGF), 153
Platinum-based
  chemotherapy, 77, 195, 257
  neoadjuvant chemotherapy, 77
Point mutations and deletion, 97
Polarity, 35, 36, 40
Poly(ADP-ribose) polymerase, 78
Polymorphisms, 56, 59, 180
Polyposis coli, 36, 37
Polyterpenoids, 231
Pomegranates, 242
Post-translational modifications, 135, 155
Potent
  biomarkers, 17
  prognostic biomarker, 76
  therapeutic vulnerabilities, 33
Precancerous
  lesions, 3, 41, 165, 166
  tumors, 39
Precursor
  lesions treatment, 8
  miRNA, 175
Premalignant dysplasia, 161
Primary cervical
  cancer tissues, 97
  carcinoma biopsies, 109
Primary-stage malignancy, 268
Pro-apoptotic
  chemicals, 125
  effects, 227
  efficacies, 126
  properties, 228
  protein, 163, 224
    actions, 11
    expression, 127
    kinase, 194
Profound stromal invasion, 184
Prognostic biomarkers, 183, 184
Programmed cell death 4 (PDCD4), 182
Progression-free survival (PFS), 258, 264
Pro-inflammatory
  cytokines, 137, 139
  signaling pathway, 137
Proliferation, 11, 18, 19, 34, 35, 37, 41, 52, 71, 75, 76, 99, 118, 138, 144, 154, 159, 197, 221, 222, 225, 226, 232, 235, 237, 244
Prophylactic vaccines, 64
Prostaglandin E2 (PGE2), 228
Prostate
  cancer, 52, 72, 73, 79, 159, 162
  liver, 165
Protein
  inhibitor, 155, 157
  kinase A (PKA), 240
  phosphatase 2, 76
  tyrosine
    kinase (PTK), 156, 162
    phosphatases (PTPs), 157, 158
Proteolytic
  breakdown, 135
  cleavage, 91, 92, 110
Protospacer-adjacent motif, 271, 272
Protumorogenic effect, 137

Pseudomonas aeruginosa, 54
Pseudosubstrate, 157
Putative biomarkers, 17
Pycnanthus angolensis, 230

Q

Quercetin, 227

R

Rabdosia rubescens, 236
Racial minorities, 1, 21
Radiation, 33, 41, 77, 78, 137, 194, 244, 245, 257
Radioresistance, 37
Radiotherapy, 6, 125, 161, 194, 215, 244, 245, 257, 258
Radixin, 156
Randomized controlled trials (RCTs), 13
Ranunculaceae, 237
Rapamycin, 77
Ras homolog gene family member A (RHOA), 36, 182
Raspberries, 242
Rat embryo fibroblasts, 100
Rb protein, 165, 166
Receptors, 49
Rel homology domain (RHD), 135, 137
Renal cell carcinoma, 72
Reproductive variables, 215
Research experimental findings, 73
Resveratrol, 243, 244
Rheumatoid arthritis, 136
Ribose nucleic acid (RNA)
  induced silencing complex (RISC), 175, 196
  polymerase enzyme dicer, 175
Ribosomal protein S6 kinase-1 (S6k-1), 71
Runt-related transcription factor 3, 36

S

Salvia miltiorrhiza, 232
Screening, 1–5, 8, 13, 21, 22
  programs, 1, 2, 8, 22
Scutellaria baicalensis, 222
Secondary
  metabolites, 216, 237, 240
  preventive strategies, 1
Serum sickness, 267
Sesterterpenoids, 231
Sexually transmitted infection, 21
Signal
  transducer and activator of transcription (STAT), 153, 155–157, 159
    mediated transcription, 159
  transduction, 153, 154, 160, 165, 183, 198, 258
Signaling pathway, 11, 20, 33–37, 40, 41, 50, 51, 55, 62, 64, 65, 71–77, 96, 109, 125, 126, 141, 144, 145, 155, 156, 158, 160, 179, 193, 195, 197, 216, 221, 223–225, 228, 229, 240, 243
Silibilin treatment, 125
Silibinin, 225
Silybum marianum, 225
Single nucleotide polymorphism, 54
Skin mucosa, 12
Small interfering RNA (SiRNA), 161, 163, 164, 196
Socio-economically disenfranchised, 1
Sophora flavescens, 239, 240
Squamous
  carcinomas patient samples, 143
  cell carcinoma (SCC), 9, 54, 62, 75, 142, 163, 195, 229
  columnar junction (SCJ), 8
  intraepithelial lesions, 76
Src 2 homology, 156
Stem cell maintenance, 35, 40, 153
SUMOylation process, 157
Sunitinib, 264
Superficial squamous cells, 19
Suppressors of cytokine signaling (SOCSs), 155–157, 160, 165, 166
  3 (SOCS3), 157, 160, 165, 243
  proteins, 165, 166
Surgical intervention, 268
Survivin, 38, 237
Synthetic nucleic acid molecules, 196
Systemic/targeted drug delivery systems, 267

T

T cell
  inflammatory activity, 269
  lymphoblastic leukemia, 93
  mediated immune response, 64

Tangerines, 224
Tanshinone IIA, 232, 235
Telomerase, 11, 226
  activation, 183
Terpenoids, 231, 233
Tetraterpenoids, 231
The Cancer Genome Atlas (TCGA), 5, 8, 97, 159
Therapeutic
  biomarkers, 198, 199
  drugs, 266, 267
  efficiency, 41, 43
  implications, 93
  properties, 216, 221
  techniques, 77, 109, 125
  vaccination, 266
  vaccine, 63
Threonine, 37, 71, 76, 96
Time-responsive manner, 225
Tissue
  homeostasis, 37, 52, 117
  metalloproteinase-1 inhibitor, 231
  regeneration, 35, 40
Toll-like receptor (TLR), 49–54, 64
  ligand interaction, 52
  mediated inflammatory response, 52
  signaling, 35
  TLR-9, 140
Topoisomerase II protein (TOP2), 19
Transactivation domain, 139, 143, 155
Transcriptional
  activation, 155
  repressor, 92, 139
Transformation zone
  cells, 140
  epithelial cells, 140
Translation suppression, 176
Transmembrane
  sequence, 92
  subunit, 91
Triterpenoids, 231
Tumor
  advancement, 142
  cell
    growth inhibition, 144
    membrane, 77
  development, 62, 165, 235
  expression necrosis factor-associated receptor factor 1 (TRAF1), 229
  formation, 11, 62, 101
  inducing potential of NF-kB, 142
  induction, 138
  infiltrating lymphocytes (TILs), 269
  mediated immune suppression, 268
  microenvironment (TME), 34, 42, 49, 136, 138, 140, 179, 264, 266, 268
  necrosis factor (TNF), 49–53, 62, 92, 127–129, 136, 140, 141, 164, 221–223, 239
    alpha converting enzyme (TACE), 92
    induced apoptosis, 128
    receptor-associated death domain (TRADD), 127, 222
    related apoptosis-inducing ligand (TRAIL), 53, 117, 125, 127, 128, 223
  neoantigens, 269
  progression, 40, 75, 94, 164, 177, 179, 182
  proliferation, 36, 165, 166
  protein p53-induced nuclear protein-1 (TP53INP1), 180, 183
  suppressor
    gene activation, 129
    miRNA (TsmiR), 182, 183, 195, 197
    proteins, 11, 19, 179, 194, 258
Tumorigenesis, 36, 94, 101, 158, 178, 183
Tumorigenic characteristics, 109
Tyrosine kinase
  activity, 153, 156
  nonreceptor-2 (TNKS2), 182

U

Ubiquitin
  ligase, 38, 40, 95, 118, 155
  proteasome pathway, 118, 128
Ubiquitination machinery, 157
Unfolded protein response (UPR), 242
Untranslated region (UTR), 98, 175, 177, 182
Upregulation, 142, 164–166, 182, 183, 193, 222
Upstream regulatory region (URRs), 13, 162
Urokinase-type plasminogen activator (u-PA), 228
US Food and Drug Administration, 264
Uterine cancer, 8

V

Vaccination, 1, 3, 4, 8, 21, 22, 266, 267
  coverage, 4
  implementation, 1
Vaccine adjuvants, 64, 65
Vaginal cancer, 12
Vascular endothelial growth factor (VEGF), 20, 38, 40, 53, 139, 144, 225, 229, 230, 235, 242, 243, 258
  splice variants expression, 258
Vasodilator-stimulated phosphoprotein (VASP), 240
Vertebrate genomes, 177
Vinblastine, 227, 237, 242
  drug-resistant KB-V1 cells, 242
Vincristine, 237
Viral
  gene expression, 10
  hepatitis, 240
  oncoproteins regulation, 164
  replication, 135
  transcription factors, 10
Virus-like particles (VLPs), 13, 62
Voltage-dependent anion channel 1 (VDAC1), 236

W

Wingless type (Wnt) & signaling system, 35
  inhibitory factor 1, 37
  ligands, 36, 37
  pathway
    activation, 37, 39
    inhibitors, 39
  signaling
    components, 37, 39
    genes, 37
    pathway, 33, 35–41, 227
Wogonin, 222
World Health Organization (WHO), 3, 21

X

Xanthones, 240
Xenograft
  animal model, 159
  tumors, 244
X-linked inhibitor of apoptosis protein (XIAP), 183, 237

Y

Y-box binding protein 1, 221

Z

Zingiberaceae family, 240